PRINCIPLES OF DRUG THERAPY IN NEUROLOGY

CONTEMPORARY NEUROLOGY SERIES AVAILABLE:

Fred Plum, M.D., *Editor-in-Chief*
Series Editors: **Sid Gilman, M.D.**
Joseph B. Martin, M.D., Ph.D.
Robert B. Daroff, M.D.
Stephen G. Waxman, M.D., Ph.D.
M-Marsel Mesulam, M.D.

PRINCIPLES OF DRUG THERAPY IN NEUROLOGY

EDITORS

MICHAEL V. JOHNSTON, M.D.

Professor and Haller Scholar of Neurology
and Pediatrics
Johns Hopkins University School of
Medicine and The Kennedy Institute
Baltimore, Maryland

**ROBERT L. MACDONALD,
M.D., Ph.D.**

Professor of Neurology and Physiology
University of Michigan Medical School
Ann Arbor, Michigan

ANNE B. YOUNG, M.D., Ph.D.

Chief, Neurology Service
Massachusetts General Hospital
Julieanne Dorn Professor of Neurology
Harvard Medical School
Boston, Massachusetts

F. A. DAVIS COMPANY • Philadelphia

Printed in the United States of America

Last digit indicates print number: 10 9 8 7 6 5 4 3 2 1

NOTE: As new scientific information becomes available through basic and clinical research, recommended treatments and drug therapies undergo changes. The author(s) and publisher have done everything possible to make this book accurate, up-to-date, and in accord with accepted standards at the time of publication. The authors, editors, and publisher are not responsible for errors or omissions or for consequences from application of the book, and make no warranty, expressed or implied, in regard to the contents of the book. Any practice described in this book should be applied by the reader in accordance with professional standards of care used in regard to the unique circumstances that may apply in each situation. The reader is advised always to check product information (package inserts) for changes and new information regarding dose and contraindications before administering any drug. Caution is especially urged when using new or infrequently ordered drugs.

Library of Congress Cataloging-in-Publication Data

Principles of drug therapy in neurology / [edited by] Michael V. Johnston, Robert L. Macdonald, Anne B. Young.
    p. cm. — (Contemporary neurology series ; CNS 37)
    Includes bibliographical references and index.
    ISBN 0-8036-5031-0 (hardback : alk. paper)
    1. Neuropharmacology.   2. Nervous system — Diseases — Chemotherapy.
I. Johnston, Michael V., 1946–   . II. Macdonald, Robert L., 1945–
. III. Young, Anne B., 1947–   . IV. Series: Contemporary neurology series ;
37.
    [DNLM: 1. Nervous System Diseases — drug therapy. W1 CO769N v. 37
/ WL 100 P9567]
RM315.P69 1991
616.8′0461 — dc20
DNLM/DLC
for Library of Congress   91-28190
                                                    CIP

PREFACE

Each year more is learned about the mechanisms responsible for neurologic diseases and the ways in which drugs can be used to treat them. Despite the current inadequacy of therapies for most serious neurologic disorders, slow but steady progress is being made. This progress is related to synergistic observations made in the laboratory and in patients, and it seems unpredictable where the next new therapeutic leads will emerge. For example, since the introduction of L-dopa for Parkinson's disease, little new therapeutic progress had been made, despite intensive laboratory investigation of dopaminergic pathways, until the serendipitous observations in patients exposed to the toxin MPTP. The excitement created by this observation is largely responsible for the recent reports that monoamine oxidase inhibition may slow the progress of naturally occurring Parkinson's disease. The potential to actually impede the progress of neurologic disease rather than simply improve symptoms is stimulating interest in therapy for a number of other degenerative disorders.

The great potential for progress in neurologic drug therapy and the unpredictability of where that progress will emerge provided the impetus for this book. We conceived this project to identify and present fundamental information that is now or soon will be directly relevant to patient care in neurology and psychiatry. We attempted to identify topics considered at the "core" of practice and the most rapid advances. Striking the right balance in the book between practical information and "basic science"—critical to the success of the enterprise—presented a challenge for the editors. Although the authors are immersed in their special areas of interest, they are each adept at balancing clinical and scientific perspectives, and this is reflected in their contributions. We hope that readers at all levels of training and experience will find this book useful for their daily practice and that it will bring to them some of the excitement and promise of the future of this field.

MICHAEL V. JOHNSTON, M.D.
ROBERT L. MACDONALD, M.D., PH.D.
ANNE B. YOUNG, M.D., PH.D.

v

CONTRIBUTORS

Jack P. Antel, M.D.
Professor and Chairman
Department of Neurology and
Neurosurgery
Montreal Neurological Institute and
McGill University
Montreal, Quebec
Canada

Alastair M. Buchan, M.D., M.R.C.P.
Assistant Professor of Neurology
University of Ottawa
Neuroscience Research
Ottawa General Civic Hospital
Ottawa, Ontario
Canada

Joseph T. Coyle, M.D.
Ebin Draper Professor of Psychiatry
and Neuroscience
Chairman of the Department of
Psychiatry
Harvard Medical School
Boston, Massachusetts

Mark S. Freedman, M.D.
Assistant Professor of Neurology
Department of Neurology and
Neurosurgery
Montreal Neurological Institute and
McGill University
Montreal, Quebec
Canada

Michael Jacewicz, M.D.
Assistant Professor of Neurology and
Neuroscience
Cerebrovascular Disease Research
Center
Cornell University Medical College
New York, New York

Michael V. Johnston, M.D.
Professor and Haller Scholar of
Neurology and Pediatrics
Johns Hopkins University School of
Medicine and The Kennedy Institute
Baltimore, Maryland

Daniel H. Lowenstein, M.D.
Assistant Professor of Neurology
Department of Neurology
University of California, San Francisco
School of Medicine
San Francisco General Hospital
San Francisco, California

Robert L. Macdonald, M.D., Ph.D.
Professor of Neurology and Physiology
University of Michigan Medical School
Ann Arbor, Michigan

Gavril W. Pasternak, M.D., Ph.D.
Professor of Neurology
Memorial Sloan-Kettering Cancer
Center
Departments of Neurology and
Pharmacology
Cornell University Medical School
New York, New York

Richard Payne, M.D.
Associate Professor and Vice Chairman
Department of Neurology
University of Cincinnati
College of Medicine, and
Chief, Neurology Service
Cincinnati Veterans Administration
Center
Cincinnati, Ohio

John B. Penney, Jr., M.D.
Professor of Neurology
Harvard Medical School and
Neurologist
Massachusetts General Hospital
Boston, Massachusetts

Stephen J. Peroutka, M.D., Ph.D.
Assistant Professor of Neurology
Department of Neurology
Stanford University Medical Center
Stanford, California

William A. Pulsinelli, M.D., Ph.D.
Professor of Neurology and
Neuroscience
Cerebrovascular Disease Research
Center
Cornell University Medical College
New York, New York

David P. Richman, M.D.
Marjorie and Robert E. Strauss
Professor of Neurological Science
Department of Neurology
The University of Chicago
Pritzker School of Medicine
Chicago, Illinois

Faye S. Silverstein, M.D.
Associate Professor of Pediatrics and
Neurology
University of Michigan Medical School
Ann Arbor, Michigan

Roger P. Simon, M.D.
Chief of Service
San Francisco General Hospital
Professor of Neurology
Department of Neurology
University of California, San Francisco
School of Medicine
San Francisco, California

Anne B. Young, M.D., Ph.D.
Chief, Neurology Service
Massachusetts General Hospital
Julieanne Dorn Professor of Neurology
Harvard Medical School
Boston, Massachusetts

CONTENTS

Chapter 1

FUNDAMENTALS OF DRUG THERAPY IN NEUROLOGY

Michael V. Johnston, M.D., and
Faye S. Silverstein, M.D.

MOLECULAR TARGETS OF DRUG ACTION IN THE NERVOUS SYSTEM
BARRIERS TO DRUG ACTION IN THE CNS
DYNAMIC FEATURES OF DRUG ACTION
TOXICITY OF NEUROACTIVE DRUGS
INFLUENCE OF AGE ON DRUG ACTION

A wide spectrum of neurologic and neurobehavioral disorders are now treatable with drugs, and the number is expanding steadily. This introductory chapter sets the stage for the chapters that follow, and highlights the basic principles that are especially relevant to drug actions in the nervous system. A glossary of abbreviations appears as Table 1 – 1.

The five issues selected for special attention in this chapter are all major determinants of the success of drug treatment in neurologic patients (Table 1 – 2).[8,20,36,65,81,86,93] *Molecular targets of drug action* in the nervous system are being defined with greater precision, and these insights are also becoming practically relevant to therapy. The facility with which drugs can be transported across the *blood-brain barrier (BBB)* also has a major impact on treatment of central nervous system (CNS) disorders. The fundamentals of drug *absorption, distribution, and metabo-*

lism have a profound effect on management of drug therapy in individual patients. In many therapeutic situations, drug *toxicity* may become a major limitation and a primary factor in selection among drugs. For some drugs, it is becoming possible to prevent morbidity by anticipating factors that predispose individual patients to toxicity. *Patient age*, the final issue considered, is increasingly recognized as an important factor that influences all the others. A drug may have a diverse spectrum of activities and toxicities depending on whether the patient is elderly, a child, or a fetus. Each of the five issues is discussed briefly, along with some practical examples from clinical practice.

MOLECULAR TARGETS OF DRUG ACTION IN THE NERVOUS SYSTEM

The major sites of action can be divided into four categories. One important target of drug action is the neurochemical synapse between neurons. A second includes other nonsynaptic targets in neurons. A third group includes actions on other cells within the nervous system such as glia and blood vessels. The fourth target is the nucleic-acid and protein synthetic machinery of

1

Table 1–1 GLOSSARY OF ACRONYMS

Acronym	Meaning
AcCoA	Acetylcoenzyme A
ACh	Acetylcholine (excitatory neurotransmitter)
AChE	Acetylcholinesterase (degradative enzyme for acetylcholine)
ACTH	Adrenocorticotropic hormone
ADP	Adenosine diphosphate
ALS	Amyotrophic lateral sclerosis
AMP	Adenosine monophosphate
APV	2-amino-5-phosphono-valerate
ARAS	Ascending reticular activating system
ATP	Adenosine triphosphate
BBB	Blood-brain barrier
Bmax	Maximal amount of ligand bound to a fixed amount of receptor
cAMP	Cyclic adenosine monophosphate
CBF	Cerebral blood flow
CCK	Cholecystokinin (a peptide neurotransmitter)
Ch1–Ch4	Groups of cholinergic cell bodies
ChAT	Choline acetyltransferase (synthetic enzyme for acetylcholine)
CNS	Central nervous system
CPP	3-[±2-carboxypiperazine-4yl] propyl-l-phosphonate
CRF	Corticotropin-releasing factor
CSF	Cerebrospinal fluid
DA	Dopamine (a neurotransmitter)
DG	Diacylglycerol
EAA	Excitatory amino acid
EKG	Electrocardiogram
GABA	Gamma-aminobutyric acid (major inhibitory neurotransmitter)
GAD	Glutamate decarboxylase (marker for GABAergic neurons)
GPC	Glycerophosphocholine
GPE	Glycerophosphoethanolamine
5-HIAA	5-hydroxyindoleacetic acid (serotonin metabolite used to measure serotonin turnover)
5-HT	5-hydroxytryptamine (serotonin)
5-HT$_1$, 5-HT$_2$	Serotonin-receptor subtypes
HVA	Homovanillic acid (an endogenous dopamine metabolite used to measure dopamine turnover)
IP$_3$	Inositol 1,4,5-triphosphate (an intracellular second messenger)
K$_D$	Equilibrium dissociation constant
M$_1$ receptors	Postsynaptic muscarinic receptor subtype
M$_2$ receptors	Presynaptic muscarinic receptor subtype
MAO	Monoamine oxidase
3-MHPG	3-methoxy-4-hydroxyphenylglycol (a norepinephrine metabolite used to measure turnover)
NADH	The reduced form of nicotinamide-adenine dinucleotide
NGF	Nerve growth factor
NMDA	N-methyl-D-aspartate (a rigid analogue of glutamate)
PC	Phosphatidylcholine (lecithin)
PCP	Phencyclidine
PE	Phosphatidylethanolamine
PGI$_2$	Prostacyclin (prostaglandin metabolite of arachidonic acid; has vasodilator actions)
PI	Phosphatidylinositol (one of the phospholipids in the neuronal membrane)
PPI	Phosphoinositides
PIP$_2$	Phosphatidylinositol 4,5-biphosphate
SRF	Sustained, [high-frequency] repetitive firing
TCA	Tricyclic antidepressants
THA	Tetrahydroaminoacridine (an AChE inhibitor)
tPA	Tissue plasminogen activator
TRH	Thyrotropin-releasing hormone
TSH	Thyroid-stimulating hormone
TXA$_2$	Thromboxane A$_2$ (platelet-derived prostaglandin)
VIP	Vasoactive intestinal peptide
VSCC	Voltage-sensitive calcium channels

Table 1–2 DETERMINANTS OF DRUG THERAPY FOR NEUROLOGIC DISORDERS

1. Molecular targets in the CNS
2. BBB transport
3. Absorption, distribution, and metabolism
4. Toxicity or adverse effects
5. Age of patient

viruses or neoplastic cells that invade the nervous system.

Neuronal Synaptic Action of Drugs

Many drugs used to treat neurologic disorders act on specific groups of synapses within the central or peripheral nervous system (Tables 1–3 and 1–4). Chemical synapses between neurons are the primary sites where interneuronal communication and information transfer in the nervous system can be modulated. Purely electrical synapses are also present in the nervous system, but drug action at these sites has not been described.

Basic components of synaptic neurochemical transmission are illustrated in Figure 1–1. Neurotransmitters are synthesized within each neuron, stored in presynaptic vesicles, and released from depolarized nerve terminals. They bind specifically to presynaptic or postsynaptic receptors, which recognize the neurotransmitter's chemical conformation. Activation of a receptor by a neurotransmitter can cause changes in a variety of effector molecules. These include alterations in ion channel permeability, stimulation of second messenger synthesis, or regulation of DNA transcription. These biochemical actions alter the electrical activity of postsynaptic neurons (Fig. 1–2).

More than 40 molecules in the mammalian brain have been identified as having neurotransmitter properties.[20] Drugs that act at synapses either enhance or block the action of these neurotransmitters. Most neurotransmitters with a prominent role in brain function, such as inhibitory and excitatory amino-acid (EAA) neurotransmitters, produce very brief receptor-mediated actions at discrete groups of synapses. However, the actions of others, especially certain peptides, may be more prolonged than the "conventional" neurotransmitters, and they may act more widely throughout the extracellular space. A single neuron may

Table 1–3 DRUGS ACTING AT SPECIFIC PRESYNAPTIC SITES

Mechanism of Action	Drug	Neurotransmitter	Clinical Use
Enhance neurotransmitter synthesis	L-dopa Tryptophan Choline	Dopamine Serotonin Acetylcholine	Parkinson's disease Sleep disorders Movement disorders
Modulate neurotransmitter release	Baclofen Clonidine Botulinum toxin Amantadine Guanidine	GABA Norepinephrine Acetylcholine Dopamine Acetylcholine	Spasticity Tourette's syndrome Focal dystonia Parkinson's disease Eaton-Lambert syndrome
Inhibit reuptake and deplete neurotransmitter	Tetrabenazine	Dopamine Norepinephrine and serotonin	Movement disorders Depression
Inactivate neurotransmitter degradation	MAO inhibitors AChE inhibitors	Catecholamines Acetylcholine	Depression Parkinson's disease Myasthenia gravis

Table 1−4 DRUGS ACTING AT SPECIFIC POSTSYNAPTIC SITES

Mechanism of Action	Drug	Neurotransmitter	Clinical Use
Receptor agonist	Benzodiazepines	GABA receptor channel complex	Anticonvulsant Anxiolytic
	Bromocriptine	Dopamine-2	Parkinson's disease Galactorrhea
	Methylphenidate	Noradrenergic	Hyperactivity Narcolepsy
Receptor antagonist	Phenothiazines	Dopamine-2	Psychosis
	Anticholinergic (muscarinic)	Cholinergic	Movement disorders
	Yohimbine	α-2 adrenergic	Autonomic failure
	Anticholinergic (nicotinic)	Cholinergic	Neuromuscular blockade

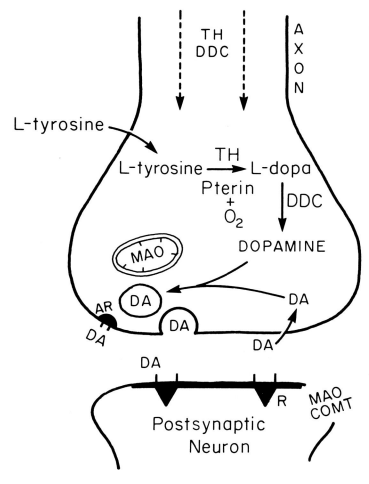

Figure 1−1. Dopamine synapse in the brain. Dopamine (DA) released from the presynaptic nerve terminal by depolarization and calcium entry interacts with postsynaptic receptors (R) and presynaptic autoreceptors (AR). Dopamine is synthesized from the amino acid L-tyrosine by the synthetic enzymes tyrosine hydroxylase (TH) and dopa decarboxylase (DDC). These enzymes are synthesized in the neuronal cell body and transported into the nerve terminal. Dopamine is removed from the synaptic cleft into the terminal or is degraded by monoamine oxidase (MAO) localized in mitochondria and on postsynaptic neuron membranes. Catechol-o-methyl transferase (COMT) also contributes to inactivation. Important sites of drug action within the dopamine synapse include depletion of dopamine stores in storage vesicles (reserpine, tetrabenazine); blockade of dopamine re-uptake (amphetamine, cocaine); inhibition of MAO (pargyline, Deprenyl); activation of presynaptic and postsynaptic dopamine receptors (apomorphine), and blockade of dopamine receptors (neuroleptic drugs).

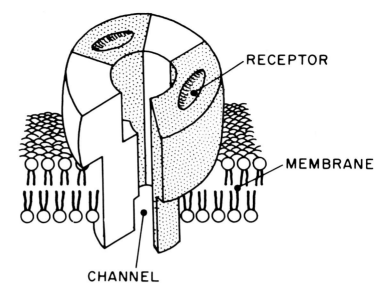

Figure   1–2. Neurotransmitter receptor channel complex lying within a phospholipid neuronal membrane. The protein structure of the channel is cut away to show the ionophore, or channel, opening. Neurotransmitter receptors or recognition sites are shown attached to the channel complex. Interaction of the neurotransmitter with the receptor causes a change in the channel conformation to open it.

contain and release more than one neurotransmitter, such as acetylcholine and a peptide (somatostatin) or gamma-aminobutyric acid (GABA) and a peptide. The combined action of both a briefly acting and a more enduring neurotransmitter produces a distinctive modulation of postsynaptic neuronal activity. To dissect the targets of drug action, effects on the nerve terminals (presynaptic) and on the neuron receiving the message (postsynaptic) are examined independently in the following section.

PRESYNAPTIC ACTIONS

The rate of neurotransmitter synthesis, and its release, reuptake into the nerve terminal, and degradation contribute to the functional synaptic activity of specific neural pathways. Selective loss or dysfunction of specific groups of presynaptic nerve terminals is a prominent feature of several important neurologic diseases. Neurons containing synthetic enzymes and/or uptake sites for a specific neurotransmitter may be most susceptible or selectively vulnerable. One of the best-characterized examples of selective

neuronal loss is in Parkinson's disease, where there is preferential damage to dopaminergic neurons. Patients with Parkinson's disease generally do not become symptomatic until there is depletion of more than 80% of striatal dopaminergic nerve terminals. When nerve terminals degenerate, both the synthetic machinery for the neurotransmitter and reuptake mechanisms that influence the duration of action of the transmitter are lost concurrently. The pathogenesis and treatment of Parkinson's disease is discussed in detail in Chapter 2.

Currently, treatments to enhance survival or regeneration of neuron cell bodies or nerve terminals are in their infancy.[43] However, pharmacologic strategies to modulate neurotransmitter synthesis, release, reuptake, and degradation to correct neurologic disorders are used regularly to attempt to restore function.

Neurotransmitter Synthesis. Substrate availability and activity of rate-limiting synthetic enzymes determine the rate of neurotransmitter synthesis. In several neurotransmitter systems, the synthetic machinery is ordinarily not saturated with substrate so that providing additional substrate enhances neurotransmitter synthesis. Both augmentation of brain levels of neurotransmitter precursors and enhancement of enzyme activity have been attempted therapeutically (Table 1–3).

Figure 1–1 illustrates the mechanisms involved in the augmentation of dopamine synthesis in dopamine nerve terminals of patients with Parkinson's disease by administration of the precursor amino-acid L-dopa, typically in conjunction with a peripheral inhibitor of L-dopa decarboxylase. L-dopa is decarboxylated to form dopamine in residual nerve terminals or perhaps, equally important, in the striatal extraneuronal space by an aromatic amino acid decarboxylase. Another example of an attempt to enhance neurotransmitter turnover in a disease state using precursor loading is the use of choline or lecithin to increase acetylcholine synthesis in tardive dyskinesia[50] or Alzheimer's disease. This approach is considered in detail in Chapter 8.

Dietary manipulation to enhance transmitter precursor availability may also increase neurotransmitter turnover in the normal brain provided that the synthetic enzyme is usually not saturated with substrate. Availability of tryptophan, the amino-acid precursor of the neurotransmitter serotonin, controls the level of serotonin synthesis. Dietary tryptophan supplementation may stimulate serotonin synthesis, and this is thought to be the mechanism by which it reduces sleep onset time in some patients with insomnia.[88] Sleep cycles in infants can be modified predictably by changing their dietary tryptophan content[107] or amount of neutral amino acids. Increasing tryptophan increases sleep; increasing the levels of neutral amino acids, which compete with tryptophan for membrane transport across the BBB, has the opposite effect.

Another approach to normalizing or augmenting brain levels of a specific neurotransmitter is to stimulate neurotransmitter synthetic enzyme activity. There are two unusual groups of patients in whom this approach has been attempted. In children with inherited defects in biopterin metabolism, severe neurodevelopmental abnormalities evolve in infancy along with a variant form of phenylketonuria. Tetrahydrobiopterin is a cofactor required for hydroxylation in the synthesis of dopamine and serotonin as well as for phenylalanine hydroxylation. In some of these children, reductions in the cerebrospinal fluid (CSF) levels of metabolites of dopamine and serotonin (homovanillic acid [HVA] and 5-hydroxyindoleacetic acid [5-HIAA], respectively) have been detected. It is uncertain to what degree these abnormalities in neurotransmitter synthesis account for the neurologic deficits. However, in several reported cases, treatment with biopterin normalized CSF levels of HVA and 5-HIAA and appeared to improve neurologic development.[55]

In another small group of children, intractable seizures responded dramatically to treatment with large doses of pyridoxine (vitamin B_6). Although initial reports described pyridoxine-dependent seizures predominantly in the neonatal period, it appears that this disorder may also present later in infancy or in early childhood. Requirements for supplemental pyridoxine may persist. In the CNS pyridoxine is a cofactor for glutamate decarboxylase (GAD), which catalyzes synthesis of the inhibitory neurotransmitter GABA.[20] No specific neurotransmitter deficiency or enzyme defect has been delineated in these children. It has been hypothesized that GABA synthesis is reduced because a molecular defect in the GAD enzyme results in its having a low affinity for pyridoxine. This abnormality presumably is overcome by administration of pharmacologic doses of the cofactor.

Neurotransmitter Release. The amount of neurotransmitter released into the synaptic cleft is determined by the neuronal firing rate, the quantity of transmitter in the nerve terminal, and the cumulative regulatory actions of excitatory and inhibitory neurotransmitters on presynaptic nerve terminal receptors. Several drugs modulate neurotransmitter release by actions mediated at presynaptic receptors, which are classified as either autoreceptors or heteroreceptors (Table 1–3). Autoreceptors recognize the endogenous neurotransmitter released from the same nerve terminal and exert a feedback regulatory effect that is typically inhibitory. Presynaptic heteroreceptors respond to different neurotransmitters released from other nerve terminals. Each nerve terminal contains multiple autoreceptors, heteroreceptors, or both.

Drugs that stimulate inhibitory neurotransmitter receptors may exert an effect on the nervous system by diminishing the release of neurotransmitters from nerve terminals. Gamma-aminobutyric acid is the major inhibitory neurotransmitter in the brain, and there are two major subgroups of GABA receptors, postsynaptic $GABA_A$ receptors and $GABA_B$ receptors, concentrated on presynaptic nerve terminals. Agonist action at $GABA_B$ receptors suppresses neurotransmitter release. Baclofen, a synthetic analog of GABA commonly used to treat spasticity, is a selective $GABA_B$ receptor agonist. Baclofen's therapeutic efficacy has been attributed in part to inhibition of excitatory neurotransmitter release, primarily in the spinal cord where both monosynaptic and polysynaptic activation of motor neurons is inhibited.[23] Similarly, the clinical efficacy of Progabide, a novel anticonvulsant with agonist properties at both $GABA_A$ and $GABA_B$ receptors, may result in part from suppression of excitatory transmission at $GABA_B$ receptors.

Clonidine, a drug used to treat hypertension, opiate withdrawal, and Tourette syndrome, may also act in part by an inhibitory presynaptic mechanism. Clonidine is an agonist at alpha-2 noradrenergic receptors, which are concentrated predominantly on presynaptic noradrenergic nerve terminals (autoreceptors) in the peripheral nervous system and inhibit norepinephrine release. Yohimbine, also an alpha-2 noradrenergic agonist, has been used experimentally to treat autonomic failure.[74] In the brain, the distribution and functional actions at alpha-2 receptors are less well defined. Clonidine's therapeutic efficacy has been attributed to suppression of norepinephrine release from brainstem locus ceruleus noradrenergic neurons. However, the drug's effects are likely considerably more complex and may act through postsynaptic alpha-2 receptors.

Opiates are another group of clinically important drugs that may act by inhibition of neurotransmitter release. A major mechanism of action of opioid agonists in the nervous system is presynaptic inhibition of transmitter release, mediated by hyperpolarization of the nerve terminal. Experimental evidence suggests that opiate-induced analgesia involves presynaptic inhibition of primary afferent sensory nociceptive neurons in the substantia gelatinosa of the spinal cord. Opiate pharmacology is discussed in detail in Chapter 9.

Recently, a unique approach to inhibiting neurotransmitter release in the peripheral nervous system has been devised. Direct local injection of botulinum toxin into a muscle leads to prolonged but reversible paralysis. The toxin binds to presynaptic sites at the neuromuscular junction, and prevents release of acetylcholine when the neuron is depolarized. Botulinum toxin has been used experimentally to treat focal dystonias (e.g., blepharospasm and strabismus). A single injection may eliminate muscle spasm for up to 3 months.[10]

In contrast with the preceding examples of drug-mediated inhibition of release, a few clinically useful drugs stimulate neurotransmitter release. Amantadine, an antiviral drug sometimes helpful for treatment of parkinsonism, may act by increasing release of dopamine. Another drug, 4-aminopyridine, has been used experimentally to treat disorders of neuromuscular transmission. Although systemic side effects limit the drug's clinical utility, it augments release of acetylcholine at the neuromuscular junction, presumably by enhancing calcium ion influx during depolarization of the nerve terminal.[72] Guanidine may also benefit patients with Eaton-Lambert syndrome and botulism, disorders in which weakness is attributed to decreased presynaptic release of acetylcholine at the neuromuscular junction.[84]

Neurotransmitter Reuptake. Actions of neurotransmitters in the synaptic cleft are terminated either by reuptake into the nerve terminal or by enzymatic degradation and diffusion away from the synaptic cleft. Reuptake processes are energy dependent and relatively substrate specific. Drugs may block reuptake or act as false substrates for reuptake systems and thereby influence the amount of neurotransmitter that is available for neurotransmission (see Table 1–3).

Reuptake blockers have dual effects. Initially, neurotransmitter accumulates in the synaptic cleft, causing acute agonist effects of the drug. Amphetamine or cocaine administration illustrates this response. These drugs inhibit reuptake of catecholamines, causing CNS stimulation with concurrent peripheral sympathomimetic actions.

With continued chronic administration of reuptake blockers, a paradoxic depletion of transmitter may occur. Clinical experience with reserpine, a drug used in the past to treat hypertension, demonstrated the consequences of this effect. Reserpine blocks reuptake at catecholamine and serotonin nerve terminals, causing depletion. Many patients treated with reserpine developed a depressive syndrome, which was attributed to CNS catecholamine depletion as a result of reuptake blockade. Both reserpine and tetrabenazine, another agent that depletes dopamine from nerve terminals, are useful for treating hyperkinetic movement disorders.[49] They may help to balance the action of overactive dopamine re-

ceptors by reducing the amount of dopamine released into the synaptic cleft.

Drugs that partially block catecholamine neurotransmitter reuptake may be effective antidepressants (see Chapter 7). Imipramine and related tricyclic antidepressants inhibit reuptake of norepinephrine and serotonin, but the mechanism underlying the clinical efficacy of these drugs for treatment of depression remains controversial. No clear abnormality of biogenic amino metabolism has been identified in untreated patients with depression.[95] Stimulant medications such as methylphenidate and dextroamphetamine are effective treatments for narcolepsy in part because of the same mechanism.[30,64,67]

Reuptake sites are only relatively selective. Drugs may gain access to specific nerve cell bodies by endogenous uptake mechanisms. Structural analogs of biogenic amines may be effective substrates for these reuptake systems; they may be taken up and stored in the nerve terminal. Consequences include subsequent release of a "false" neurotransmitter that is biologically inert or damage to the nerve terminal if the compounds taken up are neurotoxic.

Neurotransmitter Degradation. Another way to regulate the level of neurotransmitter is to influence the rate of chemical degradation. No currently available drugs stimulate these degradative enzymes, but several important drugs inhibit catecholamine, acetylcholine, or GABA degradative metabolism.

The monoamine oxidases (MAOs) are a group of enzymes that inactivate catecholamines and serotonin by oxidation. MAO inhibitors block oxidative deamination of biogenic amines; treatment with these drugs results in marked increases in brain concentrations of norepinephrine, serotonin, and dopamine. These neurotransmitters accumulate both within the nerve terminals and secondarily in the synapses. MAO inhibitors are used clinically to treat selected patients with depression. A major risk of treatment, which results from peripheral actions of MAO inhibitors, is abrupt development of hypertension. This adverse reaction occurs after ingestion of foods containing tyramine, a catecholamine agonist, which may accumulate at peripheral sympathetic synapses. Deprenyl, a selective MAO inhibitor that reduces activity of one type of MAO called *MAO type B*, is currently under evaluation for treatment of Parkinson's disease. The drug has at least two potential modes of action at dopaminergic synapses. One action is to prolong the efficacy of released dopamine by inhibiting its degradation; another potential therapeutic mechanism is to block the production of possible neurotoxic metabolites.[60] This therapeutic strategy is discussed in detail in Chapter 2.

Acetylcholinesterase, the major degradative enzyme for acetylcholine, is another target for a number of enzyme inhibitors used in clinical neurology.[28] Drugs that block activity of this enzyme, such as pyridostigmine, augment the efficacy of released acetylcholine in the neuromuscular junction. Anticholinesterase drugs that penetrate the BBB have been used experimentally in attempts to enhance cholinergic transmission in patients with dementia (see Chapter 8).

Other drugs may also act by inhibiting the degradation of the inhibitory neurotransmitter GABA. Treatment with the anticonvulsant valproate increases brain levels of GABA, possibly by inhibiting its enzymatic degradation. Vigabatrin is an experimental anticonvulsant believed to act in a mode similar to valproate to raise levels of GABA in the CSF.[12] Acting as a "suicide substrate," this GABA analogue is transformed by GABA transaminase to an intermediate that covalently binds to the active site of the enzyme and irreversibly inhibits its activity. The term *suicide substrate* refers to the ability of the specific substrate to inactivate its enzyme.

Other Presynaptic Effects. A number of endogenous molecules, classified collectively as trophic factors, are essential for maintenance and survival of CNS neurons and their terminals. For example, nerve growth factor (NGF) is a protein that supports the survival of cholinergic neurons, and stimulates the activity of the synthetic enzyme for acetylcholine, choline acetyltransferase. Intrathecal NGF infusion has been suggested as a potential treatment for early Alzheimer's disease (see Chapter 8).[43] This type of trophic therapy may be useful in the future to reverse or prevent the degeneration of neuronal terminals in certain neurologic disorders.

POSTSYNAPTIC AND
RECEPTOR-MEDIATED
EFFECTS OF DRUGS

Drug Receptors and Effectors. Some of the most widely used drugs in neurologic practice are agonists or antagonists at specific neurotransmitter receptors (see Fig. 1–2). These drugs generally mimic or block the actions of endogenous compounds (receptor ligands) at specific membrane-bound molecules or receptors (Table 1–4). A *receptor* is a molecule located on a cell membrane that selectively binds to a restricted group of endogenous neurotransmitters or drugs.[20] Receptors are sometimes referred to as a *recognition site* because they recognize a limited group of similar chemicals used to transfer information in the brain. Receptors are linked to effector molecules, either membrane channels which admit ions to the neuron, or enzymes, which generate intracellular second messenger molecules. The effector is activated when the receptor is occupied by an appropriate agonist, or deactivated when the receptor is occupied by an antagonist. Agonist activation of a receptor allows the neurotransmitter's message or drug action to be translated into information to which the neuron responds, such as changes in membrane electrical potential, intracellular calcium, or gene expression. Together, neurotransmitter receptors and effectors are among the most im-

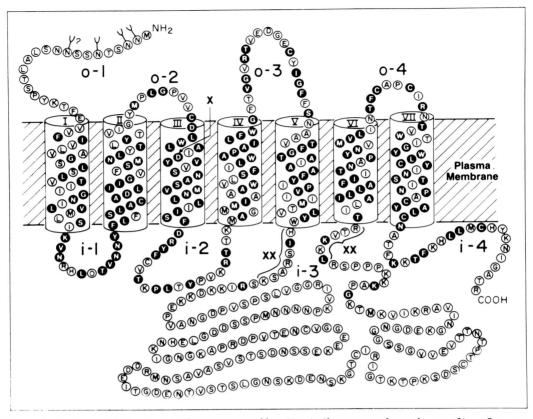

Figure 1–3. A predicted amino acid sequence and location in the neuronal membrane of type 2 muscarinic receptor M_2 based on sequencing of the cloned gene. Extracellular (o) and intracellular (i) domains of the protein are indicated. "X" marks a membrane site believed to be important in muscarinic agonist and antagonist binding. Portions of the protein marked "XX" are possible binding sites for the G proteins that link the muscarinic receptor to second messengers. (From Goyal, RK: Muscarinic receptor subtypes: Physiology and clinical implications. N Engl J Med 321:1022–1028, 1989, with permission.)

portant targets for drug action in neurology.

A number of pharmacologically relevant neurotransmitter receptor and receptor-effector complexes have been characterized during the past decade. The DNA material coding for a few receptors has been cloned (Fig. 1–3) so that their total composition and conformation can be studied. However, the most common method for characterizing neurotransmitter receptors involves ligand-binding techniques. In these experiments, brain tissue or solubilized purified receptor is equilibrated in a buffer solution with specific neurotransmitter chemicals or drugs (ligands) usually labeled with a radioiso-

tope. After a period of equilibration, free ligand is separated from receptor-ligand complexes, and measured to characterize the receptor.

Receptors are evaluated in the receptor-binding assays and in related physiologic experiments to identify the three major properties of binding to a true receptor: saturability, specificity, and reversibility. These three properties of a neurotransmitter receptor are directly relevant to the drug action that it transmits. All three follow from the *law of mass action* describing the interaction between a drug or neurotransmitter and a receptor (Fig. 1–4). The kinetic terms used in the mathematic expression of the law of mass action are com-

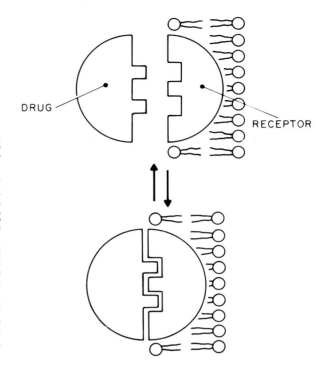

Figure 1–4. The simplest, most common model used to make quantitative estimates of drug action. This model is the basis for assumptions made in Figures 1–5, 1–6, and 1–7. The model includes only two molecules, a drug (ligand), and a receptor. At any point the amount of drug bound to the receptor is related to the rate at which drug and receptor associate (downward arrow) and dissociate (upward arrow). In reality, drug receptor interactions are often more complicated. For example, several related receptor subtypes may be present in the brain, making the graphic curves shown in Figures 1–5, 1–6, and 1–7 more complicated. Another common complication is an effect of an associated effector (e.g., ion channel), or receptor binding which is not shown here. The receptor lies within a phospholipid bilayer.

monly used to describe a drug's action in the nervous system. A working knowledge of these terms is useful for comparing drugs used in clinical practice.

Kinetics of Drug-Receptor Interaction. The law of mass action describes the interaction of pure drug or other ligand and a single population of receptors:

$$[drug] + [receptor] \rightleftharpoons [drug:receptor]$$

If drug = D, receptor = R and drug:receptor = DR, the quantitative relationship is described by:

$$[DR] = \frac{[D]\,[DRmax]}{K_D + [D]}$$

where: DRmax = drug bound to receptor at saturation
D = free drug (unbound)
K_D = equilibrium dissociation constant

DR is commonly referred to as B or bound drug. Substituting B for DR,

$$[B] = \frac{[D]\,[Bmax]}{K_D + [D]}$$

This is identical to the equation used to describe the interaction between an enzyme and substrate (Michaelis-Menton equation). Graphically, the relationship is shown in Figure 1–5.

Bmax and K_D are important terms that describe the characteristics of a receptor. Bmax describes the capacity of a receptor to bind drugs, in moles per weight of tissue or protein.

Bmax = maximal amount of ligand bound to a fixed amount of receptor

A population of drug receptors is saturable, and has a finite capacity to bind ligands that it recognizes. This feature distinguishes receptor molecules from a

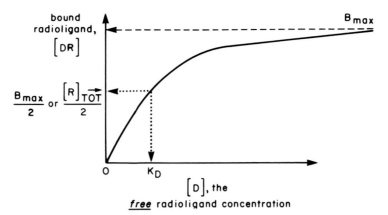

Figure 1–5. The simplest mathematical relationship between free drug (in this case a radioactive ligand) in the incubation buffer and the amount of drug bound to a specific receptor (bound radioligand) in brain tissue. The graph is based on the bimolecular model shown in Figure 1–4. The model is identical to the one used to describe interaction between an enzyme and its substrate. The equation describing this interaction is called the Michaelis-Menton equation. Increasing concentrations of unbound or free drug, [D], eventually lead to saturation of the receptor at a point defined by B_{max} (equal to $[R]_{TOT}$), the maximal possible concentration of drug/receptor complexes (maximal [DR]). The point on the curve at which half the available receptors are occupied (Bmax/2 or [R]TOT/2) is produced by a free drug concentration equal to the K_D or dissociation constant for the drug and receptor.

host of other bonding sites in the nervous system. In receptor-binding experiments, *specific* interaction with receptors is distinguished from *nonspecific* binding to nonreceptor molecules such as lipids. In contrast to specific drug-receptor interactions, nonspecific binding is usually not saturable but may be virtually limitless.

Estimation of nonspecific binding is critical to accurate determination of drug receptor–binding characteristics. Nonspecific binding is determined by measuring binding of a drug in the presence of another drug that competes at the same receptor. As shown in Figure 1–6, unlike specific binding, binding to nonspecific sites (e.g., lipid membranes) is generally linear with increasing ligand concentration and does not saturate.

The K_D or *equilibrium dissociation constant* describes the affinity or "tightness" with which a drug binds to the receptor. The K_D is expressed in moles (concentration), and a small number (e.g., 10^{-9}mol/L) indicates a higher affinity of the receptor for a drug

compared to a larger number (e.g. 10^{-3}mol/L).

Bmax and K_D are generally determined from linear graphs of the Michaelis-Menton equation reformulated as:

$$\frac{[DR]}{[D]} = \frac{1}{K_D} \cdot [DR] + \frac{Bmax}{K_D}$$

This is a linear equation in the form $y = mX + B$ where m is the slope of the line (Fig. 1–7). This linear graph is called a Scatchard plot. It can be withdrawn with the x and y coordinates reversed and then it is called an *Eadie-Hofstee plot*. As a Scatchard plot, the Bmax is determined from the x intercept and the K_D is determined from the slope where $m = -1/K_D$. For the Eadie-Hofstee plot, the Bmax is the y intercept and the slope $= K_D$.

Another way to think about the K_D that may make more intuitive sense is based on the rates at which a drug associates and dissociates with a receptor. The K_D reflects the rate of dissociation

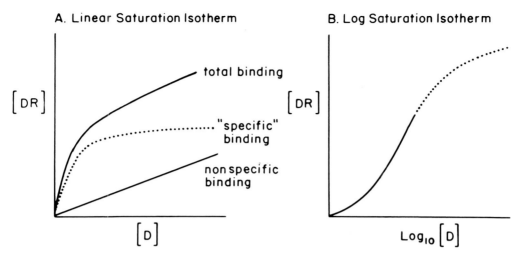

A. Linear Saturation Isotherm

B. Log Saturation Isotherm

Figure 1–6. To determine characteristics of drug receptors in the brain, tissue is incubated with buffer containing increasing concentrations of free drug [D], and the drug bound to receptors is calculated [DR]. In (A), the top curve represents the total amount of binding to the tissue. The bottom solid line represents nonspecific binding, for example, binding to lipids in the brain or to glass in the test tube used for the experiment. Nonspecific binding does not saturate at the drug level used in this experiment. Subtraction of nonspecific binding from "total" binding yields the dotted curve, which shows specific binding to a single population of receptors. Replotting the specific binding data using a logarithmic scale for [D] yields a standard, familiar pharmacologic dose response shown in (B). In this case it is called a saturation isotherm because it plots the progressive saturation of the receptor with increasing drug concentration plotted logarithmically. Provided that a drug receptor interaction follows all the assumptions outlined (e.g., single drug, single receptor population) and the receptor produces a specific identifiable clinical response, the log saturation isotherm shown here and the pharmacologic dose response shown in Figure 1–9 are very similar.

Figure 1–7. The Scatchard plot for binding data in which receptor bound drug/free drug ([DR]/[D]) is plotted versus bound drug ([DR]). The K_D, or dissociation constant, is used to estimate the affinity of a drug for its receptor and can be calculated from the slope of the line. The straight line is produced by a single drug interacting with a single population of receptors; other situations produce curved lines.

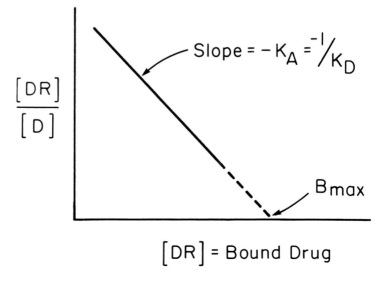

of the drug-receptor complex divided by the rate of association:

$$D + R \underset{K_2}{\overset{K_1}{\rightleftarrows}} DR$$

$$K_D = \frac{K_2}{K_1}$$

The affinity of a drug for a receptor (K_D) can be calculated directly from the rate constants for association (K_1) and dissociation (K_2). This can be done in an experiment as shown in Figure 1–8, where the time for drug-receptor complex formation and dissociation is directly measured. These "on times" and "off times" are used to calculate the rate constants and the K_D. Intuitively, it can be seen that a high affinity "tight fit" is characterized by a slow "off time," a fast "on time," or both.

For many drugs, it is also useful to have a quantitative term to compare their activity as competitive inhibitors of binding of other drugs to a receptor.

This term, the K_i, or equilibrium dissociation constant of the competitive inhibitor with respect to a given ligand and receptor, is calculated from the relationship:

$$K_i = \frac{IC_{50}}{1 + [L]/K_D}$$

where: IC_{50} = concentration of inhibitor producing 50% reduction in binding
$[L]$ = the liquid concentration in the experiment
K_D = equilibrium dissociation constant of L for the receptor

This is also called the *Cheng-Prusoff equation*.

Replotting receptor-binding data as shown in Figures 1–6 and 1–9 gives a more familiar saturation response curve or *saturation isotherm*. The "S" shape is identical to sigmoidal log dose-response curves familiar from classical pharmacology. Note that in these

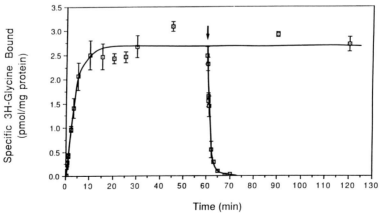

Figure 1–8. Data from an experiment to demonstrate the time course of association and dissociation between the amino acid neurotransmitter glycine and a specific receptor in the hippocampus. Radioactive glycine was added to the reaction mixture bathing the brain tissue at the "O", and the amount of radioactivity bound to the brain tissue was measured at frequent intervals over the first 30 minutes. The data demonstrate that the receptors bind glycine over the first 10 minutes but then become saturated. At 60 minutes, the concentration of radioactive glycine is rapidly lowered to a very low level so that the rate of dissociation can be measured. The rate constant for dissociation divided by the rate constant for association equals the K_D for the glycine receptor. In this case, the rate of dissociation is much more rapid than the rate of association. (From McDonald, JW, Penney, JB, Johnston, MV and Young, AB: Characterization and regional distribution of strychnine-insensitive 3-glycine binding sites in rat brain by quantitative receptor autoradiography. Neuroscience 35:653–668, 1990, with permission.)

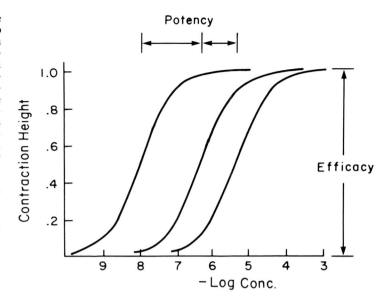

Figure 1–9. Dose response curves show the relationship between the dose (expressed in log to base 10) and a physiologic effect (in this case smooth muscle contraction) in response to epinephrine analogue drugs. In cases where drug binding to a specific receptor is directly related to its physiologic effect, the drug receptor isotherm (Fig. 1–6) will resemble its physiologic or clinical dose response curves. The figure shows the difference between potency, the dose required to produce a half-maximal response; and efficacy, the dose needed to produce a maximal effect. In this case, all three drugs have the same efficacy or intrinsic activity but have a different potency.

curves, the dose is expressed as a logarithm. Ideally, dose-response curves for a biologic effect of a drug (e.g., anxiolysis with diazepam) acting at a neurotransmitter receptor resembles the drug's binding saturation isotherm for the receptor. However, pharmacokinetics and other factors that determine the drug's access to the receptor may alter this relationship. These include absorption, metabolism penetration across the BBB, and receptor-effector coupling. Large differences between the clinical dose response and receptor-binding data may indicate that the receptor under study is irrelevant to the clinical effect.

Drugs can be compared by assessing both log dose-response curves in assays of biologic activity and by using saturation isotherms. Their relative potency and efficacy can be compared using data shown in Figure 1–9. *Potency* is the measure of the dose at which the effect or binding is half maximal, while *efficacy* is the dose at which the drug produces a maximal effect. Potency is the more useful measure of the effect of drugs because it applies to submaximal doses.

Detailed kinetic and pharmacologic analysis of receptors has revealed considerable complexity. Several receptor subtypes have been identified for common neurotransmitters such as acetylcholine, GABA, and dopamine (see Chapter 7). In addition, individual receptor subtypes commonly have two states that preferentially bind agonists or antagonists. The GABA benzodiazepine receptor has been examined extensively using a multisite model (see Chapter 3).[34]

Receptor-Effector Coupling. Receptor coupled effector mechanisms such as channels and enzymes play an equally important role in neurotransmitter and drug action (Fig. 1–10). Effector mechanisms for a number of neurotransmitter systems have been characterized including those for dopamine, acetylcholine, GABA, benzodiazepines, and EAAs.

The response to a single neurotransmitter is quite complex because it depends on the combination of receptor subtypes and effectors that are activated in each region of the brain. For example, acetylcholine may activate multiple types of muscarinic receptors in the heart, gut, or brain, and these receptors in turn are coupled to several ion channels and second messenger

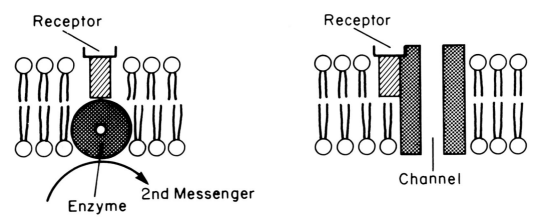

Figure 1 – 10. Neurotransmitter receptors are coupled to two types of effector molecules which transfer messages across the neuronal membrane. Receptor stimulation of enzyme activity (*left*) increases production of second messengers. Receptor stimulation of channels (*right*) changes ionic movement across membranes.

systems (Fig. 1 – 11). Second messengers that mediate the response to neurotransmitter activation include cyclic adenosine monophosphate (cAMP), inositol 1,4,5-triphosphate (IP$_3$), diacylglycerol (DG), and calcium.[106] These multiple effector mechanisms may also interact or "cross talk." For example, activation of the second messenger systems regulated by cAMP and phospholipase C (phosphoinositol turnover) appears to produce mutual interactions and competing actions at the cellular level. Often these discrete systems are organized in a regionally complementary fashion.[106] The complexity of the biochemical cascade stimulated by neurotransmitters provides a rich substrate for drug actions in the nervous system.

Excitatory Amino-Acid Receptor-Effector Mechanisms. One important neurotransmitter system, which demonstrates the variety of receptor-effector mechanisms in the brain, is the EAA system (Fig. 1 – 12). Excitatory amino-acid neurotransmitters such as glutamate mediate more than half the neuronal information flow in the brain. Interest in the pharmacology of EAA synaptic transmission is high because of the possibility that these systems are involved in the pathogenesis of neuro-

degenerative diseases, epilepsy, and neuronal injury from a variety of causes including hypoxia-ischemia and head injury. The receptor and effector mechanisms used by EAA pathways provide good examples of the diversity of ionic and metabolic actions that are triggered by a single neurotransmitter. These actions are determined to a large extent by regional differences in organization of these systems. Regions such as the cerebellum have EAA receptor and second messengers organized differently from the basal ganglia or hippocampus.

The excitatory responses of glutamate are mediated by several receptor subtypes that may be classified into two broad categories as either N-methyl-D-aspartate (NMDA) or non-NMDA-type EAA receptors (Fig. 1 – 12). NMDA maximally activates a glutamate receptor that is linked to an ion channel. Together the receptor and its channel are referred to as the NMDA receptor/channel complex (Fig. 1 – 13). The NMDA channel is permeable to cations such as sodium and calcium, and at normal membrane potential, the channel is blocked by magnesium ions. Partial depolarization of the membrane potential is necessary for the magnesium block to be removed. As a result, the NMDA receptor/channel complex is not gener-

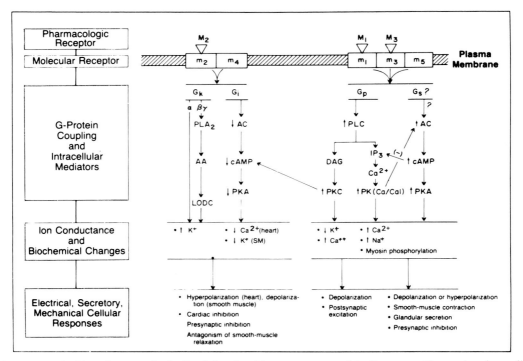

Figure 1–11. The pharmacologically defined subtypes correspond to the respective molecular subtypes. M_2/m_2 and m_4 are mainly coupled with G_k and G_i ("G proteins"), whereas M_1/m_1, M_3/m_3, and m_5 are coupled with G_p and possibly with G_s, although the latter is doubtful. G_k is so named because it is coupled with potassium (K^+) channels; G_i and G_s are coupled with adenylate cyclase (AC), which they inhibit and stimulate, respectively. G_p is a family of putative G proteins that are coupled with phospholipase C (PLC). The intracellular mediators involved depend on the type of G protein activated. The changes in the mediators lead to ion conductance and biochemical changes and subsequently to electrical, secretory, and mechanical cellular responses. There is an interaction between the products of PLC stimulation and those of AC stimulation. α and β refer to subunits of G_k; PLA$_2$ denotes phospholipase A$_2$; Abbreviations: AA = arachidonic acid; LODC = lipooxygenase-derived compounds; PKA = protein kinase A; DAG = diacylglycerol; PKC = protein kinase C; IP$_3$ = inositol 1,4,5 triphosphate; PK (Ca/Cal) = protein kinase that is sensitive to calcium and calmodulin; SM = smooth muscle. (From Goyol, RK: Muscarinic receptor subtypes: Physiology and clinical implications. N Engl J Med 321:1022–1028, 1989, with permission.)

ally involved in ordinary rapid impulse flow.

A number of antagonists of the NMDA receptor/channel complex have been developed, some of which block the NMDA receptor (competitive NMDA antagonists) and others of which block its effector, the cation channel (noncompetitive antagonists). Drugs such as CPP (3-[±2-carboxypiperazine-4yl] propyl-l-phosphonate) and APV (2-amino-5-phosphono-valerate) are noncompetitive blockers at the NMDA receptor. The channel-binding site is commonly referred to as the phencyclidine (PCP) receptor; two drugs that noncompetitively block the channel are MK-801 and PCP. The NMDA receptor/channel complex also includes several regulatory subunits. One receptor is specific for the simple amino acid glycine. Unlike the inhibitory glycine site in the spinal cord, this site is not sensitive to strychnine, and its activation facilitates opening of the NMDA channel by glutamate. Recognition sites for zinc and polyamines also appear to regulate NMDA receptor/channel complex activ-

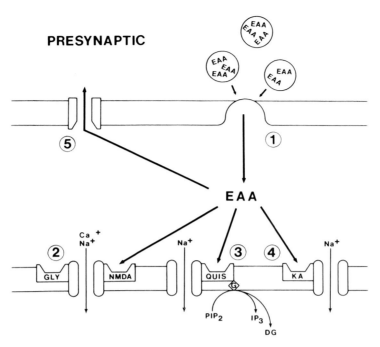

Figure 1 – 12. A diagram of important features of excitatory amino acid (EAA) neurotransmission in the brain. EAAs such as glutamate can interact with at least three types of EAA receptors. These receptors and effectors are distributed differently in different brain regions. Steps in excitatory neurotransmission include (1) Glutamate and related EAAs are released from presynaptic neuronal terminals in a calcium-dependent process by depolarization of the presynaptic neuron; (2)–(4)Once released into the synaptic cleft, glutamate can depolarize the postsynaptic neuronal membrane binding to at least 3 subsets of EAA receptors; Activation of (2) the NMDA receptor channel complex, (3) quisqualate receptors (QUIS), or (4) kainate receptors (KA) can produce cationic fluxes through receptor associated ionophores. Alternatively, a subset of quisqualate receptors are linked with phospholipase C, which activates phosphoinositol hydrolysis and generates the second messengers inositol triphosphate (IP₃) and diacylglycerol (DG); The distribution of these subtypes of EAA receptors in brain can be examined with radiolabeled ligands specific to each receptor subtype; (5) The excitatory actions of glutamate on postsynaptic membranes are inactivated by a presynaptic, high-affinity, energy-dependent transport process. (From McDonald and Johnston,[66] p 42, with permission.)

ity. NMDA receptor and channel-blocking drugs are under active investigation for a variety of neurologic disorders.

Non-NMDA receptors have been identified that are preferentially activated by the glutamate analogues quisqualic acid and kainic acid (Fig. 1 – 12). Kainic acid was identified a number of years ago as a very potent neurotoxic and convulsant compound in the adult brain. Two different subtypes of the quisqualate receptor have been identified. One type is linked to an ion channel that admits sodium primarily. The ion channel linked to the quisqualic receptor is responsible for much of the fast excitatory activity in the nervous system. In contrast, a quisqualate-type glutamate receptor that is coupled to phospholipase C activates breakdown of membrane phosphoinositol lipids such as phosphatidylinositol 4,5-biphosphate (PIP₂) leading to generation of the second messengers IP₃ and diacylglycerol DG. Antagonists have been identified that block the quisqualate re-

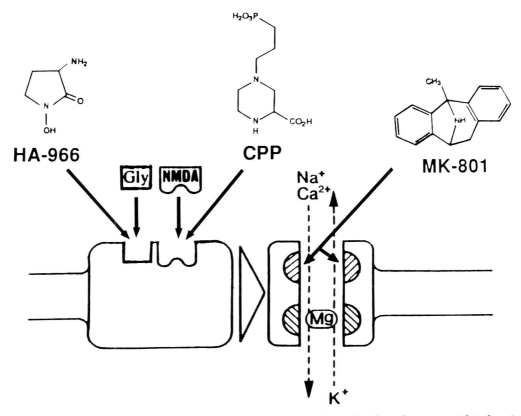

Figure 1–13. The components of the NMDA receptor/channel complex, based on current biochemical and electrophysiologic evidence. The NMDA recognition site is coupled to a cationic channel that is permeable to both Ca^{2+} and Na^+. A glycine modulatory site (distinct from the classical inhibitory glycine site) is closely associated with the NMDA receptor; glycine is required for channel activation and enhances NMDA responses. The NMDA channel is also referred to as the "PCP channel" because phencyclidine (PCP) binds within the pore. Mg^{2+} blocks the channel in a voltage-dependent manner; at relatively negative membrane potentials, Mg^{2+} blocks the channel and blockade is relieved by depolarization. Thus NMDA receptor channel activation requires both NMDA and glycine receptor activation and concomitant membrane depolarization. Also, Zn^{2+} (not illustrated) reduces NMDA responses by binding to a site on the external face of the membrane. NMDA responses can be blocked pharamacologically in at least three ways: Competitive NMDA antagonists such as CPP or APV compete for binding at the NMDA recognition site; competitive glycine receptor antagonists such as HA-966 block the glycine site and reduce NMDA-mediated responses; and noncompetitive NMDA receptor antagonists such as MK-801, PCP, and dissociative anesthetics (ketamine) bind within the ionophore and prevent ion fluxes. (From McDonald and Johnston,[66] p 43, with permission.)

ceptor linked to the ion channel but none have been identified that recognize the phosphoinosital-linked (metabotropic) receptor.

A key action of IP_3 generated from glutamate stimulation of phosphoinositide (PPI) hydrolysis is to regulate and increase intracellular free calcium. Intracellular calcium levels are critical regulators of neuronal function, and calcium metabolism is a major target for drug action in the nervous system. Several other groups of drugs also influence intracellular calcium metabolism. Systemically administered calcium channel antagonists have multiple actions; in the brain, these drugs may act on blood vessels, neurons, or both. The intracellular effects of calcium are closely linked with the regulatory protein calmodulin. Calcium has an impact on a variety of protein kinase enzymes and on gene expansion.

A major goal of neuropharmacology is to provide highly specific therapy. If a drug's action can be targeted for a specific neurotransmitter receptor or receptor-linked effector mechanism, this specificity and selectivity may be achievable. Further progress in biochemistry and molecular genetics of synaptic neurotransmitter mechanisms is likely to provide new insights for drug therapy.

Neuronal Actions on Cell Membranes and Metabolism

Many drugs that modulate neuronal function directly do not exert their effects at the synapse. Neuroactive drugs may have nonselective effects on cell membranes and energy metabolism as well as on DNA, RNA, or protein synthesis.

EFFECTS ON CELL MEMBRANE PROPERTIES

A number of drugs exert potent effects through as yet undetermined actions on neuronal membranes. For example, anesthetics produce profound reversible impairment of consciousness and analgesia, but their mechanisms of action are unknown. Anesthetic agents do not share a single chemical structural class, but they share common features including lipid solubility and the ability to inhibit both conduction of the action potential and synaptic transmission. Anesthesia is attributed to changes in the physicochemical properties of neuronal cell membranes. Proposed primary sites of action of anesthetics are the lipid matrix of the membrane and the hydrophobic region of specific membrane-bound proteins. Anesthetics modify the actions of neurotransmitter receptors by changing the membranes in which they are embedded.

Several novel therapeutic agents may protect membranes from toxic destruc-

tion. Neurotoxic free radicals derived from membrane lipid peroxidation may contribute to the evolution of neuronal damage from hypoxia, ischemia, and prolonged seizures. In the period of reperfusion after ischemia, oxygen-derived free radicals may contribute to the progression of injury by direct neuronal toxicity and indirect effects on cerebral blood flow. If normal intracellular scavenging systems fail, intracellular oxidative reactions that generate free radicals may also be detrimental to neuronal survival.[56] Vitamin E and several other antioxidant compounds show promise as neuroprotective drugs in experimental models. Allopurinol, which blocks xanthine oxidase activity in vivo, may also have potential to limit reperfusion injury. Other free-radical scavengers and antioxidants are under development (see Chapter 4).

EFFECTS ON NEURONAL METABOLISM

Drugs that stimulate or suppress neuronal metabolism might be clinically useful in several situations. Normal production of neurotransmitters and cellular proteins depends on an active neuronal metabolism. Stimulation of cerebral metabolism or improved efficiency of substrate utilization could benefit patients with neurodegenerative disorders, for example, in which metabolism is defective. The effects on cognition of neurotropic drugs, which are nonspecific activators of cerebral metabolism, are currently being evaluated (see Chapter 8).

Neuronal energy metabolism is also disrupted in inherited abnormalities of carbohydrate and fat metabolism. Administration of vitamins and cofactors such as carnitine may be beneficial for treatment of several rare inherited disorders of fat metabolism. Carnitine is an endogenous compound normally synthesized from lysine; its metabolic role is the transport of long-chain fatty acids into mitochondria for oxidation. A group of inborn errors of metabolism are attributed to systemic and/or muscle carnitine deficiency. Carnitine deficiency may also arise secondarily to abnormalities of organic acid metabolism. Clinical manifestations of systemic carnitine deficiency may include acute hepatic encephalopathy, progressive weakness, and early death. The myopathic forms are characterized primarily by progressive weakness. Recent experience indicates that supplementation with large doses of L-carnitine orally can arrest progression of the neurologic syndromes and, in some cases, can restore normal neurologic functioning.[6]

Drug Actions on Nonneuronal Elements

Many drugs used to treat neurologic disorders exert their effects primarily at nonneuronal sites, including cerebral blood vessels, glia, inflammatory cells, or the choroid plexus.

Drugs may influence cerebral blood flow differentially in the normal and the injured brain. The factors that regulate cerebral blood flow are complex. In clinical practice, perhaps the most common indication for therapy with drugs influencing cerebral blood flow has been in the treatment of migraine (see Chapter 5). Neurotransmitters, including serotonin, dopamine, and the neuromodulator adenosine, may contribute to regulation of cerebral blood flow. Pharmacologic management of cerebral blood flow by manipulation of these neurotransmitters and voltage-sensitive calcium channels[35] is discussed in Chapter 4.

Cerebral edema is another important target for drug therapy. Cerebral edema is classified as a vasogenic or cytotoxic increase in brain water content.[32] Vasogenic edema results from disruption of the integrity of the BBB and increased brain capillary endothelium permeability. Clinical settings where vasogenic edema is prominent include brain tumors, abscesses, and intracerebral hematomas. Cytotoxic edema results from increased intracellular fluid accumulation as a result of failure of the Na^+ $-K^+$ membrane pump; the most common initiating event is an hypoxic-ischemic insult. Corticosteroids are commonly used to treat vasogenic cerebral edema, but are of little use for cytotoxic edema. Their potential benefits include stabilization of capillary vascular endothelium and suppression of phospholipase-A_2-induced release of prostaglandin precursors. Steroids may also be useful, along with acetazolamide, in pseudotumor cerebri, although their mechanism of action is unclear.

Acute and chronic demyelinating disorders are a major cause of neurologic morbidity, but no available drugs are specifically targeted to act on glial cells or on the myelin sheath. Anti-inflammatory and immunosuppressive drugs currently are the mainstay of treatment of demyelinating disorders; approaches to treatment are discussed in detail in Chapter 6.

Effects on DNA, RNA, or Protein Synthesis

A number of drugs used in neurology to treat neoplasms or viral infections act on DNA, RNA, or protein synthesis. Their lack of effect on the brain is an advantage for selectively destroying invading organisms or tumor cells.

Viruses that invade the CNS may use some host-cell synthetic pathways for replication; the viral DNA may be incorporated into the host-cell genome. Effective drugs for treatment of viral infections of the nervous system will prevent viral replication without disrupting neuronal integrity. The mode of action of the drug acyclovir illustrates this approach. Acyclovir is currently the most effective drug available for the treatment of herpes infections. Acyclovir can be classified as a *prodrug*, that is, a drug administered in inactive form that is activated in vivo in target cells. This guanine nucleoside analogue is phosphorylated preferentially by viral thymidine kinase since the viral enzyme binds acyclovir with much higher affinity than the mammalian form of the enzyme. Acyclovir triphosphate is incorporated into replicating DNA and blocks DNA synthesis. Treatment with acyclovir reduces the mortality and morbidity of herpes encephalitis, and the drug has no significant neurotoxicity.[103]

Similar principles apply in the analysis of the therapeutic actions of azidothymidine (AZT). Currently, this is one of the few drugs that may be of benefit in the treatment of patients with CNS acquired immune deficiency syndrome. AZT is a synthetic analog of thymidine; it is incorporated into the viral DNA by reverse transcriptase and blocks DNA synthesis, but it has considerably less inhibitory effect on mammalian DNA synthesis.[83]

BARRIERS TO DRUG ACTION IN THE CNS

The BBB limits the exchange of molecules between the systemic circulation and the brain, and is a unique determinant of the effect of CNS drugs. Optimizing drug delivery to the brain is a major goal of investigation in clinical neuropharmacology.

The functional features of the barrier are attributable primarily to the ultrastructure of brain capillary endothelial cells (Fig. 1 – 14). The endothelial cells

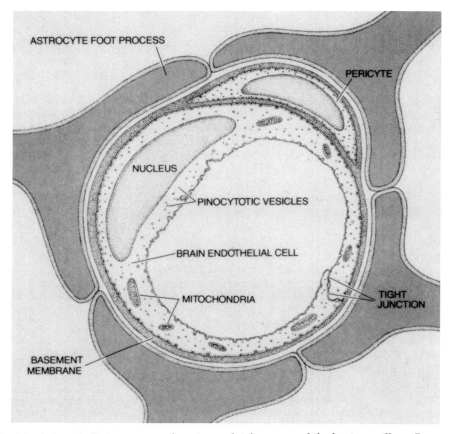

Figure 1 – 14. Astrocyte foot processes almost completely surround the brain capillary. Because of this relation it was once thought that the astrocytes form the blood brain barrier. It is now known that the endothelial cells constitute the barrier. Endothelial cells selectively transport nutrients into the brain, and their many mitochondria probably provide energy for transport. The endothelial cells of the brain have few pinocytotic vesicles. In other organs such vesicles may provide relatively unselective transport across the capillary wall. (From Goldstein, G and Betz, AL.[37] Copyright © 1986 by SCIENTIFIC AMERICAN, Inc. All rights reserved.)

are connected by continuous intercellular tight junctions, which are impervious to drugs. Other functional components of the barrier include the foot processes of astrocytes, which are closely apposed to endothelial cells, and the choroid plexus, where active removal of metabolites and drugs from cerebrospinal fluid occurs.[37]

The rate at which drugs reach the brain through the BBB is determined primarily by their blood concentrations, protein binding, lipid solubility, and polarity. Other factors are listed in Table 1–5.

Solutes are transported across the BBB either by diffusion through capillary endothelial cells or by facilitated transport. The diffusion rate is determined by the drug's solubility (Fig. 1–15). For example, after systemic admin-

Table 1–5 FACTORS INFLUENCING RATE OF DRUG TRANSPORT THROUGH THE BBB

Blood concentration of drug
Protein binding of drug
Lipid solubility of drug
Polarity of drug
Size of capillary surface area
Affinity and density of transport carriers
Possible enzymatic modification within endothelial cells

istration of the chemotherapeutic agent methotrexate, steady-state concentrations in spinal fluid are only 3% of plasma concentration. In patients with CNS diseases such as tumors and infections, however, the integrity of the barrier may be diminished, and poorly

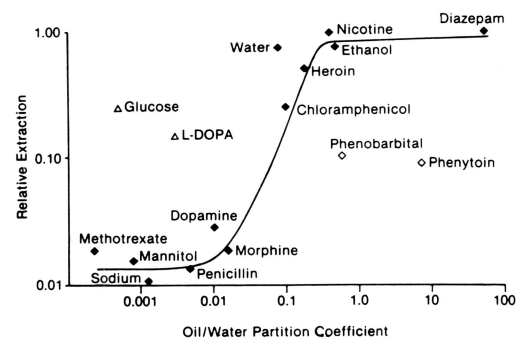

Figure 1–15. Relationship between lipid solubility and brain uptake of selected compounds. The distribution into olive oil relative to water for each test substance serves as a measure of its lipid solubility. The brain uptake is determined by comparing the extraction of each test substance relative to a highly permeable tracer during a single passage through the cerebral circulation. In general, compounds with higher oil-to-water partition coefficients show increased entry into the brain. Uptake of the two anticonvulsants, phenobarbital and phenytoin, is lower than predicted from their lipid solubility partly because of their binding to plasma proteins. This explains the slower onset of anticonvulsant activity of these agents compared with diazepam. Uptake of glucose and L-dopa is greater than predicted by their lipid solubility because specific carriers facilitate their transport across the brain capillary. (From Asbury, AK, McKhann, GM, and McDonald WI [eds]: Diseases of the Nervous System. WB Saunders, Philadelphia, 1986, p 177, with permission).

soluble drugs may penetrate more efficiently.

Facilitated transport by specific carriers in the luminal and antiluminal surfaces of the endothelial cell is highly selective, stereospecific, and saturable. Currently, few clinically useful drugs have affinity for these carrier systems. One example is the transport of L-dopa across the BBB (Fig. 1–16). Neutral amino acids compete for this transport carrier as they do in the gastrointestinal tract. Their ingestion in dietary protein may reduce the effectiveness of therapy for Parkinson's disease (see Chapter 2).

Enhancing Transport Across the BBB

A number of approaches are being used to deliver drugs beyond the BBB. These include administration of drugs directly into brain or CSF [76,96] and disruption of the BBB.

Drugs injected via lumbar puncture or through an Ommaya reservoir attached to a catheter in the lateral ventricles are commonly used to treat CNS malignancies or infections. This ap-

proach has major limitations, however. The distribution of the drug within the brain is nonuniform after intrathecal infusion. There is often a coincident increase in the drug's toxicity in brain regions adjacent to the ventricle. For example, when methotrexate is administered intrathecally, measured brain tissue concentrations are extremely high adjacent to the ventricles and fall rapidly at more distant sites. Brain regions adjacent to the ventricle exposed to peak tissue levels are especially susceptible to neurotoxicity. Other limitations of the intrathecal route include the rate of diffusion through brain tissue, extent of absorption into the systemic circulation, and prolonged half-life in CSF because of slower degradation.

New technology may enable better titration of intracranial drug delivery.[41] Catheters attached to a subcutaneously implanted pump can be placed into the epidural space or directly into the ventricles. Several pumps have been designed to include a medication reservoir from which drug is continuously released. This approach has been used experimentally to deliver anticholines-

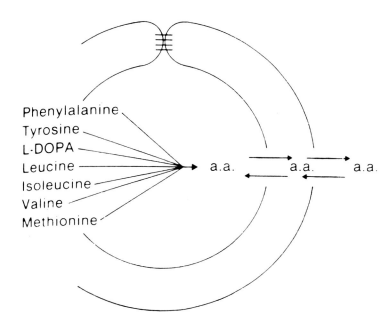

Figure 1–16. Transport of large neutral amino acids across the brain capillary. A single type of transport carrier mediates the transcapillary movement of structurally related amino acids (a.a.). As a result, these compounds must compete with each other for entry into the brain and an elevation in the plasma level of one may inhibit entry of the others. This schematic diagram shows a partial list of amino acids for which the uptake would be reduced under these circumstances. (From Asbury, AK, McKhann, GM and McDonald, WI [eds]: Diseases of the Nervous System. WB Saunders, Philadelphia, 1986, p 179, with permission.)

Phenylalanine
Tyrosine
L-DOPA
Leucine
Isoleucine
Valine
Methionine

a.a.   a.a.   a.a.

terase drugs in patients with Alzheimer's disease and for other therapies.

The intrathecal route has also been evaluated for administration of peptides. One potential application is the delivery of neurotrophic factors to enhance survival of injured or degenerating neurons.[43] Attempts have been made to administer intrathecal thyrotropin-releasing hormone (TRH) chronically to patients with amyotrophic lateral sclerosis (ALS) using constant infusion pumps.[71] Although TRH does not appear to be beneficial for ALS, the clinical studies demonstrated the feasibility of the approach.

Another method used in clinical trials to bypass the barrier is osmotic disruption. Experimentally, intracarotid injection of a hypertonic solution has been used to open the BBB before systemic administration of drugs targeted for the CNS. This method is controversial, and is limited by differential effects of osmotic agents on normal and abnormal tissue. Recent data suggest that in subjects with brain tumors, intracarotid injection of hypertonic solutions can enhance transport of drugs into normal brain tissue but not into the tumor tissue.[102]

Potential Strategies to Penetrate the BBB

Several methods hold promise for improving delivery of systemically administered drugs to the CNS, but have not yet been used in humans. The most promising strategies include enclosing drugs in liposomes, linking the drugs to an interconvertible salt carrier, or attaching the drug to a protein or other carrier molecule that can pass through the brain capillary endothelial cells by endocytosis.[96]

Liposomes are lipid-coated vesicles produced by vigorous mixing of aqueous suspensions of phospholipids. The vesicles have a hollow core which can be filled with large polar compounds entrapped within the artificial lipid bilayer. Currently available liposomes are relatively unstable, and after systemic administration they are rapidly degraded. However, addition of selected surface molecules may enhance the efficiency of liposome transport into the brain.[100] For example, attachment of a sulfatide moiety to the outer surface of the liposome may improve BBB permeability.

Another approach was recently suggested by Boder and Simpkins,[7] who described a novel redox brain-specific delivery system based on an interconvertible dihydropyridine-pyridium salt carrier. In this approach, a polar drug is covalently bound to lipophilic dihydropyridine carriers for transport into the brain where oxidation occurs. The oxidized carrier then becomes less soluble in lipid membranes and is trapped within the brain. When the compound is hydrolyzed, drug is separated from the carrier providing sustained release. Successful use of this approach required that the carrier be nontoxic.

Broadwell and colleagues[11] described another so called transcytotic pathway through brain capillary endothelial cells that may also be exploited as a method for delivering drugs to the brain. The mechanisms of transcytosis include capillary endothelial endocytosis, subsequent intracellular transport and processing, followed by exocytosis into brain interstitial fluid. Selected proteins and other large molecules enter the brain in this fashion. For proteins, passage into the brain can occur via receptor-mediated transcytosis (e.g., insulin) or by absorption (e.g., cationized albumin). Chimeric peptides can be formed when a transportable peptide is covalently coupled to a nontransportable peptide via a bond that can be broken in the brain (e.g., disulfide).[76,78] The disulfide bond is particularly convenient because it is relatively stable in plasma and is cleaved in brain tissue by disulfide reductases. One group of researchers[78] used cationized albumin coupled to endorphin to study this approach. Both in vitro studies, in isolated brain capillaries, and in vivo studies, after injection of the peptide-endorphin complex into the carotid artery, demonstrated passage of normally excluded endorphin into brain tissue.

A similar mechanism may enable cationized ferritin to act as a transporter. Ferritin enters the cell by absorptive endocytosis after which it is directed to the Golgi complex and packaged for exocytosis across the luminal surface of capillary endothelial cells.[11] Molecules internalized in endocytic vesicles are directed to endosomes (i.e., prelysomal compartment) and then may either complete transcytosis through the cell or be directed to the Golgi complex for further processing. Other molecules that could act as transporters for drugs normally excluded from the brain include lectins such as wheat germ agglutinin. Lectins bind to cell surface polysaccharides and are taken up into capillary endothelial cells. The major practical limitation of this approach for clinical practice is the lengthy transport time (hours) for such molecular complexes.

DYNAMIC FEATURES OF DRUG ACTION

Drug Delivery to the Bloodstream

GASTROINTESTINAL
ABSORPTION

Most drugs used to treat neurologic disorders are administered orally, and factors that influence drug absorption by this route may have a major impact on the success of therapy. Characteristics of drug absorption into plasma are determined by the physicochemical properties of the drug and its vehicle and by biologic variability among subjects receiving the drug (Table 1–6).

The amount of drug transferred from the gastrointestinal tract into plasma, or *bioavailability*, is determined by several biochemical factors. Most drugs are relatively small molecules which

Table 1–6 FACTORS INFLUENCING DRUG ABSORPTION

PROPERTIES OF DRUG AND DRUG VEHICLE
Solubility
Molecular size
Polarity
Bioavailability
Bioequivalency

INTERSUBJECT PHYSIOLOGIC VARIABILITY
Age
Diet
Other drugs ingested concurrently
Gut integrity, motility, and blood flow

are absorbed primarily by passive diffusion. Drugs with larger molecular weights (>900) are absorbed to a larger extent by vesicular pinocytosis. Absorption of water-soluble drugs is limited by the molecular size, whereas the absorption of most of the drugs used in neurology depends more heavily on the relative solubility of the compound in lipid membranes (Fig. 1–17). By determining the ratio of the charged to uncharged form of the drug, pH influences lipid solubility. In the stomach, the high concentration of hydrogen ions enhances the lipid solubility of weak acids by reducing the amount of ionized, water-soluble drug. This effect may be outweighed, however, by the effect of pH on drug solubility. For example, phenytoin with a pK_a of approximately 8, is predominantly ionized in the stomach but is so insoluble at that pH that very little absorption takes place. Although the pH of 7 in the duodenum causes more phenytoin to be ionized, the drug's greater solubility at neutral pH allows more absorption.

The *excipient*, or material with which the active drug is mixed, may influence absorption, and this may change the drug's relative ability to yield similar concentrations of drug in blood and tissues. For several anticonvulsants, including carbamazepine and phenytoin, clinically significant discrepancies in blood levels attained have been detected with administration of different formulations. These differences appear to be attributable to the

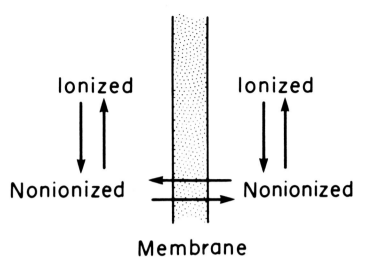

Membrane

Figure 1–17. Absorption of drugs is dependent on both their lipid solubility in the nonionized form and the amount of drug in the nonionized state.

effects of the drug excipient on absorption efficiency.[68]

Concurrent administration of food also unpredictably influences oral absorption of some drugs. Food tends to increase the absorption of water-insoluble drugs. For certain drugs, gastric-emptying time (altered by the fat content of the meal or by disorders such as diabetes) may be important. Administration of drugs along with tube feedings may sometimes result in reduced bioavailability. Food increases the systemic availability of drugs with a high hepatic extraction fraction, but the mechanism for this response is uncertain.

An interesting, clinically important drug/food interaction has been recently delineated for absorption of the amino acid L-dopa. L-dopa is absorbed from the gut primarily by a saturable carrier-mediated transport process. Neutral amino acids derived from ingested proteins compete with L-dopa for the carrier sites, and a high-protein diet reduces the bioavailability of L-dopa. A portion of the fluctuations observed in the efficacy of L-dopa resulting in the "on-off phenomenon" is attributable to protein-induced variation in the amount of drug absorbed.[53,73,79] To overcome this limitation, dietary protein restriction or a standardized diet

may be helpful. Development of effective sustained-release preparations can also help overcome this problem (see Chapter 2).[52]

Concurrent administration of multiple drugs, age, and specific systemic illness may also influence gastrointestinal absorption. Diseases associated with decreased cardiac output, malnutrition, and malabsorption may reduce the bioavailability of neurologic drugs. Age may also influence the efficiency of absorption. One important example is provided by experience with oral phenytoin administration in infancy; poor absorption of phenytoin after oral administration makes chronic use of this drug impractical in the first year of life.[75]

OTHER DRUG DELIVERY METHODS

Intravenous and intramuscular routes are often used in acute situations for loading with medication or when oral administration is impossible. The intravenous route is generally preferred because of pain and the potential unreliability of the intramuscular route for drugs such as phenytoin. Refinements of intravenous drug delivery methods have been introduced for drugs that require stabilized blood levels for optimal therapeutic effect, such as opioid analgesics. Patient-controlled analgesia uses a programmed intravenous pump to allow patients to deliver a small fixed dose as needed to reduce pain (see Chapter 10).[97] The program prevents readministration too frequently. This system appears to produce less sedation and more consistent analgesia than conventional bolus injections. A similar computerized pump has been used to deliver continuous infusions of opiates such as alfentanil during surgery.

Parenteral drug delivery methods are often quite useful, but disadvantages include their expense, cumbersomeness, and the possible increase in adverse reactions from initial high blood levels. Several more unusual methods for drug delivery are being developed to overcome these problems. They may become alternatives to chronic oral administration and find wider application in neurologic practice.

Transdermal Drug Delivery. Transdermal drug delivery systems make use of a drug-containing membrane held against the skin by an occlusive adhesive sheet (Fig. 1–18). Drugs can be delivered by this route if they are potent, highly soluble in water and oil,

and not irritating to the skin. When successful, this method delivers a steady amount of drugs into the blood, with few peaks and valleys. Transdermal patches for scopolamine (for motion sickness) and clonidine are used in neurologic practice. A preparation that delivers fentanyl for postoperative analgesia is undergoing clinical trials and appears to be useful. In addition to its convenience and comfort, the system may reduce variations in metabolism caused by the "first pass effect" seen when a large drug bolus is released into the bloodstream from parenteral delivery. A variation of the transdermal method uses iontophoresis to electrically charge drug molecules that do not pass through the stratum corneum easily.

Transmucosal Delivery Methods. Certain drugs may be administered through oral and nasal mucous membranes, providing a rapid onset and a more stable blood level. A relatively high lipid solubility is required for these routes to be effective, however. Lipid-soluble opioids such as fentanyl and methadone can be absorbed by the sublingual route, and morphine can be absorbed from buccal administration (Fig.

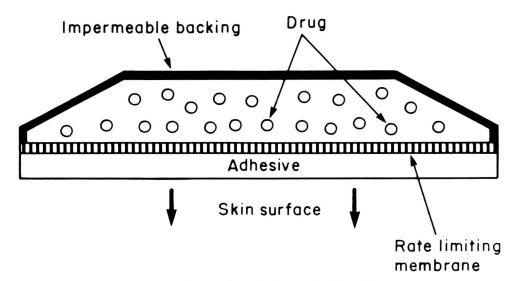

Figure 1–18. Schematic diagram of a transdermal (skin patch) drug delivery system. (From Streisand and Stanley,[97] p 458, with permission.)

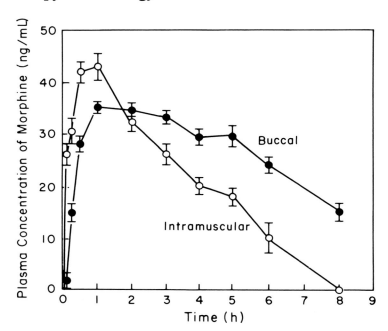

Figure 1–19. Plasma concentrations of morphine after intramuscular (*open circles*) and buccal (*filled circles*) administrations. (From Streisand and Stanley,[97] p 460, with permission.)

1–19). An investigational system incorporating fentanyl into a lozenge on a stick appears to produce sedation and anxiolysis when used as a premedication for surgery in children. The opioid sufentanil has been administered to children in nasal drops, and butorphanol, a synthetic morphine analogue, has been administered nasally to women for postcesarean section pain. This method reportedly produces longer-lasting analgesia than the intravenous route.

Rectal administration is becoming more popular as a convenient route for rapidly delivering certain drugs. Rectal administration of diazepam reportedly produces a rapid blood level of drug with few serious side effects. Although not commercially available in the United States, rectal suppository preparations in Europe are used to prevent seizures in febrile children. Reports of clinical trials suggest that this will be a useful alternative to parenteral administration of benzodiazepines.[1,16] Anticonvulsants such as valproate and paraldehyde also may be administered efficiently and effectively through the rectal mucosa. Suppositories containing morphine have also been designed; although this route has drawbacks such as potentially erratic absorption, progress in drug formulation may make it more useful for certain indications.

Drug Distribution

After absorption into the systemic circulation, distribution of a drug into tissue is an important determinant of the rapidity of onset and duration of its action (Fig. 1–20). The rate and differential distribution of a drug depends on its physicochemical properties (Table 1–7). The apparent volume of distribution, or the ratio of the amount of drug in the body to the serum concentration of the drug, is relatively large in highly tissue-bound drugs.

Protein binding in plasma is a major factor influencing drug distribution throughout the body. Many drugs, as well as endogenous compounds, bind reversibly to albumin and to a lesser extent to other serum proteins such as alpha-1 acid glycoprotein. Competitive displacement of highly bound drugs (e.g., phenytoin) from protein-binding

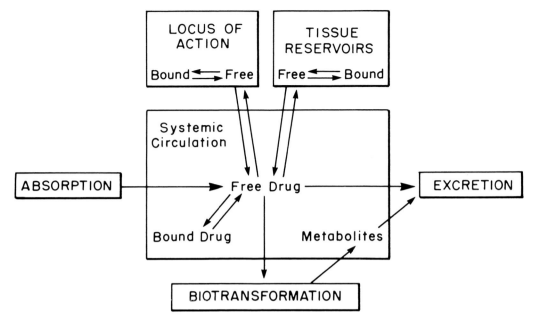

Figure 1–20. Drug distribution within the body, biotransformation, and excretion. (Adapted from Benet, LZ, Mitchell, JR, and Sheiner, LB: Pharmacokinetics: The dynamics of drug absorption, distribution, and elimination. In Gilman, AG, Rall, TW, Nies, AS and Palmer, T [eds]: Goodman and Gilman's The Pharmacological Basis of Therapeutics, ed 8. Pergamon Press, New York, 1990, p 3.)

sites by other drugs or endogenous substances may cause rapid changes in free drug levels. The extent to which drugs compete for albumin sites is difficult to predict. For example, carbamazepine is predominantly protein bound, but it does not displace drugs such as phenytoin to a significant extent. The effect of disease or other drugs on therapeutic effect may also be unpredictable. For example, renal failure often lowers albumin levels in plasma but poor protein binding causes the free level of phenytoin to remain higher, producing a compensatory therapeutic effect.

Changes in the body composition may alter the distribution and therapeutic effect of neurologic drugs. One of the best clinical examples of the impact of body composition changes in drug distribution is pregnancy. An expansion of the volume of distribution in pregnancy generally leads to lower serum levels of drugs such as anticonvulsants, and frequent monitoring is necessary to maintain a therapeutic level. Drugs that are lipid soluble and poorly protein bound are most likely to cross the placenta and be distributed in the fetus. Postpartum drug distribution to breast milk is highest for lipid-soluble drugs that are alkaline and not protein bound.

Fat may become a reservoir for lipid-soluble neuroactive drugs, and obesity may alter the clinical response. Redistribution of ultrashort-acting barbiturate anesthetics from fat may be prolonged, lengthening recovery from anesthesia. The volume of distribution

Table 1–7 FACTORS INFLUENCING DRUG DISTRIBUTION INTO TISSUES

Physicochemical properties
  Lipid solubility
  Tissue binding
  pK_a
  Molecular weight
Protein binding
Concurrently administered drugs or disease
Intersubject variations in blood volume, body fat
BBB permeability

for drugs such as benzodiazepines and phenytoin increases markedly in very obese subjects. The mechanism for this observed effect does not appear to be fully explained by the lipophilic properties of the drugs.

Drug Metabolism

The lipid-soluble drugs most commonly used for neurologic disorders are generally metabolized to create more polar, less active compounds, which can be eliminated more efficiently by the kidney. Hydroxylation, oxidation, dealkylation, and deamination reactions are the most common metabolic transformations. These so-called phase I reactions are sometimes followed up by conjugation to compounds, such as glucuronic acid or an amino acid, that enhance water solubility (phase II reactions). The liver is the major site of metabolic transformations, but the lung, gut, and kidney may also contribute. As an example, the metabolism of phenytoin is depicted in Figure 1–23.

Oxidative drug metabolism is mediated predominantly by the mixed-function hepatic cytochrome P-450 oxygenases, but other mixed-function oxidases also participate. Multiple enzymes may contribute to metabolism of a single drug. The genetic control of activity of these enzymes is complex, and may account for clinically important variability in these reactions.[19,47] Age, systemic illness, and concurrent use of other drugs that induce biotransforming enzymes may alter drug metabolism. For example, phenobarbital is metabolized more rapidly in infants than in adults, so that the dose per kilogram needed in infants is more than twice as high.[75] Powerful enzyme inducers such as phenobarbital increase the activity of P-450 oxidases in liver, which in turn stimulates the metabolism of many other drugs. For example, in transplant patients receiving phenobarbital as an anticonvulsant, the dose of the immunosuppressive drug cyclosporine required to attain therapeutic levels increases dramatically. Another example

is the ability of valproate to increase serum phenobarbital levels by an average of 50% when the two drugs are given concurrently.[13]

Biotransformation reactions can also enhance the therapeutic efficacy of a drug. For example, the major pathway for metabolism of the anticonvulsant carbamazepine is formation of a 10,11 epoxide by P-450 mixed-function oxidase; this epoxide metabolic also has anticonvulsant properties. Carbamazepine generally induces its own metabolism (autoinduction). After several weeks of treatment, the efficiency of degradation increases, and the dose may need to be increased to maintain a therapeutic level.

Drugs that block drug metabolism are occasionally clinically useful. The aromatic amino-acid decarboxylase inhibitor carbidopa can markedly reduce the amount of L-dopa that is metabolized peripherally so that more is available to cross the BBB. Carbidopa itself does not cross into the brain, allowing the decarboxylase activity to transform L-dopa into dopamine. Another example is disulfiram, which produces hypersensitivity to ethanol by blocking the metabolism of acetaldehyde to acetate. Disulfiram is an inhibitor of mixed-function oxidase activity, and inhibits aldehyde dehydrogenous activity by competing with nicotinamide adenine dinucleotide.

Drug Elimination

The kidney is the major organ responsible for elimination of unchanged polar drugs or lipophilic drugs that have been metabolized to make them less hydrophobic (Table 1–8). The concept of

Table 1–8 FACTORS INFLUENCING DRUG ELIMINATION

Renal blood flow and glomerular filtration rate
Protein intake
Renal tubular secretion efficiency
Multiple drugs administered concurrently
Kidney or liver disease

clearance of a specific compound is used to describe the efficiency of drug elimination, and is expressed as the volume of blood cleared of drug per unit time. Typically a constant fraction of the drug is removed from the plasma by the kidney (first-order or exponential kinetics).

Passive filtration and secretion both contribute to renal drug clearance. For drugs eliminated mainly by filtration, renal blood flow and the glomerular filtration rate are the major determinants of clearance rates. In patients with renal failure, multiple pathophysiologic mechanisms including reductions in glomerular filtration rates, low plasma albumin levels, concurrent administration of a large number of medications, and treatment with dialysis all influence drug clearance rates. Experience with phenytoin metabolism in uremic patients demonstrates the issues that must be considered in analyzing the effects of renal failure on drug clearance.[8] For a given dosage, total serum phenytoin levels are generally lower in uremic patients, but free serum phenytoin levels rise because of decreased protein binding. There is no change in the clearance of the unbound fraction, and free levels remain relatively stable. Reduced clearance of hydroxylate pheny-

toin may contribute a modest anticonvulsant effect.

Pharmacokinetics

Absorption, distribution, metabolism, and elimination together determine each drug's pharmacokinetic features. Both drug and host factors determine the plasma level of drug attained, the duration of sustained peak drug levels, and the magnitude of fluctuations in drug levels over time.

An appropriate dosage range for administration of each drug is typically derived from population studies. Mathematic models, based on experimental data, are used to predict drug disposition (Fig. 1–21). First-order kinetics describes responses in which there is direct proportionality between the amount of drug administered and its rate of metabolism (Table 1–9). This pattern is commonly encountered for neuroactive drugs in the therapeutic dose range. This model does not apply when one or more mechanisms of drug disposition are saturated (e.g., biotransformation, active transport, protein binding, or secretion). Zero-order kinetics describe the pattern of drug disposition in which the rate of metabo-

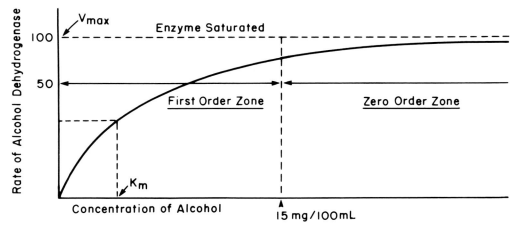

Figure 1–21. Drug metabolism kinetics, using ethyl alcohol as an example. Up to blood levels of approximately 15 mg/100 mL, ethyl alcohol is metabolized according to first-order, exponential kinetics. Above this level, alcohol dehydrogenase becomes saturated so that ethyl alcohol is metabolized by zero-order kinetics following Michaelis-Menton kinetics.

Table 1–9 DRUG KINETICS TERMINOLOGY

Term	Definition
Pharmacokinetics	The relationship between drug dosage and resulting plasma concentration of the drug.
Pharmacodynamics	The relationship between plasma concentration and physiologic drug effects.
First-order kinetics	The direct proportionality between the amount of drug administered and its rate of metabolism.
Zero-order kinetics	The pattern of drug disposition in which rate of metabolism is fixed and independent of drug concentration.
Half-life ($t_{1/2}$)	The time period over which a drug's plasma concentration falls to 50% of peak level after a single dose.

lism is fixed and independent of drug concentration.

Mathematic models can be used to estimate the appropriate dosages and frequency of administration for acute and chronic drug therapy. The half-life of a drug is the time period during which its plasma concentration falls to 50% of the peak level after a single dose (Fig. 1–22). The half-life can be measured experimentally with repeated sampling in individual patients, or alternatively it can be estimated from fewer repeated measurements in a large group of patients. Computer programs have been developed to calculate half-life; sophisticated pharmacokinetic models may take into account a variety of factors that determine plasma levels, including volume of distribution, tissue binding, and clearance. The half-life is a good in-

dicator of the amount of time required to reach steady-state drug levels with maintenance drug dosages; after initiation of therapy, steady-state levels are attained after four to five half-lives.

The pharmacokinetic features of phenytoin disposition are interesting. Phenytoin metabolism is generally partially saturated at blood levels used to treat epilepsy (Fig. 1–23). As the dose is increased, plasma concentrations rise, and the apparent half-life increases because of a shift from first-order to zero-order kinetics. This pattern is an example of Michaelis-Menton kinetics. Small increments in dosage can lead to abrupt rises in serum levels into the toxic range. When blood levels reach the toxic range, the rate of decline of levels back into the therapeutic range is correspondingly prolonged.[27]

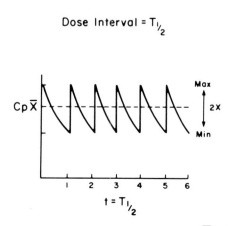
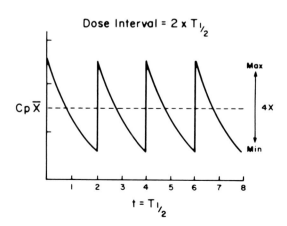

Figure 1–22. Blood concentration ($Cp\overline{X}$) of a drug given (*left*) once every half-life, or (*right*) once every other half-life.

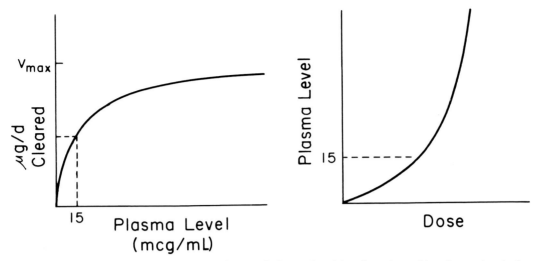

Figure 1–23. The relationship between dose and plasma level for phenytoin. At a plasma level of approximately 15 µg/mL, the enzyme begins to saturate (*left*) and the amount of drug cleared plateaus (zero-order kinetics). In this case, 15 µg/mL is the K_m concentration, or the concentration at which the enzyme is at half its capacity. The result (*right*) is that additional drug given when the serum level is above the K_m produces a greater incremental change than when the level is lower. Unexpected increases in serum level into the toxic range may result.

Therapeutic Drug Monitoring

There is significant intersubject variability in drug concentrations attained after administration of routine drug dosages. An equally important source of variability in the therapeutic efficacy of a drug is the relationship between drug concentration and physiologic drug effects (pharmacodynamic actions) in individual patients. The most readily available measure of pharmacokinetic drug parameters is the blood level attained, but this number provides little information about pharmacodynamic variability in response. This concept is important when interpreting drug levels that may be associated with a "therapeutic" or "toxic" effect that does not correspond to the "therapeutic values" provided by the laboratory.

When appropriate assays are available, indications for measuring drug levels include establishing steady-state concentrations, and determining the impact of a new drug formulation, dosage changes, or addition or elimination of other drugs. Measurement of drug levels may be especially valuable for drugs with a narrow therapeutic range. Other indications include reemergence of symptoms, kidney or liver disease, and evaluation of possible toxicity. Timing of sampling will influence results obtained; peak levels may be most helpful for assessment of toxicity while trough levels may provide more predictable information about steady-state levels.

Routinely, when drug levels are measured, values reflect the total serum concentration, which includes both protein-bound and free drug. In most cases, these measures accurately reflect free drug levels. In patients with unexpected drug toxicity or lack of efficacy, however, or in diseases in which serum protein abnormalities are found, measurement of free drug levels may be helpful.

TOXICITY OF NEUROACTIVE DRUGS

Many drugs prescribed for treatment of neurologic disorders cause neurologic dysfunction and systemic toxicity.

Adverse drug reactions may occur while a patient is receiving therapeutic or subtherapeutic drug dosages or as a result of accidental or intentional overdosage (see Chapter 10). Often, adverse effects are an important determinant of the usefulness of drugs in individual patients. The *therapeutic index*, the relationship between the therapeutic dose and the toxic dose, is used to describe this relationship.

Within a group of patients receiving the same drug at the same dose, there is significant variation in the frequency and severity of adverse reactions. Toxicity may be predictable and dose related or idiosyncratic. An idiosyncratic response occurs unpredictably in a small minority of patients. Genetic factors may account for enhanced susceptibility to certain adverse reactions. This section examines some common clinical syndromes of neurologic dysfunction and systemic toxicity. Although precise information about mechanisms of many toxic effects is lacking, some proposed mechanisms are presented.

Neurologic Disorders Attributable to Drug Therapy

MENTAL STATUS CHANGES

The most prevalent adverse effects of neuroactive drugs are alterations in mental status. Some adverse responses are commonly encountered, while in other instances only a small minority of patients are affected. Furthermore, the functional disturbances resulting from such symptoms (e.g., sedation) vary considerably. Clinical experience indicates that it is often difficult to anticipate which patients will be most susceptible to such adverse reactions.

Acute Effects. Patients may manifest significant mental status changes soon after introduction of a new therapeutic agent, especially if therapy is initiated with a loading dose of the drug. The most common acute adverse drug reaction is sedation. In the setting of an acute illness or exacerbation of a chronic neurologic disorder, it may be difficult to distinguish the effects of illness or emotional response to illness from drug-induced responses. More dramatic acute adverse effects include hallucinations and disorientation. Anticholinergics are particularly prone to produce delirium or psychosis in elderly patients who may have subclinical abnormalities in cholinergic innervation of the cerebral cortex (see Chapter 8).[57]

A high index of suspicion is essential to establish the link between drug administration and mental status changes, especially for drugs in which adverse effects are unexpected. For example, the anticonvulsant carbamazepine is commonly considered to have positive psychotropic effects, yet in occasional patients carbamazepine may produce an acute behavioral disorder with psychotic features.[91]

Patients with certain systemic disorders may be at increased risk for the development of acute drug-induced encephalopathies. For example, in liver-transplantation patients, cyclosporine appears to cause an acute encephalopathy in about 20%; patients with low total serum cholesterol levels are at highest risk.[24] The mechanism for this effect is not known.

Chronic Effects. Special attention is needed to detect subtle adverse effects on cognition, mood, or behavior. Perhaps the greatest concern about potential adverse effects on cognition arises with chronic administration of anticonvulsants, especially in children. Declines in cognition may reflect sedation, poor sustained attention, or memory deficits. In adults, objective testing has demonstrated that phenobarbital selectively impairs short-term memory.[62] In children, it is often difficult to distinguish the adverse effects of drugs from the learning disabilities attributable to poorly controlled seizures or underlying neurologic disorder. Yet both anecdotal reports and more formal studies suggest that barbiturates and other anticonvulsants can impair learning. Recent results of trials comparing the psychologic and behavioral effects of phenobarbital and valproate in children and adults with epilepsy indicated that specific aspects of neuropsychologic functioning and behavior were adversely affected by phenobarbital.[80,101] In addition, phenobarbital-induced changes in mood, behavior, and sleep patterns in young children are commonly recognized. An interesting example of biologic predisposition to specific adverse drug reactions is provided by a recent report of phenobarbital-induced depression in children with a family history of major affective illness.[9] Although barbiturates are known to act at the inhibitory GABA-benzodiazepine complex, the mechanism for these effects is not known.

Major tranquilizers such as phenothiazine, prescribed for treatment of psychiatric disorders, may also have significant adverse effects on behavior. Selected patients may be especially susceptible to these drug-induced disorders. One study[70] described 15 patients with Tourette's syndrome who abruptly developed school or work avoidance syndromes when treated with low doses (mean = 2.5 mg/d) of haloperidol for short periods; phobic syndromes resolved with reduction in dosage or discontinuation of treatment.

COMA

Coma may result either from the direct toxic effects of a drug on the brain or from metabolic derangements caused by the drug. The most common setting for drug-induced coma is accidental or intentional drug overdose of sedative drugs such as barbiturates (see Chapter 10). These drugs act by stimulating inhibitory neurotransmitter receptors (e.g., the GABA-benzodiazepine receptor complex) or by mechanisms that produce anesthesia (see Chapter 3). An example of drug-induced systemic metabolic abnormality is hyperammonemia-induced mental status changes seen in some children treated with valproate.[21] It is unknown if these children are at greater risk for more severe valproate-induced hepatotoxicity.[24]

STROKE

Drugs prescribed for treatment of neurologic or systemic disorders may predispose patients to cerebrovascular accidents. Pathophysiologic mechanisms include acute hypertension leading to intracranial hemorrhage, arteritis, thrombosis associated with a hypercoagulable state, or hemorrhage attributable to clotting deficiencies or increased fibrinolysis. Sympathomimetic compounds, including both over-the-counter medications such as ephedrine and phenylpropanolamine and drugs of abuse such as cocaine and amphetamine, have been recognized as predisposing factors for stroke and intracranial hemorrhage.[54,61] Focal arteritis and systemic hypertension may contribute to the pathogenesis of stroke in this setting.

L-asparaginase, a chemotherapeutic agent commonly used in treatment of acute lymphocytic leukemia, may cause hemorrhagic or thrombotic strokes in a small minority of patients. L-asparaginase produces deficiencies in proteins contributing to both coagulation and fibrinolysis; arterial infarction, intracerebral hemorrhage, and venous thrombosis have been described.[31]

SEIZURES

In many critically ill patients, toxic ingestions[3] or drugs used to treat their systemic illnesses may cause seizures and mental status changes; concurrent metabolic derangements may contribute to lowering the seizure threshold. Antibiotics implicated as epileptogenic include penicillins and related drugs such as imipenem, a new betalactamase, broad-spectrum antibiotic used for serious hospital-acquired infection.[15] An important mechanism for these effects is suppression of inhibitory neurotransmitter systems (see Chapter 3). In immunosuppressed transplant patients, the onset of seizures may indicate CNS infection; however, recent experience suggests that cyclosporine, an integral component of immunosuppressive therapy in these patients, may precipitate seizures and encephalopathy.[24]

Anticonvulsants may paradoxically provoke seizures in patients with epilepsy. Concurrent treatment with valproate and clonazepam may precipitate status epilepticus, as may abrupt withdrawal of barbiturates. Use of carbamazepine to treat children with some types of generalized seizures may increase seizure frequency dramatically.[89] Lorazepam has also been reported to produce paradoxic seizures.[26] Many drugs (e.g., phenothiazine and methylphenidate) have the potential to lower the seizure threshold. Treatment with such drugs poses a theoretic risk in epileptics. In most of these patients, however, judicious treatment with such drugs is well tolerated. The mechanisms for these effects is poorly understood.

MOVEMENT DISORDERS

Neuroactive drugs may produce a wide spectrum of acute and/or chronic movement disorders. Antihistamines, anticonvulsants, and antidepressants all may cause extrapyramidal syndromes in certain patients. The biologic basis for increased susceptibility to these adverse drug reactions is uncertain, but the drugs are presumed to act at specific types of neurotransmitter synapses in the basal ganglia (see Chapter 2).

Drugs that antagonize dopamine in the nigrostriatal pathway cause clinically significant extrapyramidal syndromes.[99] Phenothiazine, butyrophenones, and related neuroleptic drugs may cause acute and chronic movement disorders. Acute dystonic reactions may occur at any time during treatment with dopamine antagonists; in some cases, these reactions occur after a single dose. Focal tonic muscle spasms, typically involving the eyes, neck, and/or trunk, develop abruptly and are readily relieved by treatment with anticholinergic drugs (e.g., diphenhydramine [Benadryl]). Antiemetics with dopamine-blocking properties (e.g., metaclopromide [Reglan]) may also elicit this distressing reaction. The neurochemical mechanism underlying this response is uncertain; the manifestations are suggestive of activation rather than blockade of dopamine receptors. Of interest, elderly patients appear to be considerably less likely to develop neuroleptic-induced dystonia than younger age groups.

Drug-induced parkinsonism, characterized by bradykinesia, rigidity, and, less commonly, tremor, can result from treatment with dopamine antagonists. Older patients appear to be more susceptible; the movement disorder is most common in the first few months of treatment or if concurrent anticholinergic therapy is discontinued abruptly. Patients improve if dopamine antagonists are discontinued or anticholinergic drugs are added.

Drugs without anticipated effects on dopamine metabolism may provoke a similar range of movement disorders. Flunarizine and cinnarizine, calcium channel blockers used outside the United States to treat disorders such as migraine and vertigo, may elicit parkinsonism, akathisia, and dystonic reactions.[69] These drugs presumably act by antagonizing dopamine receptors. Drug-induced acute choreoathetosis is less common. In young children, more so than in other age groups, phenytoin toxicity may be manifested solely by abrupt onset of choreiform movements. Anticonvulsant-induced orofacial dyskinesias have also been described.[51] Tourettism or Tourette's syndrome also may be precipitated by dopamine-agonist medication in susceptible individuals.[92]

Perhaps the most serious drug-induced chronic movement disorder is tardive dyskinesia, which develops in 10% to 20% of patients treated with dopamine antagonists for more than 1 year and is irreversible in some cases.[50,99] Typical manifestations include rapid facial and lingual tics or dystonic facial movements, akathisia, and choreoathetoid limb movement. The underlying neurochemical abnormalities are uncertain; both dopamine-receptor supersensitivity and secondary changes at GABAergic synapses have been implicated. Epidemiologic data indicate that there is variation in susceptibility to development of tardive dyskinesia; elderly patients and female patients appear to be at highest risk. Important unresolved issues include the effects of dosage, drug holidays, and the nature of the underlying disease on the development of tardive dyskinesia. When phenothiazines are discontinued, transient withdrawal dyskinesia may occur. The involuntary movements are the same as in tardive dyskinesia but, by definition, the symptoms resolve spontaneously within 3 months. Tardive dyskinesia is considered in more detail in Chapter 7.

ATAXIA

Drug-induced ataxia may arise from cerebellar dysfunction or sensory neuropathy. Although it is uncommon for neuroactive drugs to produce chronic ataxia when administered in the therapeutic dose range, acute ataxia commonly results after rapid introduction of new drugs, especially anticonvulsants such as phenytoin and primidone. With acute phenytoin toxicity, nystagmus and ataxia are common. Before routine monitoring of drug levels was available, progressive ataxia sometimes evolved in patients treated with high doses of phenytoin for many years. Both cerebellar dysfunction and sensory neuropathy contributed to the deficit.

VISUAL SYMPTOMS

Blurred vision, diplopia, and abnormal eye movements may be manifestations of adverse drug reactions. Blurred vision may arise with a wide variety of drugs including carbamazepine, tricyclic antidepressants, and other drugs with anticholinergic properties. Diplopia is a common complaint in patients with mild carbamazepine toxicity, although often no abnormality of extraocular movements can be detected clinically. The mechanism is uncertain. Nystagmus has been ascribed to treatment with a variety of drugs, most commonly phenytoin and more rarely carbamazepine and lithium.[105]

PERIPHERAL NEUROPATHY AND NEUROMUSCULAR JUNCTION ABNORMALITIES

Although many drugs cause peripheral neuropathy, relatively few drugs used commonly to treat neurobehavioral disorders have been implicated.[5] Drugs may damage the axon and cell body or the myelin sheath. In most cases, the onset of motor and/or sensory deficits is insidious. For some drugs (e.g., vincristine), peripheral neuropathy is a predictable consequence of therapy. For other drugs, there is considerable host variation in individual susceptibility to neuronal injury. Electrophysiologic evidence of neuropathy may be considerably more pronounced than the clinically detectable deficit. A recent report[2] highlights the neurotoxic properties of a seemingly benign vitamin, pyridoxine (vitamin B_6). Two patients developed an acute, severe, predominantly sensory neuropathy after receiving massive doses of pyridoxine for treatment of mushroom poisoning.

Similarly, drug-induced suppression of neuromuscular transmission has been recognized in a variety of settings.[4] The neuromuscular-blocking effects of aminoglycoside antibiotics have been characterized;[17] patients such as myasthenics, who have underlying disorders of the neuromuscular junction, may be at highest risk for this adverse response.

Systemic Disorders Attributable to Drug Therapy

Drugs used to treat neurologic or behavioral disorders can also have adverse effects on other organ systems. A major practical issue for maintenance therapy with many neuroactive drugs is deciding how to monitor most effectively for systemic toxicity.

HEMATOLOGIC DISORDERS

Many drugs occasionally produce bone marrow suppression involving one or multiple cell lines and, rarely, aplastic anemia. Myelosuppression may be related to the dose of drug administered, or it may represent an idiosyncratic response. There is no evidence that routine monitoring of blood counts is effective in decreasing the incidence of drug-induced aplastic anemia.

Experience with the anticonvulsant carbamazepine demonstrates the wide range of drug-induced hematopoietic toxicity and the problems inherent in drug monitoring.[42] Aplastic anemia occurs in fewer than 1/50,000 patients treated with this drug; it may be more common in elderly patients. However, in about 10% of patients in the first few months of carbamazepine therapy, neutrophil counts decline. Although neutropenia may herald agranulocytosis or aplastic anemia, in most patients, white cell counts return to normal; thus, unless the neutrophil count falls to less than 1500 cells/mm², most physicians do not alter therapy. About 2% of patients treated with carbamazepine develop persistent neutropenia, but the majority of these patients remain asymptomatic. Anemia or thrombocytopenia are occasionally seen in these patients, but the responses are usually transient and dose related. Until recently, very frequent and costly monitoring of blood counts was recommended. Since no clear-cut benefit accrued from this approach,[42] suggestions in the package insert for monitoring were revised to recommend an initial hematologic screening and subsequent monitoring at the physician's discretion.

Hemolysis or thrombocytopenia also may result from drug-induced autoimmune responses. Eosinophilia and lymphadenopathy may reflect hypersensitivity reactions to drugs such as phenytoin. Macrocytic anemia may rarely result from anticonvulsant-induced folate deficiency. Platelet dysfunction may result from valproate therapy. Recently, a disorder of severe myalgia and eosinophilia was reported in patients taking L-tryptophan.[90] This may be attributable to a contaminant in processing this amino acid.

HEPATOTOXICITY

Many drugs may rarely and unpredictably cause hepatic necrosis. Genetic factors may predispose a small minority of patients to development of liver damage from a specific drug. For example, an inherited deficit in arene oxide metabolism may predispose a small number of patients to phenytoin hepatotoxicity.[94]

Of drugs currently used in neurologic practice, perhaps the greatest concern about hepatotoxicity has been elicited by experience with valproate. Enthusiasm for use of valproate, a highly effective anticonvulsant for generalized seizures, has been tempered by reports of lethal hepatotoxicity. Two forms of valproate-induced hepatotoxicity have been observed. The more common form is reversible and dose related. Findings include liver enzyme elevation with occasional clinical correlates of abdominal pain, mental-status changes, or both. Rarely, administration of valproate results in acute, irreversible hepatic failure; this response is not dose-dependent or predictable (i.e., it is an idiosyncratic reaction).

In a review[29] of all cases of fatal hepatotoxicity coincident with valproate therapy from 1978 to 1987 reported in the United States, it was estimated that more than 400,000 patients were treated and 37 hepatic fatalities were identified. All but one of these had other medical conditions such as mental retardation, congenital abnormalities, or other neurologic disease. The primary risk of fatal hepatic dysfunction (1/500) was found in children 0 to 2 years of age receiving valproate in conjunction with other anticonvulsants. The risk declined with age and was low overall in patients receiving valproate monotherapy (1/37,000). No fatalities occurred in patients older than age 10 receiving valproate monotherapy. Although 73% of fatal cases occurred within the first 3 months of therapy, monitoring of liver-function tests did not prevent fatal cases presumably because of their abrupt onset. Of note, a recent report of experience with valproate in Germany yielded a different risk pattern: 14 of 16 children who died while receiving valproate were older than age 3; 6 of 16 were on valproate monotherapy.[87] The effect of concurrent administration of other anticonvulsants may be explained in part by the observation that phenobarbital stimulates hepatic formation of toxic metabolites of valproate.[82]

HYPERSENSITIVITY REACTIONS

Cutaneous Reactions. Drug-induced skin reactions vary widely in their manifestations and severity. Urticaria, morbilliform eruptions, exfoliative dermatitis, photosensitivity responses, and, rarely, toxic epidermal necrolysis or Stevens-Johnson syndrome may result from prescribed drugs.[85]

Of patients treated with phenytoin, 5% to 10% develop a rash, varying in severity from mild morbilliform to life-threatening toxic epidermal necrolysis. It is often difficult to determine the risk of progression to the more severe reactions; thus, in practice, almost any rash should lead to discontinuation of the medication.

Some patients may be particularly susceptible to development of severe cutaneous reactions. For example, a recent report[25] identified an important high-risk group: erythema multiforme or Stevens-Johnson syndrome developed in eight patients with brain tumors who were treated prophylactically with phenytoin while receiving cranial irradiation. Other features common to these patients were the concurrent withdrawal of steroids and the observation that their rashes typically started on the scalp. The authors suggested that prophylactic anticonvulsants posed a significant risk and were not warranted in this setting.

Drug-Induced Systemic Lupus Erythematosus. Several anticonvulsants, including phenytoin and ethosuximide, have been implicated in the pathogenesis of drug-induced systemic lupus erythematosus. In patients with a recent onset of seizures in whom anticonvulsant therapy is initiated, it may be difficult to determine retrospectively if these seizures represented the initial manifestation of the autoimmune disorder or whether anticonvulsant therapy represented an initiating event.

In some cases, the only manifestations of a drug-induced autoimmune disorder are detected on serologic testing; typical clinical features include fever, myalgias, arthralgias, pleurisy, and pericarditis. It has been suggested that CNS and renal abnormalities are absent in drug-induced lupus.[44]

NEUROLEPTIC MALIGNANT SYNDROME

This disorder is the most serious acute complication of neuroleptic therapy. Clinical features include abrupt onset of muscular rigidity, hyperthermia, depressed consciousness, and autonomic dysfunction, typically occurring soon after initiation of treatment with neuroleptics. However, treatment with other drugs and unusual drug interactions (e.g., with concurrent administration of synthetic narcotics and MAO inhibitors and withdrawal of L-dopa therapy) have also been implicated in its causation.[33,40]

The neuroleptic malignant syndrome represents an idiosyncratic response; it is not related to toxic drug levels or to duration of treatment. Leukocytosis, elevated creatinine-kinase levels, and myoglobinuria are commonly detected, but no laboratory test is diagnostic. The pathogenesis of this life-threatening reaction is uncertain; dopamine receptor blockade may contribute. Patients may respond favorably to treatment with the dopamine agonist bromocriptine or dantrolene.[39]

CARDIAC TOXICITY

In the therapeutic dose range, few neuroactive drugs induce cardiac abnormalities in patients with normal hearts. In overdoses, however, cardiac arrhythmias may be a major mechanism for the toxicity of phenytoin and tricyclic antidepressants. The clinical setting in which cardiac toxicity of these drugs is of greatest practical concern is in rapid administration of loading doses of anticonvulsants. Significant arrhythmias may occur with rapid intravenous administration of phenytoin, and loading doses should be administered cautiously with continuous electrocardiogram (ECG) monitoring. Rapid administration of large doses of barbiturates also may lead to depression of cardiac function and hypotension.

Drugs that prolong the QT interval (e.g., tricyclic antidepressants and phenothiazine) may increase the risk of spontaneous arrhythmias. In patients with Tourette's syndrome treated with the neuroleptic agent pimozide, prolongation of the QT interval may occur in the therapeutic dose range, and regular ECG monitoring is recommended during the course of treatment.

NUTRITIONAL DISORDERS

Drugs may influence appetite directly, and also may alter the absorption or metabolism of specific nutrients. Although drug-induced alterations in appetite are commonly encountered, the underlying pharmacologic mechanisms are poorly understood. Two drugs that stimulate appetite, often resulting in significant weight gain, are the anticonvulsant valproate and the antimigraine agent cyproheptadine. Weight gain also may accompany treatment with antidepressants and phenothiazine. There is no obvious unifying neurochemical mechanism to account for the stimulation of appetite by these drugs.

Poor appetite may reflect systemic disease, depression, or the effects of drug therapy. Some drugs such as lithium produce anorexia because they distort taste. Several drugs may also alter nutrient absorption or metabolism. Anticonvulsants promote catabolism of vitamin D metabolites and cause a relative vitamin D deficiency. This biochemical deficiency is only occasionally a practical concern, but a small minority of patients develop osteomalacia during treatment with phenytoin or phenobarbital.

COSMETIC CHANGES

The most common changes in physical appearance that may result from neuroactive drug therapy (other than rashes and weight changes as mentioned earlier) include changes in hair distribution and facial features. These responses are puzzling and the underlying mechanisms are not understood.

Valproate may produce hair loss in a minority of patients; hair regrows if the drug is stopped. In contrast, phenytoin may produce hirsutism. Phenytoin may also produce gingival hyperplasia, and in some patients, prolonged treatment may lead to a coarsening of facial features. These changes may result from phenytoin-induced alterations in collagen metabolism.

Adverse Drug Interactions

When several drugs are prescribed concurrently, there is a relatively high incidence of drug interactions, including inhibition or stimulation of metabolism, alterations in free drug levels and protein binding, as well as cumulative effects on level of consciousness, learning, and memory.[36,81,93] Drug interactions may also result from unanticipated concurrent use of over-the-counter medications. Interactions between anticonvulsants and other drugs are common, and the frequency of interactions among anticonvulsants is one of the major rationales for advocating monotherapy.[58] Phenobarbital is an effective inducer of microsomal enzymes and enhances the metabolism of many concurrently administered drugs. Other drugs may also alter anticonvulsant metabolism. Administration of erythromycin to patients receiving carbamazepine may cause abrupt elevation of carbamazepine levels, accompanied by clinical toxicity,[18] as may coadministration of verapamil.[63] Similarly, unexpected valproate toxicity may be induced by administration of acetylsalicylic acid, which in antipyretic doses displaces valproate from albumin and interferes with its metabolism.[38]

INFLUENCE OF AGE ON DRUG ACTION

Geriatric Neuropharmacology

Elderly patients, especially those older than age 70, are considerably more susceptible to the adverse effects of many neuroactive drugs than are younger patients. The basis for this increased sensitivity is uncertain.[81,93] The use of multiple drugs concurrently in this age group may contribute to the risk for adverse drug reactions. In some instances, drug distribution may be different because of changes in body composition. In elderly individuals, the volume of distribution appears to be lower for water-soluble drugs and higher for lipid-soluble agents for albumin-bound drugs, the free fraction is generally increased. Variable reductions in phase-1

metabolism have been reported, but no consistent changes in phase-2 reactions have been detected.

These changes have been reported to have an impact on the disposition of benzodiazepines in the elderly. In one study of a group of 33 healthy men,[104] the elimination half-life of diazepam increased linearly fourfold to fivefold from age 15 to 82, prolonging it from 20 to 90 hours. This change appeared to be related in part to an increase in the drug's volume of distribution with age. Also, the appearance of the dealkylated desmethyldiazepam metabolite is delayed in elderly subjects. These changes might contribute to the sensitivity of older patients to benzodiazepines. Age-related changes in receptor mechanisms also could be contributing factors.

In the elderly patient, it is important to minimize the number of drugs prescribed, to be aware of the risks of drug interactions, and to determine the minimal therapeutic dosage. Even in otherwise healthy elderly patients, drugs such as benzodiazepines and other sedatives are more likely to cause sedation and depression than in younger individuals.

Pediatric Neuropharmacology

A number of issues need to be considered when prescribing drug therapy for children. These include altered drug metabolism, risks of adverse effects on brain maturation and learning, and the limited ability of the patient to communicate adverse subjective responses.[8,65,86] In neonates, reduced drug absorption and metabolism, an increase in free drug levels secondary to decreased plasma proteins, and diminished excretion rates may all influence drug requirements. Oral absorption of phenytoin, which is reasonably predictable in children and adults, is erratic in infancy. Phenytoin can rarely be used successfully to treat babies in the first year of life.[75] An unusual feature of phenobarbital kinetics in neonates is that the drug's half-life is highly variable. Typically the initial half-life is very long; then the half-life declines at an unpredictable rate during the first few weeks of treatment.

In infants, intercurrent illness or fever alters drug metabolism to a greater degree than is observed in older age groups. Infants also may be especially susceptible to CNS drug toxicity because of low plasma protein binding coupled with immaturity of the BBB. For anticonvulsants, generally in children the kinetics are highly variable, and close monitoring of blood levels is essential for optimal therapy.[26]

Teratogenesis

Drugs prescribed for treatment of neurologic disorders in pregnant women may be detrimental to the fetus. Transplacental drug transport depends on molecular weight, ionization, lipid solubility, and protein binding; the same features that enhance drug transport into the brain promote passage into the fetal circulation. A drug may exert direct toxic effects on the fetus or may cause indirect effects secondary to changes in the placenta, the uterus, or in the maternal circulation.[45,46] The nature of teratogenic effects depends on the timing of exposure. First trimester exposure may disrupt organogenesis, whereas later exposures influence histogenesis and maturation processes.

The teratogenic potential of anticonvulsants, especially phenytoin and valproate, has elicited concern. The incidence of congenital malformations in children born to epileptic mothers is about three times that in nonepileptic women (6% of drug-treated epileptics vs. 4% of untreated epileptics and 2% of nonepileptics). A fetal hydantoin syndrome has been described in infants exposed to phenytoin in utero. This syndrome includes intrauterine growth deficiency, mild mental retardation, a broad nasal bridge, coarse hair, hypoplastic nails, and occasional major

anomalies of the heart and palate. The full blown syndrome may occur in 5 to 10% of exposed infants. The risk may be up to eight times higher if a combination of phenobarbitol and phenytoin is used, and there appears to be overlap between the hydantoin syndrome and other anticonvulsant-induced disorders.[45,46]

Although the mechanism for the fetal effects of phenytoin and related compounds is not understood, some evidence suggests that a toxic arene oxide metabolite may play a role.[98] Arene oxides are oxidative intermediates in the metabolism of phenytoin, barbiturates, and carbamazepine. In a study of 24 children exposed to phenytoin in utero, lymphocytes from each child were exposed to phenytoin metabolites generated by a murine liver microsomal drug-metabolizing system.[98] There was a good correlation between the 14 children whose lymphocytes were killed by the phenytoin metabolites and those who had major birth defects and other signs of the hydantoin syndrome. The children with positive lymphocyte cytotoxic assays also had one parent with positive results, suggesting a genetic disorder in their ability to detoxify arene oxide metabolites. The results support the hypothesis that lymphocytes from affected patients are deficient in the enzyme epoxide hydrolase that normally detoxifies oxidative products of anticonvulsant metabolism. This hypothesis was tested more directly in a study that measured epoxide hydrolyase enzyme activity in cells removed from amniocentesis in 100 pregnant women.[14] Enzyme activity was distributed in a trimodal fashion, and activity less than 30% of normal was associated with clinical findings in the fetus compatible with fetal hydantoin syndrome. These results suggest that certain infants are predisposed to fetal anticonvulsant teratogenesis because of genetic defects in mechanisms for inactivating toxic metabolites (Fig. 1–24). The results also suggest that infants at increased risk may be identifiable using amniocentesis.

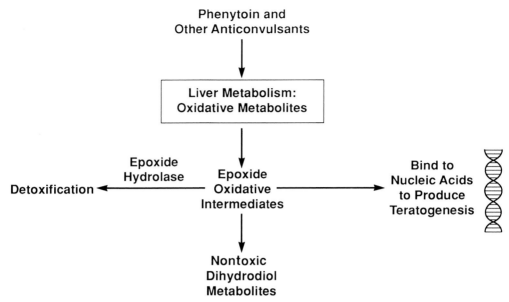

Figure 1–24. Possible mechanisms of actions of phenytoin and other anticonvulsants to produce teratogenesis.

Although valproate initially was considered to have a lower risk of teratogenicity than other anticonvulsants, more recent studies describe fetal anomalies attributed to this drug. In one study of 14 infants exposed to valproate monotherapy, four were born with major malformations including skeletal defects, meningomyelocele, and heart defects.[48] Seven had a distinctive pattern of craniofacial and digital anomalies; the median number of minor anomalies was four times higher than in a control group of infants exposed to other anticonvulsants. The incidence of fetal distress also appeared to be high in the valproate-treated group. Pharmacokinetic studies in the cohort suggested that the teratogenic effect might be dose related. Consideration of other population-based studies, especially those from Europe, suggests that valproate is associated with a relative risk for neural tube defects of 1% to 2%, which is elevated even when controlled for the effect of maternal epilepsy.[59] Valproate also may cause a pattern of minor facial anomalies, but some studies cast doubt

on its role in producing other developmental disabilities.[59] Although valproate has been shown to cause neural tube defects in animal teratogenicity studies, the mechanisms for the effect remain uncertain.

In addition to obvious effects of intrauterine drug exposure on physical features, there is increasing interest in the behavioral teratogenicity of neuroactive drugs. These concerns are based on animal studies that demonstrate long-lasting behavioral effects from perinatal exposure to drugs such as benzodiazepines. Experimental data suggest that prenatal or perinatal exposure to psychotropic drugs can have long-lasting effects on behavior and learning and may also result in measurable neurochemical changes that persist in adulthood.[22] Some drugs may have unexpected effects on brain development because certain neurotransmitter receptors play a role in neuronal development.[66] The possibility of pregnancy must be kept in mind when drugs are used in any female adolescent or woman of childbearing age.

CONCLUSION

This introduction has considered the five major determinants of drug therapy for neurologic disorders. Each of the themes is developed in greater detail in the disease-oriented chapters that follow. Progress in understanding the molecular actions of drugs goes hand in hand with progress in neuroscience and understanding basic disease mechanisms; this is reflected in the variation in the content of these chapters. The conceptual framework and methodology available to address the basic mechanisms of drug action varies from one group of disorders to another. For example, the present capacity to examine molecular actions of antiepileptic drugs on neuronal membranes is considerably greater than the ability to understand the actions of drugs that protect against ischemia. Current progress in molecular biology of the nervous system promises to narrow these gaps in our understanding, however, and to stimulate therapeutic discovery.

REFERENCES

1. Albano, A, Reisdorff, EJ, and Wiegenstein, JG: Rectal diazepam in pediatric status epilepticus. American Journal of Emergency Medicine 7:168–172, 1989.
2. Albin, RL, Albers, JW, Greenberg, HS, Townsend, JB, Lynn, RB, Burke, JM, and Alessi, AG: Acute sensory neuropathy—neuropathy from pyridoxine overdose. Neurology 37:1729–1732, 1987.
3. Alldredge, BK, Lowenstein, DH, and Simon, RP: Seizures associated with recreational drug abuse. Neurology 39:1037–1039, 1989.
4. Argov, Z, and Mastalgia, FL: Disorders of neuromuscular transmission caused by drugs. N Engl J Med 301:409–413, 1979.
5. Argov, Z and Mastalgia, FL: Drug-induced peripheral neuropathies. Br Med J 1:663–666, 1979.
6. Ashbrook, DW: Carnitine supplementation in human carnitine deficiency. In Borum, PR (ed): Clinical Aspects of Human Carnitine Deficiency. Pergamon Press, New York, 1987, pp 120–156.
7. Bodor, N and Simpkins, J: Redox delivery system for brain specific sustained release of dopamine. Science 221:65–67, 1983.
8. Boreus, LD: Principles of pediatric pharmacology. Churchill Livingstone, New York, 1982.
9. Brent, DA, Crumrine, PK, Varma, RR, Allan, M, and Allman, C: Phenobarbital treatment and major depressive disorders in children with epilepsy. Pediatrics 80(6):909–917, 1987.
10. Brin, MF, Fahn, S, Moskowitz, C, Friedman, A, Shale, HM, Greene, PE, Blitzer, A, List, T, Lange, D, and Lovelace, RE: Localized injections of botulinum toxin for the treatment of focal dystonia and hemifacial spasm. Movement Disorders 2(4):237–254, 1987.
11. Broadwell, RD, Balin, BJ, and Salcman, M: Transcytotic pathway for blood-borne protein through the blood-brain barrier. Proc Natl Acad Sci USA 85:632–636, 1988.
12. Browne, TR, Mattson, RH, Penry, JK, Smith, DB, Treinan, DM, Wilder, BJ, Ben-Menachem, E, Napoliello, MJ, Sherry, KM, and Szabo, GK: Vigabatrin for refractory complex partial seizures. Neurology 37:184–189, 1987.
13. Bruni, J, Wilder, BJ, Perchalski, CJ, Hammond, EJ, and Villareal, HJ: Phenobarbital metabolism is inhibited by therapeutic levels of VPA. Neurology 30:94–97, 1980.
14. Buehler, BA, Delimont, D, Van Waes, M, and Finnell, RH: Perinatal prediction of risk of the fetal hydantoin syndrome. N Engl J Med 322:1567–1572, 1990.
15. Calandra, G, Lydick, E, Carrigan, J, Weiss, L, and Guess, H: Factors predisposing to seizures in seriously ill infected patients receiving antibiotics: Experience with imipenem/cilastatin. Am J Med 84(5):911–918, 1988.
16. Camfield, CS, Camfield, PR, Smith, E, and Dooley, JM: Home use of rectal diazepam to prevent status epilepticus in children with convulsive disorder.

Journal of Child Neurology 4:125–126, 1989.

17. Capute, AJ, Kim, YI, and Sanders, DB: The neuromuscular blocking effects of therapeutic concentrations of various antibiotics on normal rat skeletal muscle: A quantitative comparison. J PEt 217:369.

18. Carranow, E, Kareus, J, and Co, S: Carbamazepine toxicity induced by concurrent erythromycin therapy. Arch Neurol 42:1878, 1985.

19. Clark, DW: Genetically determined variability in acetylation and oxidation. Therapeutic implications. Drugs 29(4): 342–375, 1985.

20. Cooper, JR, Roth, RH, and Bloom, FE: Biochemical Basis of Neuropharmacology, ed 5. Oxford, 1986.

21. Coulter, DL and Allen, RJ: Hyperammonemia with valproic acid therapy. J Pediatr 99(2):317–319, 1981.

22. Cuomo, V: Perinatal neurotoxicology of psychotropic drugs. TIPS 8:346–350, 1987.

23. Davies J: Selective depression of synaptic excitation in cat spinal neurons by baclofen: An iontophoretic study. Br J Pharmacol 72:373–384, 1981.

24. De Groen, PC, Aksamit, AJ, Rakela, J, Forbes, GS, and Krom, RA: Central nervous system toxicity after liver transplantation. The role of cyclosporine and cholesterol. N Engl J Med 317:861–866, 1987.

25. Delattre, JY, Safai, B, and Posner, JB: Erythema multiforme and Stevens-Johnson syndrome in patients receiving cranial irradiation and phenytoin. Neurology 38:194–198, 1988.

26. Dimario, FJ and Clancy, RR: Paradoxical precipitation of tonic seizures by lorazepam in a child with atypical absence seizures. Pediatric Neurology 4:249–251, 1988.

27. Dodson, WE: Nonlinear kinetics of phenytoin in children. Neurology 32: 42–48, 1982.

28. Drachman, DB, McIntosh, KR, De-Silva, S, Kunci, RW, and Kahn, C: Strategies for the treatment of myasthenia gravis. Ann NY Acad Sci 540:176–186, 1988.

29. Dreifuss, FE, Santilli, N, Langer, DH, Sweeney, KP, Moline, KA, and Menander, KB: Valproic acid hepatic fatalities: A retrospective review. Neurology 37:379–385, 1987.

30. Faull, KF, Guilleminault, C, Berger, PA, and Barchas, JD: Cerebrospinal fluid monoamine metabolites in narcolepsy and hypersomnia. Ann Neurol 13(3):258–263, 1983.

31. Feinberg, WM and Swenson, MR: Cerebrovascular complications of L-asparaginase therapy. Neurology 38:127–133, 1988.

32. Fishman, R: Cerebrospinal Fluid and Diseases of the Nervous System. WB Saunders, Philadelphia, 1980.

33. Friedman, JH, Feinberg, SS, and Feldman, RG: A neuroleptic malignant like syndrome due to levodopa therapy withdrawal. JAMA 254(19):2791–2795, 1985.

34. Gardner, CR: Functional in vivo correlates of the benzodiazepine agonist-inverse agonist continuum. Prog Neurobiol 31(6):425–476, 1988.

35. Gelmers, HJ, Gorter, K, De Weerdt, CJ, and Wiezer, HJA: A controlled trial of nimodipine in acute ischemic stroke. N Engl J Med 318(4):203–207, 1988.

36. Gilman, AG, Goodman, CS, Rall, TW, and Murad, F: Goodman and Gilman's The Pharmacological Basis of Therapeutics, ed 7. Macmillan, New York, 1985.

37. Goldstein, G and Betz, AL: The blood-brain barrier. Sci Am 254(3):74–83, 1986.

38. Goulden, KJ, Dooley, JM, Camfeld, P, and Fraser, A: Clinical valproic toxicity induced by acetylsalicylic acid. Neurology 37:1392–1394, 1987.

39. Granati, JE, Stern, BK, Ringel, A, Karim, AH, Krumholz, A, Coyle, JT, and Adler, S.: Neuroleptic malignant syndrome: Successful treatment with dantrolene and bromocriptine. Ann Neurol 14:89–90, 1983.

40. Guze, BH and Baxter, LR: Neuroleptic malignant syndrome. N Engl J Med 313:163–166, 1985.

41. Harbaugh, RE, Saunders, RL, and Reeder, RF: Use of implantable pumps

for central nervous system drug infusions to treat neurological disease. Neurosurgery 23(6):693–698, 1988.

42. Hart, R and Easton, J: Carbamazepine and hematologic monitoring. Ann Neurol 11:309–312, 1982.

43. Hefti, F and Knusel, B: Chronic administration of nerve growth and other neurotrophic factors to the brain. Neurobiol Aging 9(5–6):689–690, 1988.

44. Hess, E: Drug induced lupus. N Engl J Med 318:1460–1462, 1988.

45. Hill, LM and Kleinberg, F: Effects of drugs and chemicals on the fetus and newborn (Part 1). Mayo Clin Proc 59(10):707–716, 1984.

46. Hill, LM and Kleinberg, F: Effects of drugs and chemicals on the fetus and newborn (Part 2). Mayo Clin Proc 59(11):755–765, 1984.

47. Jacqz, R, Hall, SD, and Branch, RA: Genetically determined polymorphisms in drug oxidation. Hepatology 6:1020–1032, 1986.

48. Jager-Roman, E, Deichl, A, Jakob, S, Hartmann, AM, Koch, S, Rating, D, Steldinger, R, Nau, H, and Helge, H: Fetal growth, major malformations and minor anomalies in infants born to women receiving valproic acid. J Pediatr 108(6):997–1004, 1986.

49. Jankovic, J and Orman, J: Tetrabenazine therapy of dystonia, chorea, tics and other dyskinesias. Neurology 38 (3):391–394, 1988.

50. Jeste, DV and Wyatt, RJ: Therapeutic strategies against tardive dyskinesia. Arch Gen Psychiatry 3:803–816, 1982.

51. Joyce, RP and Gunderson, CH: Carbamazepine-induced orofacial dyskinesia. Neurology 30:1333–1334, 1980.

52. Juncos, JL, Fabbrini, G, Mouradian, MM, and Chase, TN: Controlled release levodopa-carbidopa (CR-5) in the management of parkinsonian motor fluctuations. Arch Neurol 44:1010–1012, 1987.

53. Juncos, JL, Fabbrini, G, Mouradian MM, Serrati, C, and Chase, TN: Dietary influences on the antiparkinsonian response to levodopa. Arch Neurol 44: 1003–1005, 1987.

54. Kane, CS, Foster, TE, Reed, JE, Spatz, EL, and Girgis, GN: Intracerebral hemorrhage and phenylpropylamine use. Neurology 37:399–404, 1987.

55. Kaufman, S: Hyperphenylalaninaemia caused by defects in biopterin metabolism. J Inherited Metab Dis 8(Suppl 1):20–27, 1985.

56. Kontos, HA: Oxygen radicals in cerebral vascular injury. Circ Res 57 (4):508–516, 1985.

57. Kurlan, R and Casno, P: Drug induced Alzheimerism. Arch Neurol 45:356–357, 1988.

58. Kutt, H: Interactions between anticonvulsants and other commonly prescribed drugs. Epilepsia 25(Suppl 2): S118–S131, 1984.

59. Lammer, EJ, Sever, LE, Oakely, GP: Teratogen update: Valproic acid. Teratology 35:465–473, 1987.

60. Langston, JW, Irwin, I, and Ricaurte, GA: Neurotoxins, parkinsonism and Parkinson's disease. Pharmacol Ther 32(1):19–49, 1987.

61. Levine, SR, Washington, JM, Jefferson, MF, Kieran, SN, Moen, M, Feit, H, and Welch, KM: "Crack" cocaine associated stroke. Neurology 37:1849–1853, 1987.

62. MacLeod, CM, Dekaban, AS, and Hunt, E: Memory impairment in epileptic patients. Selective effects of phenobarbital concentration. Science 202: 1102–1104.

63. MacPhee, GJA, Thompson, GG, Gordon, GT, and Martin, JB: Verapamil potentiates carbamazepine neurotoxicity: A clinically important inhibitory interaction. Lancet 1:700–703, 1986.

64. Manfredi, RL and Kales, A: Clinical neuropharmacology of sleep disorders. Seminars in Neurology 7(3):286–295, 1987.

65. Maxwell, GM: Principles of Pediatric Pharmacology. Oxford University Press, New York, 1984.

66. McDonald, JW and Johnston, MV: Physiological and pathophysiological roles of excitatory amino acids during central nervous system development. Brain Res 15:41–70, 1990.

67. Mefford, IN, Baker, TL, Boehme, R,

Foutz, AS, Ciaranello, RD, Barchas, JD, and Dement, WC: Narcolepsy: Biogenic amine deficits in an animal model. Science 220(4597):629–632, 1983.

68. Melikian, AP, Strajghn, AB, Slywka, GW, Whyatt, H, and Meyer, MC: Bioavailability of 11 phenytoin products. J Pharmacokinet Biopharm 5:133–146, 1977.

69. Micheli, F, Pardal, MF, Gatto, M, Torres, M, Paradiso, G, Parera, IC, and Giannaula, R: Flunarizine and cinnarizine induced extrapyramidal reactions. Neurology 37:881–884, 1987.

70. Mikkelson, EJ, Detolor, J, and Cohen, DF: School avoidance and social phobia triggered by haloperidol in patients with Tourette's disorder. Am J Psychiatry 138:1572–1576, 1981.

71. Munsat, TL, Taft, J, and Jackson, I: Pharmacokinetics of intrathecal thyrotopin-releasing hormone. Neurology 37:597–601, 1987.

72. Murray, NM and Newson-Davis, J: Treatment with oral 4-aminopyridine in disorders of neuromuscular transmission. Neurology 37:597–601, 1987.

73. Nutt, JG, Woodward, WR, Hammerstad, JP, Carter, JH, and Anderson, JL: The "on-off" phenomenon in Parkinson's disease. N Engl J Med 310:483–488, 1984.

74. Onrot, J, Goldberg, MR, Biaggioni, I, Wiley, RG, Hollister, AS, and Robertson, D: Oral yohimbine in human autonomic failure. Neurology 37:215–220, 1987.

75. Painter, MJ, Pippenger, CE, and Wasterlain, CG: Phenobarbital and phenytoin in neonatal seizures: Metabolism and tissue distribution. Neurology 31:1107–1112, 1981.

76. Pardridge, WM: Recent advances in blood-brain barrier transport. Annu Rev Pharmacol Toxicol 28:25–39, 1988.

77. Pardridge, WM, Oldendorf, WH, Cancilla, P, and Frank, J: Blood brain barrier: Interface between internal medicine and the brain. Ann Intern Med 105:82–95, 1986.

78. Pardridge, WM, Kumagai, AK, and Eisenberg, JB: Chimeric peptides as a vehicle for peptide pharmaceutical delivery through the blood-brain barrier. Biochem Biophys Res Commun 146:307–313, 1987.

79. Pincus, JH and Barry, KM: Plasma levels of amino acids correlate with motor fluctuations in parkinsonism. Arch Neurol 44:1006–1009, 1987.

80. Prevey, ML, Mattson, RH, and Cramer, JA: Improvement in cognitive functioning and mood after conversion to valproate monotherapy. Neurology 39:1640–1641, 1989.

81. Rang, HP and Dale, MM: Pharmacology. Churchill Livingstone, Edinburgh, 1987.

82. Rettie, AE, Rettenmeier, AW, Howald, WN, and Fillie, TA: Cytochrome P-450 catalyzed formation of delta 4-VPA, a toxic metabolite of valproic acid. Science 235:890–893, 1987.

83. Richman, DD: The treatment of HIV infection. Azidothymidine (AZT) and other new antiviral drugs. Infect Dis Clin North Am 2(2):397–407, 1988.

84. Riggs, JE: Pharmacologic enhancement of neuromuscular transmission in myasthenia gravis. Clin Neuropharmacol 5(3):277–292, 1982.

85. Roberts, KD and Malis, R: Skin reaction to carbamazepine. Arch Dermatol 117:273–275, 1981.

86. Roberts, RJ: Drug Therapy in Infants: Pharmacologic Principles and Clinical Experience. WB Saunders, Philadelphia, 1984.

87. Scheffner, D, Konig, S, Rauterberg-Ruland, I, Kochen, W, Hoffman, WJ, and Unkelbach, S: Fatal liver failure in 16 children with valproate therapy. Epilepsia 29(5):530–532, 1988.

88. Schneider-Helment, D and Spinweber, D: Evaluation of L-tryptophan for treatment of insomnia: A review. Psychopharmacology (Berlin) 89:1–7, 1986.

89. Shields, WD and Saslow, E: Myoclonic, atonic, and absence seizures following institution of carbamazepine therapy in children. Neurology 33:1487–1489, 1983.

90. Silver, RM, Heyes, MP, Maize, JC, Quearey, B, Vionnet-Fuasset, M, and Sternberg, EM: Scleroderma, fasciitis and eosinophilia associated with the in-

gestion of tryptophan. N Engl J Med 322:874–881, 1990.

91. Silverstein, FS, Parrish, MA, and Johnston, MV: Adverse behavioral reactions in children treated with carbamazepine (Tegretol). J Pediatr 101 (5):785–787, 1982.

92. Singer, HS, Butler, IJ, Tune, LE, Seifert, WE, Jr, and Coyle, JT: Dopaminergic dysfunction in Tourette syndrome. Ann Neurol 12(4):361–366, 1982.

93. Spector, R: The Scientific Basis of Clinical Pharmacology. Little, Brown & Co, Boston/Toronto, 1986.

94. Spielberg, SP, Gordon, GB, Blake, DA, Goldstein, DA, and Herlong, HF: Predisposition to phenytoin hepatotoxicity assessed in vitro. N Engl J Med 305:722–727, 1981.

95. Stahl, SM and Palazidou, L: The pharmacology of depression: Studies of neurotransmitter receptors lead the search for biochemical lesions and new drug therapies. Trends Pharmacol Sci 7(9):349–354, 1986.

96. Stahl, SM and Wets, KM: Recent advances in drug delivery technology for neurology. Clin Neuropharmacol 1(1):1–17, 1988.

97. Streisand, JB and Stanley, JH: Opioids: New techniques in routes of administration. Current Opinion in Anesthesiology 2:456–462, 1989.

98. Strickler, NM, Dansky, L, Miller, MA, Senn, M-H, Anderman, E, and Spielberg, SP: Genetic predisposition to phenytoin induced birth defects. Lancet 2:764–769, 1985.

99. Tarsy, D: Movement disorders with neuroleptic drug treatment. Psychiatr Clin North Am 7:453–471, 1984.

100. Tokes, ZA, St. Peteri, AK, and Todd, JA: Availability of liposome content to the nervous system. Liposomes and the blood-brain barrier. Brain Res 188:282–286, 1980.

101. Vining, E, Mellitis, ED, Dorse, MM, Cataldo, MF, Quaskey, SA, Speilber, SP, and Freeman, JM: Psychologic and behavioral effects of antiepileptic drugs in children: A double blind comparison between phenobarbital and valproic acid. Pediatrics 80(2):165–174, 1987.

102. Warnke, PC, Blasberg, RG, and Groothuis, DR: The effects of hyperosmotic blood brain barrier disruption on blood to tissue transport in ENU induced gliomas. Ann Neurol 22:300–305, 1987.

103. Whitley, RJ: Herpes simplex virus infections of the central nervous system. A review. Am J Med 85(2A):61–67, 1988.

104. Wilkinson, GR: Effects of aging on the disposition of benzodiazepines in human beings: Binding and distribution considerations. In Raskin, A, Robinson, DS, and Levind, J, (eds): Age and the Pharmacology of Psychoactive Drugs. Elsevier, New York, 1981.

105. Williams, DP, Troost, BT, and Rogers, J: Lithium-induced downbeat nystagmus. Arch Neurol 45:1022–1023, 1988.

106. Worley, PF, Barbanan, JM, and Snyder, SH: Beyond receptors: Multiple second messenger systems in brain. Ann Neurol 21:217–229, 1987.

107. Yogman, MW and Zeisel, SH: Diet and sleep patterns in newborn infants. N Engl J Med 309(19):1147–1149, 1983.

Chapter 2

MOVEMENT DISORDERS

John B. Penney, Jr., M.D., and
Anne B. Young, M.D., Ph.D.

NEUROCHEMICAL ANATOMY OF
  THE BASAL GANGLIA
PARKINSON'S DISEASE
HUNTINGTON'S DISEASE
DYSTONIA
TREMORS
TICS
HEMIBALLISMUS
SPASTICITY
WILSON'S DISEASE
DRUG MANIPULATION OF
  TRANSMITTER SYSTEMS

Movement disorders are characterized by abnormalities in the quality and quantity of spontaneous movements. There may be too few voluntary movements or spontaneous involuntary movements. Abnormalities in the resistance of the muscles to passive stretch (tone) are common, but actual muscle weakness or paralysis are not part of a pure movement disorder. Several of the classic movement disorders, such as Parkinson's disease, Huntington's disease, and hemiballismus, have been associated with specific pathologies in the basal ganglia. Other movement disorders, such as tics and dystonia, are thought to be due to basal ganglia dysfunction, although classic neuropathologic studies have not demonstrated abnormalities in any brain region in these disorders. Essential tremor and spasticity are movement disorders that do not appear to result from basal ganglia dysfunction. They also will be discussed in this chapter.

This chapter is divided into three major sections. The first section reviews the anatomy of the basal ganglia, with special attention to the neurotransmitter systems involved. The second section outlines the clinical manifestations, neurochemical pathology, pathogenesis, and general plan of treatment for each of the major classes of movement disorder. The final section discusses rational pharmacotherapeutic approaches to manipulation of the major neurotransmitter systems involved in the treatment of movement disorders. Surgical therapy, such as the older ablative procedures and the newer experimental procedures involving transplantation of neural tissue, are not discussed in detail.

NEUROCHEMICAL ANATOMY OF THE BASAL GANGLIA

Basal Ganglia Structures

The anatomic regions of the brain important in the generation of movement include certain deep forebrain structures, the caudate nucleus and the putamen; their diencephalic projection zones, the globus pallidus and the subthalamic nucleus; the substantia nigra; and the projection pathways from the globus pallidus and the substantia nigra (Fig. 2–1).[1] The general flow of neural impulses is into the cau-

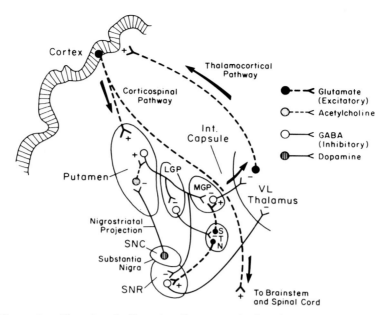

Figure 2-1. The major efferent and afferent pathways in the basal ganglia that are relevant to drug therapy for movement disorders. Excitatory pathways (axons) that use the neurotransmitters glutamate and acetylcholine are shown as broken lines; inhibitory pathways that use GABA and dopamine are shown as solid lines. A major function of the motor portion of the basal ganglia (putamen, lateral globus pallidus [LGP]; medial globus pallidus [MGP]; substantia nigra; and subthalamic nucleus [STN]) is to modulate the excitatory thalamic feedback loop to motor cortex from the ventrolateral (VL) nucleus of the thalamus shown at the right side of the diagram. Motor commands that activate the corticospinal pathways also excite inhibitory neurons (containing both GABA and substance P) in the putamen that innervate the MGP. The GABAergic output from the MGP to VL thalamus is the major output from the basal ganglia. This neuronal loop (motor cortex to putamen to MGP to VL thalamus to motor cortex) provides continuous feedback to motor cortex to adjust motor tone. This pathway appears to be stimulated by dopaminergic input to the striatum from the substantia nigra pars compacta (SNC). Its function is inhibited in parkinsonism. Dopamine neuronal activity is modulated by substance P(SP)/GABA neurons projecting from the putamen to pars compacta of the substantia nigra (SNR). This pathway participates in the control of eye movements. The other main motor control pathway in the basal ganglia goes from the cortex through enkephalin (ENK)/GABA cells of the putamen to LGP, then to the STN, which sends excitatory fibers to the MGP and the SNR. This pathway is inhibited by dopamine and has decreased activity in hemiballismus and chorea. Striatal acetylcholine and somatostatin neurons are interneurons within the putamen. The SP/GABA pathway to SNC comes from the striosomes (see Figure 2-2) and governs striatonigral feedback. To simplify the diagram, SP/GABA and ENK/GABA neurons are now shown separately but are represented by a single neuron (Based on information from Albin et al[1]).

date nucleus and putamen from the cerebral cortex and brainstem, then through the globus pallidus and substantia nigra pars reticulata to the thalamus and other regions of the brain. The afferents, the internal organization, and the efferents of each of these major regions of the basal ganglia are discussed in turn.

THE STRIATUM

The caudate nucleus and the putamen, together with the nucleus accumbens and the olfactory tubercle, have similar histologies and are collectively called the striatum.[29] The caudate nucleus and putamen are important in coordinating movement. They receive major excitatory, glutamatergic inputs from the cerebral cortex. Cortical projections to putamen emanate mainly from the primary motor and sensory cortices, whereas those to the caudate come from the association cortices. The striatum also receives excitatory projections from the intralaminar nuclei of the thalamus. There is a major dopaminergic pathway to the striatum from the substantia nigra pars compacta and ventral tegmental area. Lesser serotoninergic and noradrenergic projections also emanate from the raphe nuclei and locus ceruleus in the brainstem.

Internally, the striatum has two major organizational components — the matrix and the striosomes (Fig. 2–2).[29,62] The striosomes are 1-mm–wide interconnected patches embedded in the matrix. They were first discovered because they have low levels of the enzyme acetylcholinesterase.[29] The ma-

trix and the striosomes have different connections. The matrix compartment receives major projections from upper layers of cerebral cortex (particularly the primary motor, sensory, and association cortices) the thalamus, the ventral tegmental area, and the dorsal nigra, whereas the striosomes receive afferents from ventral nigra and deep layers of cerebral cortex, particularly the limbic cortices (see the section on striatal afferents from the substantia nigra for further details). A small percentage of striatal neurons are inter-

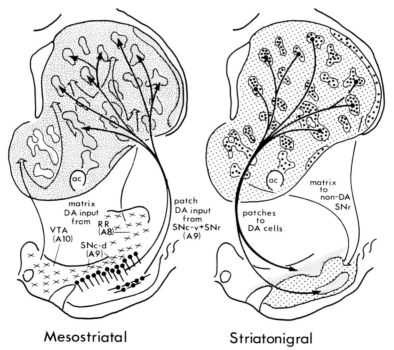

Mesostriatal   Striatonigral

Figure 2–2. The relationship between striosomes (*patch*); matrix, their inputs from dopamine cells of the substantia nigra and ventral tegmental area (mesostriatal, *left*); and their outputs to the substantia nigra (striatonigral, *right*) as established in the rat. The striosomes are 1-mm-wide, interconnected subregions of the caudate and putamen that contain low levels of acetylcholinesterase and have different connections from the surrounding matrix. Not shown are the cortical input to striosomes (*patch*) that comes from deep layer 5 and layer 6 of cortex, particularly limbic cortex, and the cortical input to matrix that comes from superficial layer 5 and layer 3 of cortex, particularly motor, sensory and association cortices.[26] Matrix also receives input from the thalamus (also not shown). The dopaminergic input to matrix comes from a set of dorsally located midbrain neurons (X) in the ventral tegmental area (VTA, A10); dorsal substantia nigra pars compacta (SNc-d, A9); and retrorubral area (RR, A8). (A8, A9, and A10 are anatomic locations assigned to these neurons based on early investigations.[39]) Dopaminergic input to the striosomes comes from ventral substantia nigra pars compacta neurons (SNc-v) and isolated groups of cells located more ventrally in substantia nigra pars reticulata (SNr). Striatal matrix neurons send outputs to the globus pallidus (not shown) and to the substantia nigra pars reticulata, avoiding regions of the SNr and SNc that contain dopamine neurons. Striosomal neurons send outputs to the regions of the dopamine neurons in SNc and SNr. (From Gerfen et al,[27] p 3932, with permission.)

neurons. These include somatostatin neurons, which are exclusively present in the matrix, and acetylcholine neurons, which occur in both matrix and striosome compartments and which send their processes from one region into the other. All other striatal neurons appear to confine their dendritic processes to the compartment where their soma resides.

The vast majority of the matrix efferent neurons appear to use gamma-aminobutyric acid (GABA) as a neurotransmitter.[29,62] Many of these GABA neurons contain enkephalin as a colocalized neuromodulator. These neurons appear to project primarily to the lateral portion of the globus pallidus. Other striatal efferents contain GABA and both substance P and dynorphin. These neurons project to the medial segment of the globus pallidus and to the substantia nigra pars reticulata. Striosomal efferent neurons include both GABA neurons and substance P/dynorphin neurons. The only currently known projection of the striosomes is to pars compacta of the substantia nigra.[26] Both dopamine D-2 and muscarinic cholinergic receptors are present in high density in the striatum (Fig. 2–3). GABA/benzodiazepine receptors are also dense in the striatum.

THE LATERAL GLOBUS PALLIDUS AND SUBTHALAMIC NUCLEUS

The lateral globus pallidus consists of large, multipolar neurons that appear to be GABAergic. The vast majority of these neurons are efferent neurons although apparently there are some interneurons. The lateral pallidal neurons send their axons to the subthalamic nucleus, which also receives projections from the cerebral cortex, particularly the motor regions. The cortical pathway is excitatory and presumably glutamatergic. The neurotransmitter used by subthalamic nucleus neurons is also thought to be excitatory and glutamatergic. Subthalamic projections go back to the lateral pallidum and

striatum and out to the medial segment of the globus pallidus and the pars reticulata of the substantia nigra. Thus, information from the GABA/enkephalin striatal matrix neurons goes to the lateral globus pallidus and is then relayed via the subthalamic nucleus to the medial segment of the globus pallidus and the substantia nigra pars reticulata. Here the information is processed along with that of the matrix substance P/dynorphin direct projections to nigra and medial pallidum.

THE MEDIAL GLOBUS PALLIDUS AND SUBSTANTIA NIGRA PARS RETICULATA

The medial globus pallidus and substantia nigra pars reticulata consist of large GABAergic neurons similar to those in the lateral globus pallidus. The medial globus pallidus appears to receive the majority of its striatal projections from the putamen. Its efferents project to the pars oralis of the ventral lateral thalamic nucleus, which in turn projects to the supplementary motor cortex.[73] This pathway joining the putamen, medial globus pallidus, thalamus, and supplementary motor cortex may be the primary route by which the basal ganglia influence spontaneous movements.

The substantia nigra pars reticulata receives the majority of its striatal afferents from the caudate, and it has a number of important projections. One is a projection to the dopaminergic pars compacta neurons, thus completing a nigral-striatal-nigral feedback loop. Another projection is to the ventral anterior and medial dorsal nuclei of the thalamus, which in turn project to the prefrontal cortex. This pathway joining the caudate, pars reticulata, thalamus, and prefrontal cortex is thought to mediate the behavioral disorders seen in basal ganglia disease. A third major pathway goes from the pars reticulata to the superior colliculus. This pathway subserves an important basal ganglia influence on eye movements.[1] Pars reticulata projections to the reticular formation may mediate basal ganglia effects on tone (muscle resistance to passive stretch).

Striatal Afferents

THE CEREBRAL CORTEX

The cerebral cortex sends large projections to the caudate and putamen.[29] The neurotransmitter of these cortical pathways is thought to be the excitatory amino acid, glutamate. Motor and sensory cortex project principally to the extrastriosomal matrix of putamen. Association and cingulate cortices project to matrix of the caudate. The posterior parietal cortex projects to the dorsolateral caudate, the dorsolateral prefrontal cortex to the central caudate, and the anterior cingulate cortex to the ventromedial caudate.

The striosomes receive projections from the medial prefrontal cortex, insulotemporal cortex, and basolateral amygdala. They also receive minor projections from deep layers of other cortical regions. The implication of these differential projections to striosome and matrix is that there may be distinct circuits for the basal ganglia modulation of limbic and motorsensory tasks. Further study is necessary for understanding how the two circuits are affected in different basal ganglia disorders.

THALAMIC PROJECTIONS TO THE STRIATUM

A major afferent pathway to the caudate/putamen arises in the thalamus. The centromedian and parafascicular nuclei of thalamus provide an excitatory input whose functional significance is as yet unknown. The transmitter of this pathway is also unknown, although substance P and acetylcholine have been ruled out. The centromedian and parafascicular projections innervate primarily the extrastriosomal matrix.

THE SUBSTANTIA NIGRA PARS COMPACTA

One of the best-studied projections to the striatum is the dopaminergic pathway from the substantia nigra pars compacta. Initially, the dopamine inputs to the striatum were thought to be rather uniform, but in the early 1970s, islands of intense dopamine fluorescence were noted in neonatal and adult rat striatum.[25] Subsequent studies on the striosomal/matrix system have shown that during development, striosomes are innervated by dopamine afferents earlier than matrix; only later are the matrix dopamine terminals evident.[29] The synaptic chemistry of dopamine neurons is discussed in Chapter 1.

Recent studies have also shown that specific pars compacta regions project preferentially to striosome rather than matrix (Fig. 2–2).[27,39] In the rat, the ventral-caudal densocellular portion and the substantia nigra pars lateralis project primarily to striosomes. In contrast, the more dorsal region of pars compacta (A8) and the ventral tegmental area project primarily to extrastriosomal matrix. Investigators are now studying whether differential loss of these subsets of dopaminergic afferents to striatum plays a role in human disease. In monkeys treated with 1-methyl-4-phenyl-1,2,3,6-tetrahydropyridine (MPTP), A8 neurons appear to be lost preferentially,[5,43] and in Parkinson's disease differential loss of pigmented substantia nigra dopamine neurons is found.[35]

BRAINSTEM PROJECTIONS TO THE STRIATUM

The serotonergic cells in the raphe nuclei send projections to the substantia nigra, the striatum, and the pallidum. The role of this pathway in modulating striatal outflow is unclear. Serotonergic dysfunction, however, has been linked to depression in patients with Parkinson's disease.[51]

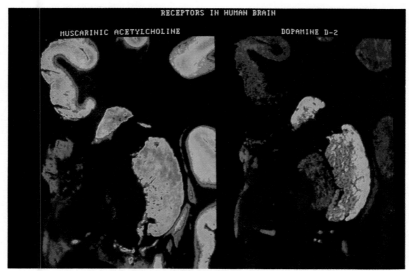

Figure 2-3.

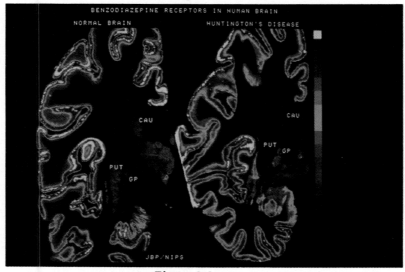

Figure 2-8.

Figure 2-3. Color transformations of receptor autoradiograms of muscarinic cholinergic *(left)* and dopamine D-2 *(right)* receptor binding in coronal sections from normal human basal ganglia. Muscarinic cholinergic receptors were measured with 1 nm [³H] quinuclidinyl-benzilate as previously described[88] and dopamine D-2 receptors were measured with 0.25 nm [³H] spiroperidol in the presence of 100 nm mianserin, as previously described.[67] Muscarinic cholinergic receptors are most dense in caudate and putamen. Relatively high densities are also present in cerebral cortex. There are very few muscarinic cholinergic receptors in lateral globus pallidus, but the external border of medial globus pallidus clearly has receptors present. Dopamine D-2 receptors are most dense in caudate and putamen. Cerebral cortex and lateral globus pallidus also have D-2 receptors, but receptors are negligible elsewhere in basal ganglia (except substantia nigra pars compacta, not shown, which has receptors). On the color scale, red and yellow indicate the highest densities, and blues, purple, and black indicate the lowest densities.

Figure 2-8. Color transformations of benzodiazepine receptor autoradiograms in coronal sections from a neurologically normal individual *(left)* and a person who died with Huntington's disease *(right)*. Benzodiazepine receptors were measured with 10 nm [³H] flunitrazepam as previously described. The color bar on the right shows that the highest density of binding is in white and red; lowest density is in blue and black. Note that in the Huntington's case, receptors are decreased in caudate (CAU) and putamen (PUT) and increased in globus pallidus (GP).

Clinical Implications

The circuitry of the basal ganglia is quite complex, and as our knowledge increases, the apparent complexity increases as well. Nevertheless, some generalizations can be made about the system that allow one to interpret the clinical symptomatology in terms of neuronal circuitry.

Two major circuits seem to be modulated by the striatum. The first is the limbic circuit, which is relatively self-contained and includes the medial prefrontal and insulotemporal cortices, the basolateral amygdala, the striosomes, and the densocellular area of the substantia nigra pars compacta. The second circuit probably modulates motor and sensory function, because it includes association, motor, and sensory cortices; matrix; pallidum; subthalamic nucleus; substantia nigra pars reticulata; thalamus; superior colliculus; and the brainstem.

This latter, larger circuit can be thought of as two separate but interconnecting circuits.[1,62] The first pathway is from cortex to matrix to medial pallidum and pars reticulata and thence to thalamus and cortex. It is probably modulated by dopaminergic input from the substantia nigra in an excitatory fashion (i.e., dopamine normally excites or stimulates this circuit). The second pathway is from cortex to matrix to lateral pallidum to subthalamic nucleus to medial pallidum/pars reticulata and thence to thalamus and cortex. This circuit is inhibited by dopaminergic inputs.

Loss of dopamine to the striatum in Parkinson's disease therefore results in underactivity of the first matrix circuit and overactivity of the second matrix circuit leading to inability to facilitate switching of motor programs and excessive suppression of spontaneous movements. In the striatum, loss of specific subgroups of neurons may lead to quite different clinical abnormalities. Loss of matrix inhibitory inputs to lateral pallidum should result in chorea, as would a subthalamic nucleus lesion (see the section on selective vulnerability in Huntington's disease for further details), whereas loss of matrix projections to medial pallidum or pars reticulata might result in akinesia or dystonia.

Future studies of basal ganglia pathophysiology will have to address the relationship between clinical symptomatology and selective striatal cell loss or selective loss of striatal afferents. Improvements in labeling specific neuronal populations quantitatively in postmortem human tissues will help in this regard. The new neuropathology presumably will consist of immunocytochemical, in situ hybridization, and receptor autoradiographic techniques.

PARKINSON'S DISEASE

Clinical Manifestations

The cardinal features of Parkinson's disease are a tremor that is greater at rest than during movement, rigidity that is usually of the cogwheel type, and bradykinesia or akinesia. Accompanying signs are a loss of facial expression (masked facies), a stooped flexed posture, and the "freeze" phenomenon, a tendency to suddenly stop moving when startled by a new sensory input. These symptoms can be caused by any process that interferes with the action of the neurotransmitter dopamine.

Classical Parkinson's disease is usually unilateral in onset and remains more severe on the initially involved side. A dementia of the Alzheimer's type appears as a late complication more frequently than would be expected on a statistical basis. There is some evidence that cigarette smokers are less likely than the general population to develop the disease. The disease must be distinguished from other parkinsonian syndromes (Table 2–1), including progressive supranuclear palsy, the Shy-Drager syndrome (olivopontocerebellar atrophy type 4), and striatonigral atro-

Table 2 – 1 PARKINSONIAN SYNDROMES

DEGENERATIVE DISEASES

Parkinson's disease
Wilson's disease
Progressive supranuclear palsy
Multiple system atrophy
   Striatonigral degeneration
   Shy-Drager syndrome
   Olivopontocerebellar atrophy
Alzheimer's disease
Creutzfeldt-Jakob disease
Hallervorden-Spatz disease
Corticodentatonigral degeneration
Huntington's disease

SECONDARY CAUSES

Infectious diseases
   von Economo's encephalitis
Toxins
   Manganese
   Carbon monoxide
   MPTP
   Parkinson's-dementia-ALS of Guam
Drug-induced
Brain tumors
Head trauma
Vascular irregularities
Metabolic irregularities
   Hypoparathyroidism
   Basal ganglia calcification
   Non-Wilsonian hepatocerebral degeneration

phy. Shy-Drager syndrome and striatonigral degeneration may be subsets of a broader clinical syndrome, multisystem atrophy. Complete lack of tremor is often an indication that one of the other diseases is present. However, the most powerful predictor that Parkinson's disease is not present is the failure to respond to dopamine precursor treatment.[47a]

The disease responds remarkably well to symptomatic therapy in its early stages,[8] but the underlying pathology, loss of substantia nigra neurons, progresses inexorably. A number of late complications of therapy may, in fact, be brought on by progression of the disease. These include drug-induced dyskinesias and the "on-off" phenomenon, which is characterized by an oscillation between a severe parkinsonian state and a more mobile state accompanied by dyskinesia.[49] Dyskinesias are of two types. More common are "peak dose" dyskinesia. These are usually not perceived as a major problem by the patient, tend to be choreoathetoid in nature, and are increased by stress. The other type of dyskinesia is biphasic, occurring at the beginning or the end of a dosing interval. Biphasic dyskinesias are much more distressing to the patient and tend to be ballistic in nature. They may become a severe problem late in the day. An extreme complication in some patients is a failure to respond to therapy at all.

Neurotransmitter and Receptor Changes

DOPAMINE

The major pathologic change in Parkinson's disease is the loss of the dopamine-producing cells of the substantia nigra and, to a lesser extent, of the ventral tegmental area. The pigmented cells of the substantia nigra are more severely affected than the nonpigmented cells.[35] There is consequently a great loss of presynaptic dopamine terminals, dopamine uptake sites, and a drop in tyrosine hydroxylase and dopamine levels in the putamen of parkinsonian patients.[36] The loss is less severe in the caudate, nucleus accumbens, and the frontal cortex, which receive innervation from the ventral tegmental area. Levels of dopamine metabolites do not decrease as much as those of dopamine, presumably because of an increased turnover in the remaining dopamine terminals.

Early studies of human postmortem material suggested that dopamine receptors of both the D-2 and D-1 subtypes were increased in untreated patients with Parkinson's disease.[44] Later studies of treated patients tended not to demonstrate such changes in receptor numbers, either because patients currently coming to postmortem examination all have received long-term dopamine treatment, or because of improvements in the techniques of measuring dopamine receptors.

NOREPINEPHRINE

Loss of the norepinephrine-containing cells in the locus ceruleus and consequent loss of norepinephrine terminals in the forebrain also occurs.[36] Some have attributed the "freeze" phenomenon to loss of norepinephrine terminals.[55] Evidence exists that suggests an increased number of norepinephrine receptors in parkinsonian brains. These receptors may largely be located on cerebral microvessels.[11]

ACETYLCHOLINE

Animals with experimental parkinsonism show evidence of increased acetylcholine turnover.[46] These changes have not been confirmed in parkinsonian patients, but Parkinson's patients respond clinically to blockade of acetylcholine receptors. Tremor is the symptom most likely to benefit.

GABA

Striatal GABA levels tend to be increased in parkinsonian patients.[36] Levels have not been measured in the different striatal output areas of the postmortem human brain. Evidence suggests, however, that GABA receptors are decreased in the lateral globus pallidus and increased in the medial globus pallidus and substantia nigra of experimental parkinsonian animals.[60] These data suggest that the striatal-lateral pallidal GABA pathway may be overactive, whereas the striatal-medial pallidal and substantia nigra pathways may be underactive in patients with Parkinson's disease.

SEROTONIN

Depletion of serotonin has been found in a number of parkinsonian patients' brains, but there is little evidence for actual loss of raphe nucleus neurons.[36] Several studies have demonstrated that cerebrospinal fluid serotoninergic markers are depleted in depressed as opposed to nondepressed patients with Parkinson's disease.[51] Antidepressant treatment aimed at manipulating the serotonin system has been proposed as the most rational way of treating the depression associated with Parkinson's disease.

OPIATES

Evidence from experimental animals of interactions between dopamine and the opiate system suggests that dopamine affects opiate neurons and opiates affect dopamine neurons. Manipulation of the opiate system may improve restless legs or akathisias in Parkinson's patients.[87]

OTHER NEUROTRANSMITTER SYSTEMS

Although the glutamatergic, substance P, neurotensin, somatostatin, and cholecystokinin systems might all be involved in Parkinson's disease, few drugs are available to manipulate these systems. There is evidence for loss of neurotensin receptors in the substantia nigra of parkinsonian brains,[84] probably because these receptors are located on the dopamine neurons themselves. If drugs to manipulate these systems become available, they might be assessed in the treatment of parkinsonian patients.

Selective Vulnerability

Two age-associated neurochemical changes in the brain may have important consequences for the pathogenesis and treatment of Parkinson's disease. The first factor is that both postmortem human data and positron emission tomography (PET) scan data suggest that humans lose dopamine neurons and dopamine terminals with age.[52,82] These data, combined with the recent experience with MPTP (see below) suggest that multiple factors contribute to the age of onset in Parkinson's disease.[11] Some people may be born with a small number of dopamine neurons. With natural aging, they will lose a sufficient number of neurons to become symptomatic. Others may simply have an accelerated rate of aging, so they lose neurons faster than normal. Another clearly documented phenomenon may be an early environmental exposure to a toxin or infectious agent that depletes the number of dopamine neurons. The normal loss of neurons with age will then inevitably lead to the production of symptoms.

The second factor that may play a role in producing the age-related loss of dopamine terminals is an increase with age in the enzyme monoamine oxidase (MAO).[69] This enzyme, which breaks down dopamine, is present in high concentration in the glia of the substantia nigra, and produces free radicals as byproducts of its reaction. Free-radical scavenging systems, glutathione, catalase, and so forth are very high in normal substantia nigra and markedly depleted in parkinsonian brains, suggesting that free-radical scavenging is an important part of the normal function of substantia nigra neurons. Its impairment may be part of the pathogenesis of Parkinson's disease.

VIRUSES

The world-wide pandemic of influenza after World War I was accompanied by occasional cases of von Economo's encephalitis. The encephalitis patients often developed a parkinsonian syndrome months to years later,[64] frequently accompanied by additional signs such as oculogyric crises. Pathologic studies of postencephalitic brains have found neurofibrillary tangles in the substantia nigra, rather than the Lewy bodies characteristic of idiopathic parkinsonism. Presumably, the virus infected substantia nigra neurons and produced symptoms of parkinsonism either immediately or as a late complication. The particular virus that caused parkinsonism recurred intermittently until the 1930s but now seems to have vanished. Occasionally, patients with other types of encephalitis will develop parkinsonism as a complication, however.

TOXINS

A number of specific toxins have been associated with the development of parkinsonism. Demographic studies suggest that living in certain environments may be associated with increases in parkinsonism. Areas implicated include farms in Saskatchewan, herbicide-using areas of Quebec, and iron-smelting regions of Sweden. Some specific parkinsonism-producing toxins are mentioned below:

Manganese. In experimental animals and in miners who are exposed to high levels of manganese, a parkinsonian syndrome has been described.[3] The pathology is characterized by loss of substantia nigra neurons. Presumably manganese is toxic to nigra neurons.

Carbon Monoxide. Carbon monoxide exposure produces a parkinsonian syndrome,[68] but the syndrome tends not to respond to L-dopa and is characterized by striatal and globus pallidus neuron loss. Thus, this syndrome may not be analogous to natural Parkinson's disease.

MPTP. MPTP has produced a parkinsonian syndrome in a number of persons, including a chemist involved in its manufacture and drug users who made or used the drug as a substitute for meperidine.[43] A single injection is now known to cause symptoms, but a number of repeated injections produces a severe parkinsonian syndrome with all the characteristics of typical Parkinson's disease.[7,42] If the drug is given to experimental animals, it will reproduce the symptoms of Parkinson's disease. Much is now known about the drug's mechanism of action. It is converted by MAO type B to an active metabolite, MPP+, which is taken up into dopamine terminals by the dopamine high-affinity transport system. MPP+ is toxic at that stage, but is stored in dopamine neurons because it binds to neuromelanin. This bound MPP+ may result in delayed toxicity.

Several persons who took MPTP are not symptomatic at present but have reduced numbers of dopamine terminals on PET scans.[11] These individuals provide a test of the aging theory of parkinsonism. If the theory is correct, they should develop parkinsonism with increasing age and loss of dopamine neurons.

Cycad Circinalis. A large number of the Chamorro people who were living on Guam in World War II have developed neurodegenerative diseases.[79] In the years immediately following World War II, many cases of amyotrophic lateral sclerosis (ALS) developed. This syndrome was later superseded by a parkinsonism/dementia complex. Current evidence suggests that these syndromes have been caused by ingestion or exposure to polstices of the cycad nut, which the Chamorros were forced to eat because of lack of other foodstuffs during the Japanese occupation. The nut contains a number of toxic substances including a compound, beta-methylaminoalanine, which appears to be neurotoxic in animals.[79] The neurotoxicity can be prevented by blockade of the N-methyl-D-aspartate (NMDA) type of glutamate receptors. Patients who developed an ALS syndrome appear to have taken very large, acute doses of the compound.[79] Those who developed the parkinsonism/dementia complex may have been exposed to lower doses and then developed parkinsonism and dementia as a delayed phenomenon. Further work attempting to delineate the pathophysiology of these presumably environmentally induced neurodegenerative disorders is in progress.

Rationale for Therapy

SYMPTOMATIC THERAPY

Precursors. The major symptoms of Parkinson's disease can be treated by replacing or substituting for the dopamine depletion in the brain (Table 2–2) In patients with the early stages of Parkinson's disease, virtually complete symptomatic relief can be achieved with intermittent use of the dopamine precursor levodopa. Intermittent ther-

apy with levodopa is associated with wide swings in the plasma levels and in the rate of delivery of levodopa to the brain.

The rate of delivery of levodopa to the brain is controlled by several factors. The rate of dissolution of the pill is determined by whether it is of the regular or "controlled-release" type (Fig. 2–4).[90] The rate of opening of the pyloric valve governs the rate of delivery to the intestine. Levodopa is absorbed from the gut by the same facilitated transfer system that is used to transport neutral and aromatic amino acids. Thus, the protein in a meal will interfere with the rate of delivery of levodopa to the blood (Fig. 2–5).[59] A similar facilitated-transport mechanism carries levodopa from the blood to the brain. Thus, amino acids present in the bloodstream after a protein meal also can interfere with the transport of levodopa across the blood-brain barrier (BBB) (Fig. 2–6).[59]

In patients with early Parkinson's disease, the therapeutic response to levodopa does not vary with the rate of levodopa delivery to the brain. Unfortunately, in patients with advanced disease, fluctuations in symptomatic control can be shown to correlate with the availability of levodopa to the brain.[59] Thus, patients who are "off" have insufficient drug available to overcome their symptoms, whereas those who are "on" have a sufficient or excessive amount of drug available to relieve symptoms. This change in response between early and late disease is probably due to continued loss of presynaptic dopamine terminals. Patients with early Parkinson's disease probably have sufficient dopamine terminals left to store levodopa. The levodopa can then be released as dopamine on neuronal demand. As the disease progresses, however, more dopamine terminals are lost, leaving insufficient terminals for patients to be able to maintain their dopamine stores from one dose interval to the next. Thus, the "wearing-off" phenomenon develops, in which the therapeutic response from a pill does not last until the next dose is due. At some point, insufficient presynaptic termi-

Table 2–2 DRUGS USED IN THE THERAPY OF PARKINSON'S DISEASE*

Drug	Mechanism of Action	Dose Range per Day	Notes
PREVENTIVE THERAPY			
Selegiline (Eldepryl, L-Deprenyl)	Monoamine oxidase type B inhibitor	5–10 mg	Possibly effective at slowing substantia nigra degeneration. Potentiates all levodopa effects including side effects.
SYMPTOMATIC THERAPY			
PRIMARY Levodopa	Dopamine precursor	450–1500 mg	Sold in fixed combinations as Sinemet and Madopar (not available in United States).
		PLUS	
Carbidopa or benserazide	Peripheral dopa decarboxylase inhibitor	150–600 mg	For patients who need a higher decarboxylase/ levodopa ratio, carbidopa has been available from the manufacturer to physicians but not to pharmacies.
ADJUNCTIVE			Adjunctive drugs are often useful as sole therapy early in the disease.
Bromocriptine pergolide lisuride	Dopamine receptor agonists	20–30 mg 3–5 mg 0.5–1.2 mg	Dose should be slowly titrated upward over months. Lisuride is water soluble but not available in the United States.
Various anticholinergics	Block muscarinic acetylcholine receptors	Vary	Benztropine (Cogentin; 1–4 mg/d) and trihexyphenidyl (Artane 2–8 mg/d) have high ratios of central-to-peripheral effects.
Tricyclics	Anticholinergics and dopamine reuptake inhibitors	25–75 mg	Selegiline (Eldepryl) may be contraindicated in patients treated with tricyclics.
Amantadine (Symmetrel)	Unknown Anticholinergic? Dopamine reuptake inhibitor? Increases dopamine release?	100–200 mg	The effects often wear off after 4–6 months, but if the drug is discontinued temporarily, its effects may be regained.
Selegiline (Eldepryl, (L-Deprenyl)	Monoamine oxidase type B inhibitor	5–10 mg	Potentiates levodopa's effects.
Apomorphine injectable	Dopamine receptor agonist	1–7 mg/dose	Must be given with domperidone.

*Descriptions of drug side effects are in the sections on the classes of drugs.

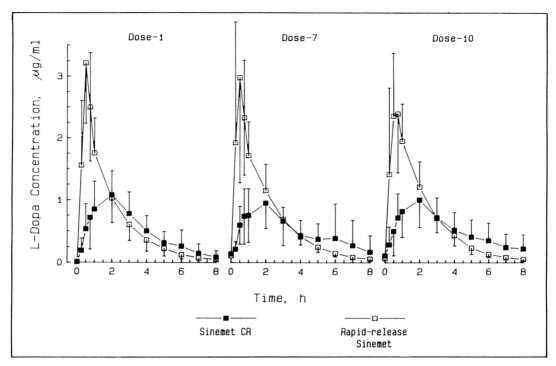

Figure 2–4. Plasma levels of levodopa in 12 healthy elderly subjects following repeated administration of 50/200 mg of "controlled-release" carbidopa/levodopa (Sinemet CR) or regular carbidopa/levodopa (Rapid-release Sinemet). Doses were given every 8 hours for 10 consecutive dosages. Doses 1, 7, and 10 are shown. Subjects had been pretreated with 50 mg of carbidopa every 8 hours for 2 days. Vertical bars represent mean ± 1 SD. The controlled-release formula does not achieve the rapid, high peak plasma level of the regular tablets. It does have a longer duration of high levels and would be expected to give a smoother therapeutic response. It must often be combined with a small first dose of the regular tablets in order for therapeutic levels to be reached quickly in the morning. (From Yeh et al,[90] p 31, with permission.)

nals are left to remove excess dopamine from synaptic clefts, so that overdose phenomena such as dyskinesias can develop.[58] As more terminals are lost, synaptic levels of dopamine become more and more dependent on the current delivery of levodopa to the brain. Thus, clinical fluctuations become more and more prominent. This situation may be further complicated by fluctuations in the sensitivity of the receptors to dopamine.[14] (For further discussion, see p 77.)

Therapy with levodopa produces more dopamine in the brain, which is metabolized by MAO. As already discussed, this reaction produces free radicals as a byproduct. It has been argued that free-radical production may accelerate the rate of disease progression.[80]

Clinical data conflict on this point. Some authors argue that levodopa therapy should be postponed as long as possible to delay accelerating the course of the disease.[18] Others argue that levodopa therapy clearly reduces morbidity and mortality and should be instituted as soon as possible.[47] It has not been possible to produce substantia nigra toxicity with levodopa in experimental animals.

Receptors. Two types of dopamine receptors, D-1 and D-2, mediate dopamine's postsynaptic effects. A third dopamine receptor (D-3), found predominantly in the brain's limbic regions, has been cloned recently (see Chapter 7). Clinical relief of parkinsonian symptoms is due primarily to stimulation of

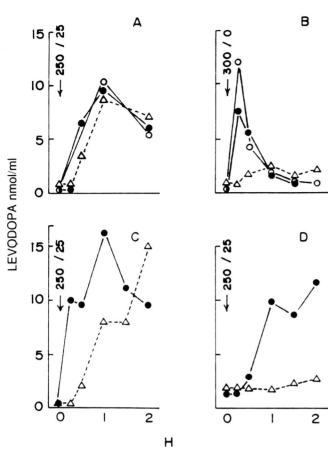

Figure 2–5. The effects of meals on the absorption of levodopa in four representative patients. The solid lines indicate plasma levodopa concentrations when the drug was given after an 8- to 12-hour fast. (Concentrations were tested twice for patients A and B.) The dashed lines indicate plasma levodopa concentrations when the drug was given after a meal. The dose of levodopa/carbidopa (mg) is shown above the arrows. A meal, particularly one containing protein, often causes a delay in (patient C) or completely blocks (patients B and D) the absorption of levodopa. (From Nutt et al,[59] p 485, with permission.)

the D-2 receptors. D-2 agonist drugs such as bromocriptine are useful by themselves as therapy for Parkinson's disease.[12] Bromocriptine is, in fact, a slight D-1 antagonist. Experimental evidence, however, suggests that some D-1 stimulation is necessary for a maximal response of the dopamine system.[88] Many patients do not get a full response from bromocriptine and must have a small dose of levodopa as well. Whether this extra response is due to D-1 stimulation is unclear, as trials of selective D-2 plus selective D-1 agonists have not shown any improvement over D-2 agonists alone.

While the use of D-2 agonists has been associated with dyskinesias in patients who have already developed dyskinesia and the "on/off" phenomenon, the development of dyskinesia and "on/off" has not been reported in patients treated solely with D-2 agonists. It is not clear whether D-1 stimulation is necessary for production of dyskinesias or whether patients who can obtain symptomatic relief from D-2 agonists alone simply have not lost enough presynaptic dopamine terminals to have dyskinesias.

Some patients lose the ability to respond to levodopa therapy. Levodopa can be converted to dopamine in presynaptic terminals other than those of dopamine, so it is not clear why such patients do not respond. Fortunately, they seem to be rare. Many more patients develop disabling side effects of levodopa therapy that prevent them from being given an adequate therapeutic dose.

In addition to stimulation of dopa-

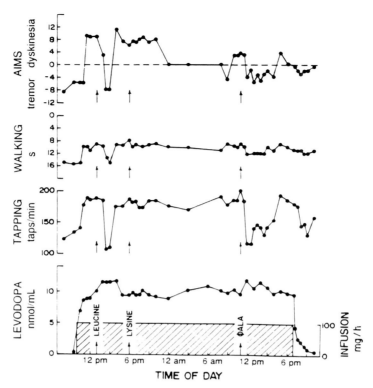

Figure 2–6. Effects of the ingestion of amino acids on the plasma levodopa concentration and various measures of clinical response during intravenous infusion of levodopa. Amino acids (100 mg/kg) were administered in solution at the times indicated by arrows. *Tapping* indicates the number of times the patient could alternately tap 2 keys 20 cm apart in 60 seconds. *Walking* indicates the time required to arise from an armless chair, walk 6 m, return to the chair, and sit down (cutoff time is 30 seconds). AIMS is the algebraic sum of dyskinesia, graded on a scale of 0 (absent) to 4 (severe), and tremor, graded from 0 (absent) to −4 (severe) in the trunk, head, and each limb (scores could range from −24 to 24). ØALA denotes phenylalanine. The ingestion of amino acids did not affect the plasma levodopa level, but ingestion of neutral amino acids did cause increased parkinsonism. This is believed to be owing to interference of neutral amino acids in the blood stream after a meal with the transport of levodopa across the blood-brain barrier. (From Nutt et al,[59] p 487, with permission.)

mine receptors, adjunctive therapy manipulating other neurotransmitter systems is useful. This is particularly true for anticholinergic drugs.

Also beneficial are drugs that increase the release of dopamine and block its reuptake, including tricyclic antidepressants and amantadine.

Theoretically, increases in the GABA system through benzodiazepine therapy might be helpful. Occasionally, mild success is demonstrated in some patients; however, such benefit is usually temporary and may simply be related to increasing sleep in parkinson-

ian patients who are known to have sleep disturbances.

PREVENTIVE THERAPY

The rationale of preventive therapy is to prevent or delay further loss of dopamine terminals in patients with symptoms and in patients who are presymptomatic for the disease. Experimental data suggest that any of several different approaches might work. One approach would be to block MAO. Another would be to increase the free-radical scavenging ability of the brain. A third might be to block NMDA receptors. At the time of this writing, trials of selegiline (Jumex, L-Deprenyl, Eldepryl), a selective MAO inhibitor, and alpha tocopherol, a free-radical scavenger, are underway. It might be logical to try other free-radical scavengers as well. The first results from these trials indicate that selegiline given to early patients can delay the time when symptomatic therapy is needed by about 1 year (Fig. 2–7).[61,83] How much of this delay is due to a symptomatic effect of the drug and how much is due to slowing of the loss of dopamine terminals is currently being studied. Data on the effects of alpha tocopherol are not yet available. If the loss of dopamine terminals really can be slowed, one would expect that

patients will be maintained in a state in which they have a good response to symptomatic therapy for a much longer period by concomitant use of "preventive" therapy.

HUNTINGTON'S DISEASE

Clinical Manifestations

Huntington's disease is a dominantly inherited, neurodegenerative disorder characterized by the onset in midlife of progressive cognitive decline and progressive involuntary movements and motor incoordination.[50] The disease was first described by Dr. George Huntington in 1872, when he observed a fa-

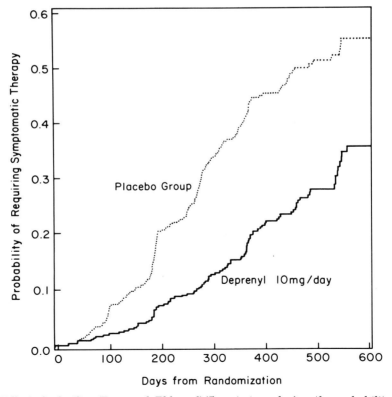

Figure 2–7. Effect of selegiline (Deprenyl, Eldepryl) (5 mg twice a day) on the probability that a patient with early Parkinson's disease who is on no symptomatic antiparkinsonian medication will reach the clinical endpoint of having disease severe enough to require symptomatic therapy with carbidopa/levodopa. Eight hundred patients were randomized to either placebo or selegiline. Selegiline delayed the average time until symptomatic therapy was required by an average of 11 months. This may represent a protective effect of selegiline on the substantia nigra degeneration in Parkinson's disease. (Modified from Parkinson Study Group.[61])

milial disorder among residents on Long Island. The prevalence of this disorder is approximately 10/100,000 population. Because of its late age of onset, about three times as many individuals are at 50% risk at any given time. The disease displays full penetrance; that is, all persons who inherit the gene will display clinical manifestations if they live long enough. The disorder affects men and women equally. The average age of disease onset is between 35 and 40 years, and there is a slight statistical tendency for those who inherited it from their mother to have about 3 years later age of onset than those who inherited it from their father.[54] Although the mean age of onset is between 35 and 40, cases starting as early as age two have been documented as well as cases whose symptoms commence after the age of 70. Approximately three fourths of those who show signs of disease before their twentieth birthday have inherited the disease from their father. Age of onset itself appears to be genetically determined; studies of monozygotic twins indicate strict concordance for age of onset, whereas the quality of the clinical manifestations can be more variable.

Huntington's disease begins insidiously, usually with personality changes and minor motor incoordination. Psychiatric symptoms and personality changes may precede the overt onset of the disorder by many years. At the time of earliest diagnosis, most persons display not only abnormal choreic movements but also slow voluntary saccades and impaired fine motor coordination.[94] As the disease progresses, memory becomes impaired, speech becomes abnormal, the amplitude and magnitude of the abnormal involuntary movement increases, the eye movement disorder worsens, and motor coordination is increasingly impaired.[15] Tone and posture are usually normal early in the disease, but increases in tone and dystonic posturing become more prominent as the disease progresses and eventually can become the predominant symptoms. The disease progresses during a

period of 15 to 20 years, and in the last years of the illness, the patient requires full-time care. Death usually occurs from secondary causes such as pneumonia.

The gene for Huntington's disease has been localized to the tip of chromosome 4,[30] but the exact genetic abnormality has not yet been determined. Because the location of the gene is known, it is possible to carry out linkage studies in families with Huntington's disease to determine who is or is not likely to be a gene carrier.[53] The current accuracy of the test is approximately 95%.

Neurotransmitter and Receptor Changes

Pathologically, Huntington's disease results in neuron loss predominantly in the caudate nucleus and putamen. Detailed analysis of several hundred cases indicates that the disease begins in the dorsal medial caudate nucleus and dorsolateral putamen and progresses ventrally.[85] Although thought initially to affect all caudate and putamen neurons equally, it is now known that there is selective vulnerability of certain striatal neuronal types. There is little pathology elsewhere in the brain, although systematic studies have shown cell loss in the globus pallidus, thalamus, and brainstem in advanced cases. There is less evidence for cortical cell loss, although neurochemical changes have been observed in cortical samples.

GABA

Early neurochemical studies of Huntington's disease reported significant losses of the amino-acid neurotransmitter GABA in the striatum.[63] Subsequent studies from numerous groups have confirmed that GABAergic neurons are severely depleted in the striatum of brains of Huntington's patients, and that GABA levels are also decreased in striatal projection regions, the globus pallidus, and the substantia nigra. Studies have indeed indicated that losses of GABA and glutamic acid decarboxylase, the enzyme that synthesizes GABA, are larger in the lateral globus pallidus than in the medial globus pallidus.

GABA receptors are also abnormal in Huntington's postmortem tissue. As measured with tritiated GABA, tritiated muscimol, and tritiated benzodiazepines, receptors all show moderate reductions in caudate nucleus and putamen (Fig. 2–8). In striatal projection areas, the density of GABA and benzodiazepine receptors is increased in the substantia nigra pars reticulata and lateral segment of the globus pallidus.[86] Receptor changes have not been documented in the medial globus pallidus. The upregulation of the receptors in striatal projection areas presumably is secondary to receptor supersensitivity after denervation.

ACETYLCHOLINE

Acetylcholine is the neurotransmitter of large aspiny interneurons in the striatum. In initial postmortem studies, choline acetyltransferase (ChAT) activity was found to be decreased in Huntington's striatum, suggesting loss of cholinergic neurons.[81] Subsequent studies have confirmed a minor loss of these neurons in Huntington's disease. Relative to the loss of GABAergic neurons, however, cholinergic interneurons are spared. Thus, the density of ChAT and acetylcholinesterase-positive neurons is relatively increased in Huntington's postmortem striatum compared to control striatum.[21]

SUBSTANCE P

Substance P is contained in many of the medium spiny neurons of the striatum, which project predominantly to the medial globus pallidus and substantia nigra. In many instances, substance P is co-localized with GABA. Measurements of substance P levels show a profound decrease in striatal substance P in postmortem tissues as well as a decrease in the substantia

nigra pars reticulata.[50,81] Immunohistochemical studies of substance P-like immunoreactivity indicate a significant loss of all substance P neurons in end-stage cases.[66] Analysis of early Huntington's cases, however, suggests a selective sparing of those substance P neurons that project to the medial globus pallidus as compared to those projecting to the substantia nigra pars reticulata, which are affected early in the disease.

OPIOID PEPTIDES

Just as substance P is co-localized with GABA in many medium spiny neurons in the striatum, so enkephalin is also co-localized with GABA in another subset of striatal neurons. Immunohistochemical studies of enkephalin-like immunoreactivity in early Huntington's striatum indicate a loss of enkephalin neurons projecting to the lateral globus pallidus.[66] A virtual loss of these cells occurs by midstage disease.

CATECHOLAMINES

There are virtually no intrinsic biogenic amine neurons in the striatum. Instead, dopamine and serotonin neurons project to the striatum from the substantia nigra pars compacta and the raphe nucleus. There is very little norepinephrine in normal human striatum. Biogenic amine markers are relatively spared in Huntington's striatum, presumably reflecting the lack of pathology in these afferent neuronal systems.[50,81] When measured in a per-gram basis, biogenic amine markers appear to be slightly increased compared with those in normal striatum, presumably due to a concentrative phenomenon.

SOMATOSTATIN

Measurements of somatostatin and neuropeptide Y levels indicate large increases in Huntington's striatum. Somatostatin levels are increased approximately fourfold to fivefold above those found in normal tissues.[2,57] Immuno-histochemical studies have demonstrated that somatostatin-positive interneurons are relatively spared in Huntington's striatum.[22] Therefore, these neurons appear resistant to the disease process.

OTHER NEUROTRANSMITTER AND RECEPTOR CHANGES

Angiotensin-converting enzyme activities are decreased in Huntington's striatum.[81] As discussed below, neurotoxic phenomena may be responsible for the selective cell death seen in Huntington's disease. Measurements of glutamate and quinolinic acid levels have shown little change in Huntington's striatum. Quinolinic acid is an endogenous neurotoxin that is synthesized as a byproduct of serotonin metabolism. The enzyme responsible for quinolinic acid synthesis is contained in glial cells and is increased approximately fivefold above normal in Huntington's striatum.[75] The enzyme responsible for quinolinate degradation is increased only 20% to 50% in Huntington's disease,[24] thus, there is a propensity for increased quinolinic acid synthesis.

Studies of excitatory amino-acid (EAA) receptors in Huntington's disease have indicated a major loss of NMDA receptors in Huntington's striatum.[93] These receptors are virtually absent in advanced Huntington's disease; major losses have even been found in several early cases examined. The loss of NMDA receptors is considerably greater than the loss of other neurotransmitter receptors in Huntington's striatum, suggesting that those neurons that possess NMDA receptors are preferentially lost in the disease.

Selective Vulnerability

Taken together, the neurochemical studies suggest that certain striatal cell types are selectively lost in Huntington's disease. Medium spiny neurons

that co-contain GABA and enkephalin and project to the lateral globus pallidus are affected very early in the disease, as are GABA- and substance-P-containing neurons that project to the substantia nigra pars reticulata. Loss of the GABA/enkephalin neurons projecting to the lateral pallidum would cause disinhibition of the lateral pallidum, which would in turn more actively inhibit the subthalamic nucleus. Inhibition of the subthalamic nucleus is likely to be responsible for the abnormal involuntary movements seen in Huntington's disease. Loss of GABA/substance P neurons projecting to the substantia nigra pars reticulata is likely to be responsible for the abnormal eye movements, as this pathway normally inhibits reticulata neurons projecting to the superior colliculus. One might speculate that these two striatal neuronal subsets contain a higher density of NMDA receptors than other striatal neurons, but this hypothesis will need to be investigated further.

Other striatal neurons appear to be affected later in the disease, either as part of the primary disease process or as a secondary transneuronal degeneration. Acetylcholine and somatostatin neurons are spared and appear less vulnerable to the primary process.

Rationale for Therapy

SYMPTOMATIC THERAPY

At the current time, there is no effective therapy for Huntington's disease. Many types of medications have been tried and have little or no effect on the overall functioning of the patients. Dopamine antagonists and neuroleptics have been used extensively to control the psychiatric symptoms and the involuntary movements. It was thought that involuntary movements reflect an imbalance of dopamine and GABAergic function in Huntington's striatum and that excessive dopaminergic activity could be blocked by neuroleptics. Significant cognitive side effects can occur from these medications, however, and there is little evidence that the overall functional capacity of the patient is improved with their use. Alternative methods of depleting striatal dopamine have included the use of tetrabenazine and reserpine, medications which have proved helpful in reducing the abnormal involuntary movements early in the disease. Cognitive side effects are rare, but these agents can induce depression. Because depression is common in patients with Huntington's disease, this side effect frequently limits the use of these agents. Late in the disease, the cells that contain dopamine receptors are lost, and dopamine antagonists have little or no therapeutic efficacy.

For the treatment of psychosis, depression, and irritability, neuroleptic, antidepressant, and antianxiety agents can be helpful,[77] but it is important to limit the use of these agents to that period when the patient is experiencing symptoms. Because of the disease progression, medications that are useful at one stage may be ineffective or detrimental at another stage.

Because of the profound decrease in GABA levels in Huntington's striatum, and the GABA-receptor supersensitivity seen in striatal projection areas, GABA agonists have been tried therapeutically in Huntington's disease. Treatment with benzodiazepines can be helpful for patients who find that stress and anxiety worsen the movement disorder and cognitive functioning. Low doses should be used, because they will have more selective effects on the denervated pallidum and substantia nigra. Larger doses simply result in sedation. Overall, most patients do very well on no medication, and no studies have indicated that medical therapy improves overall functional capacity in any patient group.

For those presenting with early-onset, rigid Huntington's disease, dopamine agonists may be tried. These appear to be of only limited benefit, however. Furthermore, L-dopa can induce or worsen myoclonus in these patients. The use of baclofen and GABAergic agents may be more helpful in reducing the increased tone in these patients.

PREVENTIVE THERAPY

Although we do not know the genetic defect in Huntington's disease, preventive therapies may ultimately prove to be the most useful. Just as in Wilson's disease, where the exact genetic defect is also unknown (see p 74), preventive treatment of the secondary effects of the disorder may result in a "cure." In this regard, the neurotoxic hypothesis of Huntington's disease is intriguing. The disease itself may cause the cell death by affecting cellular and metabolic function. At the same time, however, such a genetic defect may make certain types of neurons more vulnerable to neurotoxic damage. If this was the case, the preventive therapy with EAA antagonists might prevent the onset and progression of the disorder. Baclofen, which is thought to decrease EAA release, was administered prospectively in a group of Huntington's patients.[78] Unfortunately this trial was unsuccessful, but additional studies using EAA antagonists are being planned.

DYSTONIA

Clinical Manifestations

Dystonia has both primary and secondary causes. The clinical manifestations of these various disorders have been described in detail elsewhere.[19] The secondary dystonias in general are due to inherited metabolic disorders such as the amino acidoses and lipidoses, toxic disorders such as carbon monoxide poisoning or traumatic disorders such as stroke or subdural hematoma[10] (Table 2–3). The age of onset of the secondary dystonias and their progression are quite variable depending on the actual etiology.

The primary dystonias are inherited disorders and have a more characteristic presentation. They can be inherited as either autosomal dominant or auto-

Table 2-3 PRIMARY AND SECONDARY DYSTONIAS

I. Primary Dystonia
  A. Hereditary: Autosomal dominant, autosomal recessive, or X-linked recessive
  B. Idiopathic: Adult or childhood onset
                  Focal or generalized
II. Secondary Dystonia
  A. Hereditary neurodegenerative diseases
    1. Wilson's disease
    2. Huntington's disease
    3. Hallervorden-Spatz disease
    4. Fahr's disease
    5. Joseph's disease
    6. Familial acanthocytosis
    7. Progressive supranuclear palsy
    8. Striatonigral degeneration
  B. Enzyme deficiencies and storage diseases
    1. Ceroid lipofuscinosis
    2. GM1 gangliosidosis
    3. Leigh's disease
    4. Hexosaminidase A and B deficiency
    5. Lesch-Nyhan syndrome
    6. Metachromatic leukodystrophy
    7. Glutaric acidemia
  C. Environmental causes
    1. Trauma
    2. Infections
    3. Postinfections
    4. Perinatal hypoxia/ischemia
    5. Brain tumors
    6. Toxins and drugs: Carbon monoxide, manganese, dopamine
                         D-2 antagonists, levodopa, phenytoin

somal recessive disorders and can be divided into those that start in adulthood and those that start at age 20 or younger. Dystonia that begins in patients younger than 20 usually involves first the legs and later the trunk, neck, and upper extremities. The disorder can start in early childhood but most commonly begins about the age of 8 to 10. It progresses over several years and then usually plateaus in the early 20s. Childhood-onset dystonia usually becomes generalized and causes significant physical impairment. It is not accompanied by cognitive or intellectual decline.

Dystonia that begins in adulthood rarely generalizes and usually is segmental (involving the trunk, neck [spasmodic torticollis], or one or both upper extremities) or cranial (involving the eyes or mouth). The segmental and axial dystonias begin between the ages of 20 and 50, and the cranial dystonias most commonly occur in the 50s and 60s.

Neurochemical Pathology

Pathologic examination of patients with the primary dystonias has been normal. Neurochemical studies on a few cases have suggested an imbalance of catecholamine pathways, but only a limited number of transmitter systems have been examined in selected structures.[37] Current treatment strategies have relied completely on empiric observations.

In the secondary dystonias, the most frequent pathology has been observed in the putamen and globus pallidus. In rare cases, brainstem pathology has been demonstrated.[19]

Approach to Therapy

Many different drugs have been tried in dystonia. The most popular therapies include baclofen, anticholinergic medication, and long-acting benzodiazepines. One form of inherited dystonia, the Segawa variant, manifests diurnal variations. In these patients, L-dopa therapy appears to be particularly helpful.[19,76] For treatment of other types of dystonia, trials of different medications must be carried out, and each patient may experience only limited benefit. In early-onset dystonias, some patients appear to improve significantly with long-term, high-dose anticholinergic treatments.[20] In these patients, medication trials of at least 6 months are indicated, as some of the beneficial effects are not seen immediately after optimization of therapy.

Surgery, particularly stereotaxic thalamotomy, has been urged as a treatment for dystonia.[16] Prominent neurologists, however, feel that the 20% risk of severe dysarthria that accompanies the bilateral thalamotomies needed for generalized dystonia and spasmodic torticollis makes thalamotomy too dangerous a treatment for all but the most desperate cases.[48]

For the focal dystonias, a promising new therapy is the use of local injections of botulinum toxin every 2 to 4 months.[6,38] Injections at the motor endplates of the affected muscles cause limited but sufficient weakness in the muscles to afford relief from the dystonic contractions. Injections last weeks to months and so far have shown few side effects.

TREMORS

Clinical Manifestations

Tremors involve rhythmic flexion and extension of a limb or the head and can be divided into resting, action, and postural subtypes.[33] Resting tremors usually indicate Parkinson's disease. Action and postural tremors can occur individually or as part of another neurologic disorder. The more frequent type of action tremor is the so-called essential or familial tremor. Usually the tremor is of low amplitude and high frequency (10 to 12 cycles/sec). Such tremors can involve the extremities as well as the head, tongue, lips, and voice. When severe, they can be quite disabling. Persons with this form of tremor frequently have a first-degree relative with a similar disorder. The magnitude and distribution of the tremor can vary substantially within a family. Patients find that their tremor frequently improves after a drink of an alcoholic beverage and commonly is made worse by caffeine, stress, or hyperthyroidism. In fact, tremor will frequently develop in normal individuals taking large quantities of caffeine or medications that increase epinephrine. Certain drugs also have been associated with the development of tremor (Table 2-4).

A second form of action tremor is observed in individuals with cerebellar disorders. These tremors involve instability of the limb at a proximal muscle joint, and will dampen when the distal extremity is stabilized. Usually the differentiation between cerebellar tremors and essential tremors is not difficult. Cerebellar tremors worsen when the individual attempts to approach a target with an extremity, whereas essential tremors have basically the same amplitude and magnitude throughout the course of a given movement. Persons with cerebellar disorders have marked impairment of fine-motor coordination in addition to the tremor, whereas those patients with essential tremor usually have relatively intact fine-motor coordination.

Table 2-4 DRUGS THAT EXACERBATE TREMOR

I. Adrenergic agonists
   A. Drugs that release catecholamines (amphetamines, cocaine)
   B. Beta-adrenergic agonists (metaproterenol)
   C. Phosphodiesterase inhibitors (theophylline, caffeine, methylxanthines)
   D. Uptake inhibitors (tricyclic antidepressants)
II. Miscellaneous
   A. Lithium
   B. Sodium valproate
   C. Harmaline

Neurochemical Pathology

The neurochemical pathology of cerebellar and essential tremors is unknown. Lesions of cerebellar afferents or efferents can result in a tremor, but the specific chemical abnormalities responsible remain hidden. Furthermore, examination of the brains of patients dying with familial tremor appears normal and no specific biochemical defect has been elucidated.

Rationale for Therapy

Therapies for essential tremor have involved the use of several types of agents.[23] Probably the most useful have been beta blockers. These drugs result in a reduction in the amplitude of the tremor and in significant clinical improvement. The second group of medications found effective in the treatment of essential tremor are the benzodiazepines, which in low dosages can be helpful either alone or in combination with beta blockers. Because patients can develop tolerance to these medications, they should be used on an as-needed basis before social events or during periods of excess stress. As with benzodiazepines, alcohol can be useful in treatment of tremor, although the risk of developing alcoholism is of concern. Nevertheless, one standard alcoholic beverage prior to a meal may allow patients to eat and drink with less impairment. Finally, a recent observation has been that Mysoline in low dosages (25 to 75 mg/d) can be helpful in the treatment of essential tremor.[41] Usually this therapy is most effective when combined with beta blockers.

For people with cerebellar tremor, a variety of GABAergic agents have been tried, but these have been of limited or no utility. Several reports on the use of isoniazid in the treatment of cerebellar tremor have been published,[32] but this agent appears to be of limited clinical utility. There have been case reports of successful treatment of cerebellar tremor with clonazepam[71] and primidone.[34] One of the best therapeutic approaches for cerebellar tremor, however, has been stereotaxic surgery, rather than medication.[56]

TICS

Clinical Manifestations

Three types of tic disorder have been defined.[45] The first is the transient tic of childhood, which occurs in up to 25% of individuals younger than the age of 15. These tics involve repetitive, stereotyped contraction of several muscle groups. The movements can either be rapid or slightly sustained (dystonic). They most frequently involve the face, neck, and arm, but they can also involve the trunk and the leg. Some patients will have vocalizations or abnormal sniffing or grunting. By definition, however, the transient tic of childhood lasts less than 1 year and does not recur. The second type of tic disorder is a chronic motor tic, a single motor tic that occurs repetitively. Usually the onset occurs within the first three decades of life. These tics then remain stable through the lifetime of the person. The third type of tic disorder is Tourette's syndrome, which is defined as having (a) onset younger than the age of 15, and (b) both vocal and motor tics that wax and wane over the months but are present for the lifetime of the patient. When the tics are severe, they can become physically and socially disabling. Usually, however, they are primarily a social nuisance. Knowledge about Tourette's syndrome is rapidly increasing, and it appears to be a much more frequent disorder than had previously been believed. Probably at least 1/1000 population has this disorder. The syndrome appears to be dominantly inherited in a large number of cases; other family members may have either simple tics or obsessive-compulsive disorder as another manifestation of the illness.

Neurochemical Pathology

The brains of only a handful of persons with Tourette's syndrome have been examined, and no clear neuropathologic or neuochemical abnormality has been identified. In one case, an absence of basal ganglia dynorphinlike immunoreactivity was noted.[31]

Rationale for Therapy

Although the chemical pathology of this disease is unknown, an early observation was that tic disorders are very responsive to low doses of neuroleptics.[45] Almost all dopamine antagonists can be effective in the treatment of the disorder, although the most popular agents are haloperidol and fluphenazine. A recently released agent, pimozide, appears to have fewer cognitive side effects than haloperidol and has been found to be effective in the treatment of Tourette's syndrome.[65] The general strategy for treatment is to start with as low a dose as possible for 2 to 3 weeks and then gradually increase the dose until symptom relief is achieved or side effects occur. Because some tics are well tolerated, the goal of the therapy is not to eliminate tics completely but to make the disorder tolerable to the patient and his or her friends, school, and family. Therapy is symptomatic and does not affect the overall course of the illness. Many patients do quite well on no medication at all. For those patients who do require medication, the development of tardive dyskinesias is always of concern. The patient should be followed closely for any indication of this long-term side effect.

A second therapy for Tourette's syndrome is the use of the alpha-adrenergic agonist clonidine. Although there is some controversy as to whether this agent is effective,[15,28] it has no known long-term side effects and in a subgroup of patients may relieve both the tics and the obsessive-compulsive behavior seen in the syndrome. Again, the therapy should be started in low dosage and gradually increased until side effects appear or symptom relief is obtained. Care must be taken that the patient does not abruptly terminate the therapy, because headache and hypertension can become disabling after abrupt discontinuation of the medication.

Medicines are available for the obsessive-compulsive disorder that often accompanies Tourette's syndrome. Fluoxetine (and clomipramine, available in Europe) has been found to be quite helpful for the behavioral problems associated with Tourette's syndrome.[40]

HEMIBALLISMUS

Clinical Manifestations

Hemiballismus usually results from a structural abnormality in the subthalamic nucleus such as ischemic damage, tumor, or infection, and is rarely bilateral.[9] The disorder is manifested by large-amplitude, choreic, and ballistic movements of the limbs on one side of the body and will frequently involve dyskinesias of the face. The movements can be of such large amplitude that they are physically exhausting to the patient. Fortunately, if the acute period can be survived, the movements suppress over time and eventually are manifested only by unilateral chorea.

Pathology

Any disorder involving the subthalamic nucleus can cause hemiballism. Most commonly, the cause is ischemic disease, but tumor, infection, and demyelinating disease can also cause the disorder.

Rationale for Therapy

Although the abnormal subthalamic nucleus is downstream from the dopamine system, dopamine blockers have some beneficial effects in treatment of the ballistic movements. In addition, benzodiazepines, valproate, and barbiturates can sometimes reduce the magnitude of the movements.[9] Otherwise no specific therapy exists.

SPASTICITY

Clinical Manifestations

Spasticity is an abnormality of resistance to passive manipulation of the limbs. A velocity-dependent increase in tone is followed by a relaxation phase; the change in tone is often termed the *clasp-knife phenomenon.* Spasticity arises from chronic interruption of the corticospinal tract at any level between the cerebral cortex and the anterior horn cell. When the corticospinal tract is damaged above the cervical spinal cord, a spastic hemiparesis develops, characterized by increased flexor tone in the upper extremities and increased extensor tone in the lower extremity. Concomitant with the tone changes are other symptoms and signs such as increased deep-tendon reflexes (hyperreflexia), an extensor plantar response, and clonus. In patients with brainstem or spinal cord lesions, abnormal flexor or extensor spasms can occur spontaneously or in response to cutaneous stimulation. Lesions below the vestibular nuclei and reticular formation result in increased flexor tone in both legs and arms.

Rationale for Therapy

Because glutamic acid is the presumptive neurotransmitter of the corticospinal tract, glutamate agonists and antagonists might be expected to change tone in spastic animals. Unfortunately, no glutamate agonists that cross the BBB to any appreciable extent are available for clinical use. In addition, glutamate agonists might be neurotoxic and convulsant. Interestingly, the NMDA antagonists and NMDA channel blockers appear to reduce

muscle tone and cause ataxia in animals, but no trials of such agents have been tried in humans with spasticity.

Other descending pathways important in the control of reflex activity and tone are the descending catecholamine and serotonin pathways.[92] Animal studies indicate that catecholamines are important in regulating flexor-reflex afferent pathways and overall reflex mechanisms at the spinal cord level. In patients with lesions above the brainstem serotonin and catecholamine nuclei (raphe nuclei, locus ceruleus, and substantia nigra), the clasp-knife phenomenon and clonus are common but extensor and/or flexor spasms are rare. In these cases, the descending biogenic amine pathways may be relatively overactive, and one strategy for treating this type of spasticity has been the use of alpha-adrenergic and dopaminergic antagonists. Serotonin antagonists have not been examined.

In patients in whom the descending biogenic amine pathways are interrupted, spinal cord serotonin and catecholamine receptors are increased. Dopamine and adrenergic agonists may relieve the flexor or extensor spasms that develop in these individuals.

A number of antispasticity agents are directed toward altering reflex activity and tone at the segmental (or spinal-cord) level.[17] Baclofen was initially designed as a prodrug for GABA but has since been found to act directly at a unique group of bicuculline-insensitive GABA receptors called GABA$_B$ receptors. This drug not only produces inhibition at the postsynaptic level but also inhibits catecholamine, serotonin, and glutamate release. Baclofen has been shown to be effective in the treatment of spasticity, and is particularly helpful in reducing the frequency and severity of clonus.

GABAergic interneurons in the dorsal and intermediate gray of the spinal cord that mediate the presynaptic inhibition of primary afferent input are underactive in spasticity. GABA released from these interneurons acts primarily at bicuculline-sensitive GABA_A receptors. Benzodiazepines, which modulate GABA_A-receptor function, have been used in the treatment of spasticity. Unfortunately, GABA_A receptors are present throughout the nervous system, and benzodiazepine doses that improve clonus and reduce tone also cause ataxia and sedation.

The other major inhibitory interneuron in the spinal cord, the glycine interneuron, mediates postsynaptic inhibition, particularly the reciprocal inhibition associated with type I_A afferents. Glycinergic function is underactive in animal models of spasticity. Unfortunately, no effective glycine agonists or prodrugs are currently available for the treatment of spasticity.

In summary, either baclofen or benzodiazepines combined with biogenic amine agonists or antagonists (depending on the level of the lesion) may be the best approach for the treatment of spasticity. Therapy should be targeted at the particular disabling symptom, because for some persons a particular symptom (such as increased leg extensor tone) may actually be beneficial.

WILSON'S DISEASE

Clinical Manifestations

Wilson's disease is characterized by abnormal copper accumulation in many organs, including the brain, liver, kidney, and cornea.[72] It was described by S.A. Kinnier Wilson in 1912, and his descriptions of the disease have remained the most complete in the literature:

> It is characterized by a definite symptom-complex, whose chief features are: generalized tremor, dysarthria and dysphagia, muscular rigidity and hypertonicity, emaciation, spasmodic contractions, contractures, [and] emotionalism. There are also certain mental symptoms, either transient and such as one sees in a toxic psychosis, but not severe, or more chronic, consisting in a general restric-

tion of the mental horizon, and a certain facility or docility without delusions or hallucinations, and not necessarily as progressive as the somatic symptoms. The mental symptoms may be very slight and are sometimes absent.[89]

Wilson noted most of the clinical features of the disease, but did not believe that the liver was involved primarily and did not note abnormal pigment around the cornea (now known to be the deposition of copper in the cornea, called *Kayser-Fleischer (KF) rings*). Wilson's disease is inherited as an autosomal recessive gene localized to chromosome 13.[4] Most commonly, patients present in the second or third decade with predominant neurologic, hepatic, or psychiatric symptoms (about one third in each group). A few patients, however, present in the first decade or as late as the sixth.

Patients presenting with neurologic symptoms most commonly complain of dysarthria, dysphagia, poor fine-motor coordination, tremor, and rigidity. Occasionally, patients present with chorea, dystonia, or cerebellar ataxia. If the disease is not diagnosed readily, the patient usually deteriorates rapidly with progressive liver disease and progressive dysarthria or anarthria, dystonia, wing-beating tremor, and death. Behavioral and personality changes, depression, and emotional lability are common. Frequently, a history in the patient or a sibling of unexplained hepatitis, hemolytic anemia, or renal dysfunction exists. The diagnosis should be considered in all patients with movement disorders and dysarthria with or without psychiatric complaints, as the disease is readily treatable.

Clinical Diagnosis

In more than 90% of patients with Wilson's disease and a neurologic presentation, KF rings are detected either at the bedside (70%) or by slit lamp examination (97%).[5,72] Sunflower cataracts are also detectable in some cases.

If KF rings are present, the diagnosis will be correct in more than 99% of cases. Otherwise, laboratory tests are necessary for confirmation.

The gold standard for diagnosis (in the absence of cholestatic liver disease, which can lead to copper accumulation) is measurement of hepatic copper.[5] Values in untreated patients of greater than 250 μg/g dry weight of liver are diagnostic (normal is less than 50 μg/g dry weight).

The second most accurate test is measurement of copper incorporation into ceruloplasmin.[5,72] After ingestion of copper 64 (^{64}Cu), serum samples are measured sequentially for 48 hours. Initially the concentration of ^{64}Cu peaks at 1 to 2 hours and then falls. In normal patients, the serum concentration of ^{64}Cu then rises linearly for the next 48 hours (as the copper is incorporated into ceruloplasmin). In Wilson's disease, the secondary rise is absent even if the serum ceruloplasmin is normal. Heterozygotes show an intermediate rise in the secondary phase. Using this test, there is no overlap between patients with Wilson's disease and normal patients, although some heterozygotes have a blunted response.

Measurement of 24-hour urine copper is a simple test that usually distinguishes normal patients from those with Wilson's disease. Normal excretion in the absence of therapy is 20 to 45 μg/24 h; and in Wilson's disease, excretion is almost always greater than 80 μg/24 h. A urine copper excretion of greater than 125 μg/24 h is virtually diagnostic. If it is between 45 to 125 μg/24 h, it is possible that the patient is either a heterozygote or a homozygote. Taking the measurement during a 48-hour period may improve the accuracy of the test.

Measurement of serum ceruloplasmin concentration is the most common test employed diagnostically for Wilson's disease. In 10% of cases, however, the ceruloplasmin level is normal (>20 mg/dL). Furthermore, even in those with Wilson's disease whose ceruloplasmin levels are low (<20 mg/dL) at one point in the illness, the level can rise due to liver disease, pregnancy, or estrogen administration. Serum ceruloplasmin levels can be low in other diseases such as protein loss, copper deficiency, Menkes' syndrome, and fulminant hepatitis, and in individuals who are heterozygous for Wilson's disease.

Measurements of serum copper concentrations are most helpful for monitoring patients after the diagnosis. Normally the serum copper level in Wilson's disease is low because the ceruloplasmin level is low. In normal patients, serum copper is approximately 100 μg/dL and 90% of it is bound to ceruloplasmin. Free copper levels in normal patients are about 10 to 15 μg/dL. In Wilson's disease, free serum copper levels are greater than 25 μg/dL. To estimate free serum copper, a rule of thumb is to multiply the ceruloplasmin level times three and subtract it from the serum copper level.

From the practical standpoint, if a patient presents with a suspicious neurologic or psychiatric disorder, a slit lamp examination should be performed; if positive, the diagnosis is almost certain. A serum copper and ceruloplasmin and a 24-hour urine test should be performed to substantiate the diagnosis and to provide a baseline for monitoring therapy. If the serum or urine tests are ambiguous, liver biopsy and/or ^{64}Cu uptake tests should be performed.

Rationale for Therapy

Once a diagnosis has been established, the patient should be started on a decoppering agent (Table 2–5).[5,72] In addition, the patient should be cautioned to avoid foods with high copper content (e.g., liver, chocolate, nuts, mushrooms, and shellfish). If the source of water is a well, the copper content of the water should be checked. Patients should be monitored frequently for the first 2 months or so of therapy to assess side effects of the medication and worsening of the symp-

Table 2-5 TREATMENT OF WILSON'S DISEASE

| | Dosage | | Adjunctive Therapy | Monitor | Comments |
	Initial	Maintenance			
D-penicil- lamine	250 mg 2–3 times a day (adults) 30 min before or 2 h after meals (see text)	1 g/d in 2–4 divided doses (adults)	25 mg pyridoxine daily	24-h urine copper, free serum copper, blood and platelet count, serum chemistries, urinalysis for first 6 wk, then every 3–12 mo	Greatest experi- ence, many long-term and short- term side effects
Triethylene- tetramine hydro- chloride (Trien)	1 g/day in divided doses (adults)	1 g/d in divided doses (adults)	25 mg pyridoxine daily	Same as for penicillamine	Less experi- ence, generally effective
Zinc acetate	50 mg tid for presymp- tomatic patients	50 mg tid	—	24-h urine copper and zinc, free serum copper every 3–12 mo. Oral ^{64}Cu uptake after 6 wk of therapy or prn	Less experi- ence, not drug of choice for initial therapy

toms. Although many recommend an initial dose of 250 mg D-penicillamine four times per day 30 to 60 minutes before meals, about 10% to 30% of neurologically ill patients worsen in the first few months of therapy.[5] One possible reason for this occurrence is an initial rise in free serum copper levels due to mobilization of liver and other peripheral stores, which then damage the brain. Starting with 250 mg D-penicillamine two or three times per day with monitoring of free serum copper (to minimize any acute rise) and urine copper to effect an excretion of 2 mg/24 h may be a better strategy. The dose can then be increased to 1 g/d once the free serum copper levels and urinary excretion of copper begin to fall. Chronic monitoring should include measurements of serum copper, serum ceruloplasmin, and urine copper levels to assess compliance. Yearly slit lamp exams indicate the completeness of the decoppering.

Penicillamine has a high frequency of toxic side effects. Blood counts, differential, and platelet counts should be monitored two to three times a week and urinalysis performed once a week during the first month. The patient's temperature should be taken nightly. Penicillamine has been associated with the development of lupuslike syndromes, dermatitis, stomatitis, lymphadenopathy, thrombocytopenia, agranulocytosis, and a host of additional problems that should be monitored.

Other decoppering agents include British antilewisite, triethylene-tetramine dihydrochloride (Trien, Trientine), and zinc. Trien is usually given in doses of 1 to 1.5 g/d, and therapy should be monitored as with the use of penicillamine. Renal, bone marrow, and dermatologic toxicity are most common.

Zinc acetate (150 mg/d) has been shown to maintain the decoppered state in patients intolerant to penicillamine and/or Trien.[5] It is well tolerated systemically with very few side effects. It can be used effectively for maintenance therapy but is not recommended for initial therapy. Zinc sulfate also has been used, but the sulfate is a gastric irritant and many patients cannot tolerate the side effects. Zinc is effective in decoppering because it induces the production of metallothionein in the gut. The metallothionein chelates dietary and biliary copper and excretes it in the feces, thereby reducing absorption and reabsorption.

Many patients continue to have neurologic problems such as dysarthria, dystonia, parkinsonism, chorea, tremor, or combinations thereof. Symptomatic therapy for these movement disorders is similar to that used for the primary disorders already discussed.

DRUG MANIPULATION OF TRANSMITTER SYSTEMS

Dopamine System

AGONISTS

Dopamine agonist therapy in the movement disorders is important for the relief of parkinsonism. Lesser roles in the treatment of dystonia and spasticity have been reported. Two major problems are associated with dopamine agonist therapy: Acute side effects of medication, and abnormal movement associated with long-term use of medications. Some of the acute side effects due to stimulation of dopamine receptors outside the BBB include nausea and orthostatic hypotension. These are common problems when levodopa is used by itself. The other type of acute side effect is due to central nervous system (CNS) stimulation, where dopaminergic agents can produce confusion and hallucinations. The hallucinations are usually well-formed and can be visual, auditory, and tactile. Once established, they may persist even with extremely low doses of the medication. Occasionally, delusions develop when using dopamine agonists. These tend to respond to reduction in medication.

The movement disorders (dyskinesias) associated with long-term dopamine therapy are of two types: "peak-dose," choreoathetoid movements associated with high levels of dopamine agonists in the brain, and "biphasic," ballistic movements associated with rapid swings in brain levels of dopamine agonists.[62] The peak-dose, choreoathetoid dyskinesias respond to lowering of brain levels of dopamine agonists, whereas the biphasic, transitional, ballistic dyskinesias respond, at least temporarily, to maintaining a continued high level of agonist. Patients can then function during the day, but may have severe offset dyskinesias in the evening. These dyskinesias may be life threatening. The use of D-2 receptor agonists alone may reduce biphasic dyskinesias.

Precursors. The biosynthetic pathway of dopamine is from tyrosine, via tyrosine hydroxylase to levodopa, via L-aromatic amino acid decarboxylase to dopamine (see Fig. 1 – 1). Tyrosine has been reported to be somewhat beneficial in early parkinsonism but the major response is to levodopa, perhaps because decarboxylase activity is present in nondopaminergic nerve terminals and in blood vessels, whereas tyrosine hydroxylase is limited to dopamine terminals and neurons in the brain. Although levodopa therapy alone has been remarkably successful, its use is limited by severe peripheral side effects of nausea and orthostatic hypotension, so that many patients cannot tolerate the therapy. Therefore, carbidopa and benzeraside, inhibitors of dopa decarboxylase that do not cross the BBB, have been introduced as adjuncts to levodopa therapy. These drugs are currently marketed in fixed-dose combinations with levodopa. Sinemet (carbidopa/levodopa) is available worldwide, whereas Madopar (benzeraside/levodopa) is not available in the United States. Time-release versions of Sinemet, which may relieve some of the fluctuations in the rate of dopa delivery to the brain, are supposed to be marketed sometime in the 1990s.[90]

Unfortunately, dopa delivery to the

brain is not governed solely by concentrations of levodopa in the gut. Neutral and aromatic amino acids compete with levodopa for transport from the gut to the blood and from the blood to the brain.[59] Thus, protein in the diet has a significant effect on delivery of levodopa to the brain. Depending on the patient's clinical status, this effect can be either good or bad. If the patient is bothered by side effects such as nausea or dyskinesia, a protein load can decrease the rate at which levodopa is delivered to the brain. Some patients always take their pills with food in their stomach, and some patients have discovered that eating protein makes their dyskinesias go away. Unfortunately, many patients are "turned off" by protein in their diet and get no response from pills given with a protein meal. For these patients, it may be beneficial to reduce markedly the amount of protein in the diet during the day and to consume all the necessary proteins at the end of the day when the patient no longer needs to function.

Another problem of levodopa delivery appears to be intermittent opening of the pyloric valve, which may play some role in the seemingly random fluctuations of the "on/off" phenomenon. Continuous duodenal infusion of levodopa bypasses the pyloric valve and has been of significant benefit in a number of severely affected patients.[14,70] This improvement could be due solely to bypassing the pylorus, but continuous infusion may also improve the sensitivity of intracerebral dopamine receptors.[14]

Transport Inhibitors. Drugs that inhibit the high-affinity transport of dopamine into dopamine terminals have an adjunctive role in Parkinson's therapy, as they increase the amount of dopamine in the synaptic cleft. Such drugs include the tricyclic antidepressants, which also have a role in treating the depression associated with Parkinson's disease. Amphetaminelike compounds will both inhibit dopamine transport and increase the release of dopamine. They have been reported to have short-term beneficial effects in

parkinsonism. Unfortunately, long-term use of amphetamines is associated with psychosis.

Amantadine (Symmetrel) may work by increasing the release and perhaps blocking reuptake of dopamine, and may also have anticholinergic effects. It has a temporary, beneficial effect on parkinsonism. Stopping the drug for several months may resensitize the patient, so that occasionally it can be reused many times with success each time.

Metabolic Inhibitors. Monoamine oxidase inhibitors increase the therapeutic effect of levodopa by blocking one step in dopamine metabolism. Initially, nonspecific MAO inhibitors were used with levodopa therapy alone. They potentiated levodopa's therapeutic effect, but a number of patients died of hypertensive crisis. Use of MAO inhibitors with levodopa plus a decarboxylase inhibitor has not been associated with this problem, but clinicians have remained leery of such combinations. The specific MAO type B inhibitor selegiline (Jumex, Eldepryl, L-Deprenyl) has been used for more than 10 years in Europe as an adjunct to levodopa therapy. It increases the duration of levodopa's action. It also increases the synaptic level of dopamine and all of levodopa's side effects, including nausea, ileus, confusion, hallucinations, and dyskinesias. These side effects can be eliminated by reducing the levodopa dosage. The drug is currently undergoing trials as a preventive therapy for blocking the progression of the disease (see pp 63–64).

Receptor Agonists. Specific dopamine D-2 receptor agonists are beneficial in treating parkinsonism. These drugs do not seem to be as potent as levodopa; perhaps some D-1 stimulation is necessary as well. D-1 stimulation has been found necessary for full dopamine stimulation in animals with experimental parkinsonism. However, trials of D-1–specific drugs along with D-2 drugs have not produced any increased benefit in parkinsonian patients. Use of direct dopamine-receptor agonists may be limited by peripheral side effects such as nausea, gastrointestinal hypomotility, and orthostatic hypotension, or by central side effects of confusion, hallucinations, or delusions.

Some patients with intolerable peripheral side effects of dopamine agonists get relief of these side effects with domperidone. This drug, currently available in Canada and Europe but not in the United States, is a D-2 blocker that only minimally crosses the blood-brain barrier. Patients on domperidone maintain their central response to D-2 agonists without unacceptable peripheral side effects. In other patients, enough domperidone seems to cross the BBB to block the central, beneficial effects of D-2 agonists. The dose of the agonist may have to be adjusted if domperidone is added.

The major D-2 agonist drugs include bromocriptine (Parlodel), a D-2 agonist and a mild D-1 antagonist; pergolide (Permax), a pure D-2 agonist; and lisuride, a water-soluble D-2 agonist, which is not going to be made available in the United States. These drugs are ergot derivatives and have the potential to cause retroperitoneal and pulmonary fibrosis.[12] Erythromelalgia is reported with bromocriptine use. Other D-2 agonists having therapeutic effects include lergotrile, ciladopa, and mesulergine, but these drugs, unfortunately, are too toxic to other organ systems for use in humans. A number of new agonists are under development.

ANTAGONISTS

Antagonists are associated with the production of parkinsonism as a side effect and may blunt or block the therapeutic response to antiparkinsonian drugs in patients with Parkinson's disease. They have been used therapeutically in chorea and in some dyskinesias.

Dopamine-Depleting Agents. The *Rauwolfia* alkaloids, particularly reserpine and tetrabenazine, work by blocking the transport of catecholamines into presynaptic vesicles, thereby depleting dopamine stores. Reserpine also decreases norepinephrine and serotonin stores. These drugs decrease chorea and dyskinesias. Dopamine depletors are antihypertensives and therefore may produce low blood pressure as a side effect. They may also produce depression, although tetrabenazine has fewer side effects than reserpine. Tetrabenazine is also a dopamine antagonist in higher doses and therefore can induce tardive dyskinesia.

Receptor Antagonists. A number of drugs that are useful as antipsychotic agents, including the butyrophenones and phenothiazines, work because they block dopamine D-2 receptors. These drugs are more extensively discussed in Chapter 7. The major side effects are the production of parkinsonism and blocking the response to antiparkinsonian medications. These side effects also occur with antiemetics such as prochlorperazine (Compazine) and metaclopramide (Reglan). In addition, these drugs can produce acute dystonic reactions. These reactions usually can be relieved with intravenous diphenhydramine (Benadryl) or oral anticholinergics.

As discussed above, domperidone is a butyrophenone that crosses the BBB poorly and may be used to prevent peripheral side effects of the dopamine-receptor agonist drugs.

Acetylcholine System

AGONISTS

A number of muscarinic cholinergic agonists have been used in movement disorder therapy, usually as antichoreic and antidyskinetic drugs. They have proved to have little effect. In addition, they produce a number of major side effects due to their stimulation of peripheral muscarinic receptors.

Precursors. The rate-limiting step in acetylcholine synthesis is the availability of its precursor, choline, in the brain. Choline can be given orally to patients. Lecithin is given orally, is less malodorous than choline, and is metabolized to choline. The choline from either source will penetrate the BBB and be converted to acetylcholine. Choline and lecithin once were popular for the treatment of tardive dyskinesia and Alzheimer's disease, but neither has been shown to be very effective. Deanol (Deaner), reported to be a drug that was converted to choline, was used to treat tardive dyskinesia. It was occasionally found to be successful, but also has been found to compete for endogenous choline transported into the brain. Thus, it may actually act as an acetylcholine antagonist. Precursor therapy to enhance cholinergic activity is discussed in detail in Chapter 8.

Transport Inhibitors. No such drugs that penetrate the BBB are available for clinical use.

Metabolic Inhibitors. The anticholinesterases are the mainstay of therapy for myasthenia gravis. Only one of them, physostigmine, crosses the BBB. It will reduce chorea. It has been used with little success in the treatment of Alzheimer's disease. Tetrahydroaminoacridine has been reported useful in Alzheimer's disease, but more thorough studies are needed to assess its utility (see Chapter 8). Peripheral anticholinesterases such as pyridostigmine can be used in low doses to relieve some of the peripheral side effects of anticholinergic agents.

Receptor Agonists. Oxotremorine and arecoline are acetylcholine-receptor agonists that cross the BBB. Unfortunately, they are associated with intolerable peripheral side effects and have no therapeutic indication at this time. For these agents to become clinically useful, it will be necessary to block their peripheral effects.

ANTAGONISTS

Receptor Blockers. Anticholinergics are useful for treatment of Parkin-son's disease, particularly the tremor. They tend to aggravate chorea and dyskinesia, even if the dyskinesia is induced by a dopaminergic agonist. Side effects of these agents include the peripheral problems of dry mouth and eyes, urinary retention, constipation, and orthostatic hypotension. In addition, at high doses there are prominent central side effects with hallucinations, confusion, and recent memory loss. The drugs vary a great deal in their potency and in their tendency to have peripheral versus central effects. However, there is no drug that acts purely as either a central or peripheral agent. Thus, drugs that are advertised to increase urinary retention, such as oxybutynin (Ditropan), will have effects on parkinsonism and memory. Some of the central agents, especially ethopropazine, are reputed to have fewer effects on memory and relatively more effects on movement than the others.

In addition to their ability to block dopamine reuptake, tricyclic antidepressants also block muscarinic receptors. This tendency is most prominent with the tertiary tricyclics such as amitriptyline (Elavil).

GABAergic Systems

AGONISTS

Precursors. The immediate precursor for GABA in the CNS is glutamic acid, which does not cross the BBB. Glutamic acid in the CNS is synthesized from glutamine, which also crosses the BBB only to a limited extent. Baclofen was initially synthesized as a precursor for GABA, because it has a chlorophenyl group attached to the GABA molecule. It was hoped that baclofen would be broken down in the CNS to form GABA and it would, therefore, act as a GABA agonist. Baclofen does have potent CNS effects; however, it does not appear to act as a GABA precursor per se, but rather acts at a subgroup of GABA receptors, the bicuculline-insensitive $GABA_B$ receptors. Baclofen affects the release of several neurotransmitters from the presynaptic terminals. In addition, there are postsynaptic GABA$_B$ receptors that cause inhibition. Another agent that was initially synthesized as a GABA precursor is the drug progabide. Just like baclofen, however, it appears to have its own unique effects on the nervous system, working predominantly at GABA$_A$ receptors.

Metabolic Inhibitors. A number of drugs are available that both reversibly and irreversibly block the activity of the enzyme responsible for GABA metabolism, GABA-transaminase. These drugs include isoniazid as well as gamma-acetylenic-GABA and gamma-vinyl-GABA. Gamma-vinyl-GABA appears to be useful as an anticonvulsant in clinical trials. Isoniazid in high concentrations causes convulsions by inhibiting the enzyme glutamate decarboxylase, which synthesizes GABA from glutamate. Isoniazid competes with pyridoxine, a cofactor for both GABA-transaminase and glutamate decarboxylase. Isoniazid-induced seizures are treated by giving pyridoxine.

Receptor Agonists. There are both GABA$_A$ and GABA$_B$ types of GABA receptors in the CNS. GABA$_A$ receptors are the traditional postsynaptic receptors mediating GABA-induced chloride conductance changes in the postsynaptic membrane. GABA$_B$ receptors were defined after it was discovered that baclofen had unique functions at bicuculline-insensitive GABA receptors. A wide variety of agents are known to be GABA$_A$ agonists, but few of these agents are available clinically. Baclofen is the only known agonist at the GABA$_B$ receptor in addition to GABA.

Receptor Modulation. The GABA$_A$ receptor has been purified and studied at the molecular level.[74] The GABA receptor includes four transmembrane domains that constitute the ion channel and several extracellular and intracellular domains that bind a variety of ligands. There is an active site that binds GABA itself, and adjacent sites that bind the benzodiazepines, barbiturates, and other agents. The benzodiazepines enhance GABA binding and the physiologic actions of GABA by increasing the affinity of the GABA receptor for GABA. Thus, small dosages of benzodiazepines enhance GABAergic activity through this allosteric modulatory action. Barbiturates act at another site on the GABA-receptor complex and also enhance GABA postsynaptic effects by changing the kinetics of ion channel opening.

ANTAGONISTS

Metabolic Inhibitors. The same metabolic inhibitors that block the action of GABA-transaminase also affect GABA synthesis in higher dosages because the enzyme glutamic acid decarboxylase can be reversibly or irreversibly inhibited by a variety of drugs. In general, GABA metabolic inhibitors cause seizures, presumably due to the decrease in GABA levels.

Receptor Antagonists. The action of GABA at the postsynaptic receptor is blocked by both competitive and noncompetitive antagonists. Most of these drugs are plant alkaloids and potent convulsants. Bicuculline is a competitive GABA antagonist and is not used clinically. The GABA-receptor chloride channel is blocked by agents such as picrotoxin, which is also a potent convulsant. None of these agents have been used in human studies.

CONCLUSION

This chapter has reviewed the clinical features, neurochemistry, and neuropharmacology of the movement disorders. Except for the dystonias, rational approaches can be used on the basis of our current understanding about normal and pathologic basal ganglia functional anatomy.[1] As pharmacologic tools for manipulating the EAA and peptide systems become available, the therapies should improve. In conjunction with the development of new pharmacologic agents must come detailed studies of the neurochemical pathology of movement disorders.

ACKNOWLEDGMENTS

We would like to thank Suyin Liang and Catherine Leggieri for their secretarial assistance. Supported by US Public Health Service grants NS 19613 and 15655.

REFERENCES

1. Albin, RL, Young, AB, and Penney, JB: The functional anatomy of basal ganglia disorders. Trends in Neuroscience 12:366–375, 1989.
2. Aronin, N, Cooper, PE, Lorenz, LJ, Bird, ED, Sagar, SM, Leeman, SE, and Martin, JB: Somatostatin is increased in the basal ganglia in Huntington disease. Ann Neurol 13:519–526, 1983.
3. Barbeau, A: Manganese and extrapyramidal disorders. Neurotoxicology 5:13–36, 1985.
4. Bowcock, AM, Farrer, LA, Cavalli-Sforza, LL, Hebert, JM, Kidd, KK, Frydman, M, and Bonne-Tamir, B: Mapping the Wilson's disease locus to a cluster of linked polymorphic markers on chromosome 13. Am J Hum Genet 41:27–35, 1987.
5. Brewer, GJ, Yuzbasiyan-Gurkhan, VA, and Young, AB: The treatment and diagnosis of Wilson's disease. Current Opinion in Neurology and Neurosurgery 1:302–306, 1988.
6. Brin, MF, Fahn, S, Moskowitz, C, Friedman, A, Shale, HM, Greene, PE, Blitzer, A, List, T, Lange, D, Lovelace, RE, and McMahon, D: Localized injections of botulinum toxin for the treatment of focal dystonia and hemifacial spasm. Movement Disorders 2:237–254, 1987.
7. Burns, RS, Chiueh, CC, Markey, SP, Ebert, MH, Jacobowitz, DM, and Kopin, IJ: A primate model of parkinsonism: Selective destruction of dopaminergic neurons in the pars compacta of the substantia nigra by N-methyl-4-phenyl-1,2, 3,6-tetrahydropyridine. Proc Natl Acad Sci USA 80:4546–4550, 1983.
8. Burton, K and Calne, DB: Pharmacology of Parkinson's disease. Neurology Clinics 2:461–472, 1984.
9. Buruma, OJS and Lakke, JPWF: Ballism. In Vinken, PJ, Bruyn, GW, and Klawans, HL (eds): Handbook of Clinical Neurology, Vol 49 (Revised Series 5): Extrapyramidal Disorders. Elsevier, Amsterdam, 1986, pp 369–380.
10. Calne, DB and Lang, AE: Secondary dystonia. In Fahn, S, Marsden, CD, and Calne, DB (eds): Dystonia. Advances in Neurology, Vol 50. Raven Press, New York, 1988, pp 9–34.
11. Calne, DB, Langston, JW, Martin, WRW, Stoessl, AJ, Ruth, TJ, and Schulzer, M: Positron emission tomography after MPTP: Observations relating to the cause of Parkinson's disease. Nature 317:246–248, 1985.
12. Calne, DB, Teychenne, PF, and Claveria, LE: Bromocriptine in parkinsonism. Br Med J 4:442–444, 1974.
13. Cash, R, Lasbennes, F, Sercombe, R, Seylaz, J, and Agid, Y: Adrenergic receptors on cerebral microvessels in control and parkinsonian subjects. Life Sci 37:531–536, 1985.
14. Chase, TN, Baronti, F, Fabbrini, G, Heuser, IJ, Juncos, JL, and Mouradian, MM: Rationale for continuous dopaminomimetic therapy of Parkinson's disease. Neurology 39(Suppl 2):7–10, 1989.
15. Cohen, DJ, Young, JG, Nathanson, AA, and Shaywitz, BA: Clonidine in Tourette's syndrome. Lancet 2:551–552, 1979.
16. Cooper, IS: Dystonia: Surgical approaches to treatment and physiological implications. In Yahr, MD (ed): The Basal Ganglia. Raven Press, New York, 1976, pp 369–383.
17. Davidoff, RA: Pharmacology of spasticity. Neurology 28:46–50, 1978.
18. Fahn, S and Bressman, SB: Should levodopa therapy for parkinsonism be started early or late? Evidence against early treatment. Can J Neurol Sci 11:200–206, 1984.
19. Fahn, S, Marsden, CD, and Calne, DB: Dystonia. Advances in Neurology, Vol 50. Raven Press, New York, 1988.
20. Fahn, S: High dosage anticholinergic

therapy in dystonia. Neurology 33: 1255–1261, 1983.

21. Ferrante, RJ, Beal, MF, Kowall, NW, Richardson, EP, and Martin, JB: Sparing of acetylcholinesterase-containing striatal neurons in Huntington's disease. Brain Res 411:162–166, 1987.

22. Ferrante, RJ, Kowall, NW, Beal, MF, Richardson, EP, Jr, Bird, ED, and Martin, JB: Selective sparing of a class of striatal neurons in Huntington's disease. Science 230:561–564, 1985.

23. Findley, LJ: The pharmacology of essential tremor. In Marsden, CD and Fahn, S (eds): Movement Disorders, ed 2. Butterworths Scientific, London, 1987, pp 438–458.

24. Foster, AC, Whetsell, WO, Bird, ED, and Schwarcz, R: Quinolinic acid phosphoribosyltransferase in human and rat brain: Activity in Huntington's disease and in quinolinate-lesioned rat striatum. Brain Res 336:207–214, 1985.

25. Fuxe, K, Anderson, K, Schwarcz, R, Agnati, LF, Perez de la Mora, M, Hokfelt, T, Goldstein, M, Ferland, L, Possani, L, and Tapia, R: Studies on different types of dopamine nerve terminals in the forebrain and their possible interactions with hormones and with neurons containing GABA, glutamate and opioid peptides. Adv Neurol 24:199–215, 1979.

26. Gerfen, CR: The neostriatal mosaic: Compartmentalization of corticostriatal input and striatonigral output systems. Nature 311:461–464, 1984.

27. Gerfen, CR, Herkenham, M, and Thibauld, J: The neostriatal mosaic 2. Patch-directed and matrix-directed mesostriatal dopaminergic and nondopaminergic system. J Neurosci 7:3915–3934, 1987.

28. Goetz, CG, Tanner, CM, Wilson, RS, Carroll, VS, Como, PG, and Shannon, KM: Clonidine and Gilles de la Tourette's syndrome: Double-blind study using objective rating methods. Ann Neurol 21:307–310, 1987.

29. Graybiel, AM and Ragsdale, CW: Biochemical anatomy of the striatum. In Emson, PC (ed): Chemical Neuroanatomy. Raven Press, New York, 1983, pp 427–504.

30. Gusella, JF, Wexler, NS, Conneally, PM, Naylor, SL, Anderson, MA, Tanzi, RE, Watkins, PC, Ottina, K, Wallace, MR, Sakaguchi, AY, Young, AB, Shoulson, I, Bonilla, E, and Martin, JB: A polymorphic DNA marker genetically linked to Huntington's disease. Nature 306:234–238, 1983.

31. Haber, SN, Kowall, NW, Vonsattel, JP, Bird, ED, and Richardson, EP: Gilles de la Tourette's syndrome: A postmortem neuropathological and immunohistochemical study. J Neurol Sci 75:225–241, 1986

32. Hallett, M, Lindsey, JW, Adelstein, BD, and Riley, PO: Controlled trial of isoniazid therapy for severe postural cerebellar tremor in multiple sclerosis. Neurology 35:1374–1377, 1985.

33. Hallett, M: Differential diagnosis of tremor. In Vinken, PJ, Bruyn, GW, and Klawans, HL (eds): Handbook of Clinical Neurology, Vol 49. Extrapyramidal Disorders. Elsevier Science, New York, 1986, pp 583–596.

34. Henkin, Y and Herishanu, YO: Primidone as treatment for cerebellar tremor in multiple sclerosis—two case reports. Isr J Med Sci 25:720–721, 1989.

35. Hirsch, E, Graybiel, AM, and Agid, YA: Melanized dopaminergic neurons are differentially susceptible to degeneration in Parkinson's disease. Nature 334:345–348, 1988.

36. Hornykiewicz, O and Kish, S: Biochemical pathophysiology of Parkinson's disease. In Yahr, MD and Bergman, KJ (eds): Parkinson's Disease. Advances in Neurology, Vol 45. Raven Press, New York, 1987, pp 19–34.

37. Hornykiewicz, O, Kish, SJ, Becker, LE, Farley, I, and Shannak, K: Biochemical evidence for brain neurotransmitter changes in idiopathic torsion dystonia (dystonia musculoram deformans). In Fahn, S, Marsden, CD, and Calne, DB (eds): Dystonia. Advances in Neurology, Vol 50. Raven Press, New York, 1988, pp 157–165.

38. Jankovic, J and Orman, J: Botulinum A toxin for cranial-cervical dystonia: A double-blind placebo-controlled study. Neurology 37:616–623, 1987.

39. Jimenez-Castellanos, J, and Graybiel,

AM: Subdivisions of the dopamine-containing A8-A9-A10 complex identified by their differential mesostriatal innervation of striosomes and extrastriosomal matrix. Neuroscience 23:223–242, 1987.

40. Kurlan, R: Tourette's syndrome: Current concepts. Neurology 39:1625–1630, 1989.

41. Koller, WC and Royse, VL: Efficiency of primidone in essential tremor. Neurology 36:121–124, 1986.

42. Langston, JW, Forno, LS, Rebert, CS, and Irwin I: Selective nigral toxicity after systemic administration of 1-methyl-4-phenyl-1,2,3,6-tetrahydropyridine (MPTP) in the squirrel monkey. Brain Res 292:390–394, 1984.

43. Langston, JW, Langston, EB, and Irwin, I: MPTP-induced parkinsonism in human and non-human primates: Clinical and experimental aspects. Acta Neurologica Scandinavia 70(Suppl 100):49–54, 1984.

44. Lee, T, Seeman, P, Rajput, A, Farley, IJ, and Hornykiewicz, O: Receptor basis for dopaminergic supersensitivity in Parkinson's disease. Nature 273:59–61, 1978.

45. Lees, AJ: Tics and Related Disorders. Churchill Livingstone, New York, 1985.

46. Mao, CC, Cheney, DL, Marco, E, Revuelta, A, and Costa, E: Turnover times of gamma-aminobutyric acid and acetylcholine in nucleus caudatus, nucleus accumbens, globus pallidus, and substantia nigra: Effects of repeated administration of haloperidol. Brain Res 132:375–379, 1977.

47. Markham, CH and Diamond, SG: Modification of Parkinson's disease by long-term levodopa treatment. Arch Neurol 43:405–407, 1986.

47a. Marsden, CD: Personal communication, month, year.

48. Marsden, CD and Fahn, S: Surgical approaches to the dyskinesias: Afterword. In Marsden, CD and Fahn, S (eds): Movement Disorders. Butterworths, Boston, 1981, pp 345–347.

49. Marsden, CD, Parkes, JD, and Quinn, N: Fluctuations of disability in Parkinson's disease—Clinical aspects. In Marsden, CD and Fahn, S (eds): Movement Disorders. Butterworths Scientific, London, 1982, pp 96–122.

50. Martin, JB and Gusella, JF: Huntington's disease. Pathogenesis and management. N Engl J Med 315:1267–1276, 1986.

51. Mayeux, R, Stern, Y, Cote, L, and Williams, JBW: Altered serotonin metabolism in depressed patients with Parkinson's disease. Neurology 34:642–646, 1984.

52. McGeer, PL, McGeer, EG, and Suzuki, JS: Aging and extrapyramidal function. Arch Neurol 34:33–35, 1977.

53. Meissen, GJ, Myers, RH, Mastromauro, CA, Koroshetz, WJ, Klinger, KW, Farrer, LA, Watkins, PA, Gusella, JF, Bird, ED, and Martin, JB: Predictive testing for Huntington's disease with use of a linked DNA marker. N Engl J Med 318:535–542, 1988.

54. Myers, RH, Cupples, LA, Schoenfeld, M, D'Agostino, RB, Terrin, NC, Goldmakher, N, and Wolf, PA: Maternal factors in onset of Huntington disease. Am J Hum Genet 37:511–523, 1985.

55. Narabayashi, H, Kondo, T, Yokochi, F, and Nagatsu, T: Clinical effects of L-threo-3,4-dihydroxyphenylserine in cases of parkinsonism and pure akinesia. In Yahr, MD and Bergman, KJ (eds): Advances in Neurology, Vol 45. Parkinson's Disease. Raven Press, New York, 1986, pp 593–602.

56. Narabayashi, H: Tremor: Its generating mechanism and treatment. In Vinken, PJ, Bruyn, GW, and Klawans, HL (eds): Handbook of Clinical Neurology, Vol 49. Extrapyramidal Disorders. Elsevier Science, New York, 1986, pp 597–608.

57. Nemeroff, CB, Youngblood, WW, Manberg, PJ, Prange, AJ, and Kizer, JS: Regional brain concentrations of neuropeptides in Huntington's chorea and schizophrenia. Science 221:972–975, 1983.

58. Nutt, JG: Levodopa-induced dyskinesias: Review, observations and speculations. Neurology 40:340–345, 1990.

59. Nutt, JG, Woodward, WR, Hammerstad, JP, Carter, JH, and Anderson, JL: The on-off phenomenon in Parkinson's

disease: Relation to levodopa absorption and transport. N Engl J Med 310:483–488, 1984.

60. Pan, HS, Penney, JB, and Young, AB: GABA and benzodiazepine receptor changes induced by unilateral 6-hydroxydopamine lesions of the medial forebrain bundle. J Neurochem 45:1396–1404, 1985.

61. Parkinson Study Group: Effect of deprenyl on the progression of disability in early Parkinson's disease. N Engl J Med 321:1364–1371, 1989.

62. Penney, JB and Young, AB: Striatal inhomogeneities and basal ganglia function. Movement Disorders 1:3–15, 1986.

63. Perry, TL, Hansen, S, and Kloster, M: Huntington's chorea: Deficiency of gamma-aminobutyric acid in brain. N Engl J Med 288:337–342, 1973.

64. Poskanzer, DC and Schuab, RS: Cohort analysis of Parkinson's syndrome: Evidence for a single etiology related to subclinical infection about 1920. J Chronic Dis 16:961–973, 1963.

65. Regeur, L, Pakkenberg, B, Fog, R, and Pakkenberg, H: Clinical features and long-term treatment with pimozide in 65 patients with Gilles de la Tourette's syndrome. J Neurol Neurosurg Psychiatry 49:791–795, 1986

66. Reiner, A, Albin, Rl, Anderson, KD, D'Amato, CJ, Penney, JB, and Young, AB: Differential loss of striatal projection neurons in Huntington disease. Proc Natl Acad Sci USA 85:5733–5737, 1988.

67. Richfield, EK, Young, AB, and Penney, JB: Comparative distribution of dopamine D-1 and D-2 receptors in the basal ganglia of turtle, pigeon, rat, cat, and monkey. J Comp Neurol 262:446–463, 1987.

68. Richter, R: Degeneration of the basal ganglia in monkeys from chronic carbon disulfide poisoning. J Neuropathol Exp Neurol 4:324–353, 1945.

69. Robinson, DS: Changes in monoamine oxidase and monoamines with human development and aging. Fed Proc 34:103–107, 1975.

70. Sage, JI, Trooskin, S, Sonsalla, PK, Heikkila, R, and Duvoisin, RC: Long-term duodenal infusion of levodopa for motor fluctuations in Parkinsonism. Ann Neurol 24:87–89, 1988.

71. Sandyk, R: Successful treatment of cerebellar tremor with clonazepam. Clinical Pharmacy 4:615–618, 1985.

72. Scheinberg, IH and Sternlieb, I: Wilson's Disease. WB Saunders, Philadelphia, 1984.

73. Schell, GR and Strick, PL: The origin of thalamic inputs to the arcuate premotor and supplementary motor areas. J Neurosci 4:539–560, 1984.

74. Schofield, PR, Darlison, MG, Fujita, N, Burt, DR, Stephenson, FA, Rodriguez, H, Rhee, LM, Ramachandran, J, Reale, V, Glencorse, TA, Seeburg, PH, and Barnard, EA: Sequence and functional expression of the GABA$_A$ receptor shows a ligand-gated receptor super-family. Nature 328:221–228, 1987.

75. Schwarcz, R, Bird, ED, and Whetsell, WO: The quinolinic acid-synthesizing enzyme is increased in the brains of Huntington's disease victims. Society for Neuroscience Abstracts 13:215, 1987.

76. Segawa, M, Hosaka, A, Miyagawa, F, Nomura, Y, and Imai, H: Hereditary progressive dystonia with marked diurnal fluctuation. Adv Neurol 14:215–233, 1976.

77. Shoulson, I: Huntington's disease. In Asbury, AK, McKhann, GM, and McDonald, WI (eds): Diseases of the Nervous System. Clinical Neurobiology. WB Saunders, Philadelphia, 1986, pp 1258–1267.

78. Shoulson, I, Odoroff, C, Oakes, D, Behr, J, Goldblatt, D, Caine, E, Kennedy, J, Miller, C, Bamford, K, Rubin, A, Plumb, S, and Kurlan, R: A controlled clinical trial of baclofen as protective therapy in early Huntington's disease. Ann Neurol 25:252–259, 1989.

79. Spencer, PS, Nunn, PB, Hugon, J, Ludolph, AC, Ross, SM, Roy, DN, and Robertson, RC: Guam amyotrophic lateral sclerosis-parkinsonism-dementia linked to a plant excitant neurotoxin. Science 237:517–522, 1987.

80. Spina, MB and Cohen, G: Dopamine turnover and glutathione oxidation: Implications for Parkinson's disease. Proc

Natl Acad Sci USA 86:1398–1400, 1989.

81. Spokes, EGS: Neurochemical alterations in Huntington's disease. Brain 103:179–210, 1980.

82. Tedroff, J, Aquilonius, SM, Hartvig, P, Lundqvist, H, Gee, AG, Uhlin, J, and Langstrom, B: Monoamine reuptake sites in the human brain evaluated in vivo by means of ^{11}C-nomifensine and positron emission tomography: The effects of age and Parkinson's disease. Acta Neurologica Scandinavia 77:192–201, 1988.

83. Tetrud, JW and Langston, JW: The effect of deprenyl (selegiline) on the natural history of Parkinson's disease. Science 245:519–522, 1989.

84. Uhl, GR, Whitehouse, PJ, Price, DL, Tourtelotte, WW, and Kuhar, MJ: Parkinson's disease: Depletion of substantia nigra neurotensin receptors. Brain Res 308:186–190, 1984.

85. Vonsattel, JP, Myers, RH, Stevens, TJ, Ferrante, RJ, Bird, ED, and Richardson, EP: Neuropathological classification of Huntington's disease. J Neuropathol Exp Neurol 44:559–577, 1985.

86. Walker, FO, Young, AB, Penney, JB, Dorovini-Zis, K, and Shoulson, I: Benzodiazepine receptors in early Huntington's disease. Neurology 34:1237–1240, 1984.

87. Walters, A, Hening, W, Chokroverty, S, and Fahn, S: Opioid responsiveness in patients with neuroleptic-induced akathisia. Movement Disorders 1:119–127, 1986.

88. Walters, JR, Bergstrom, DA, Carlson, JH, Chase, TN, and Braun, AR: D1 dopamine receptor activation required for postsynaptic expression of D2 agonist effects. Science 236:719–722, 1987.

89. Wilson, SAK: Progressive lenticular degeneration: A familial nervous disease associated with cirrhosis of the liver. Brain 34:295–509, 1912.

90. Yeh, KC, August, TF, Bush, DF, Lasseter, KC, Musson, DG, Schwartz, S, Smith, ME, and Titus, DC: Pharmacokinetics and bioavailability of Sinemet CR: A summary of human studies. Neurology 39(Suppl 2):25–38, 1989.

91. Young, AB, Albin, RL, and Penney, JB: Neuropharmacology of basal ganglia functions: Relationship to pathophysiology of movement disorders. In Neural Mechanisms in Disorders of Movement. John Libbey, London, 1989, pp 17–27.

92. Young, AB and Penney, JB, Jr: Pharamacologic aspects of motor dysfunction. In Asbury, AK, McKhann, GM, and McDonald, WI (eds): Diseases of the Nervous System. Ardmore Medical, Philadelphia, 1986, pp 423–434.

93. Young, AB, Greenamyre, JT, Hollingsworth, Z, Albin, R, D'Amato, C, Shoulson, I, and Penney, JB: NMDA receptor losses in putamen from patients with Huntington's disease. Science 241:981–983, 1988.

94. Young, AB, Shoulson, I, Penney, JB, Starosta, S, Gomez, F, Travers, H, Ramos-Arroyo, MA, Snodgrass, SR, Bonilla, E, Moreno, H, and Wexler, NS: Huntington's disease in Venezuela: Neurologic features and functional decline. Neurology 36:244–249, 1986.

Chapter 3

SEIZURE DISORDERS AND EPILEPSY

*Robert L. Macdonald,
M.D., Ph.D.*

CLASSIFICATION OF SEIZURES
AND THE EPILEPSIES
CLINICAL CLASSIFICATION OF
ANTICONVULSANT DRUGS
MECHANISMS OF ACTION OF
ANTICONVULSANT DRUGS
MECHANISTIC CLASSIFICATION OF
ANTICONVULSANT DRUGS
CLINICAL USE OF
ANTICONVULSANT DRUGS FOR
CHRONIC THERAPY
THERAPY FOR STATUS EPILEPTICUS

Seizures and epilepsy are prevalent medical conditions throughout the world, and anticonvulsant drugs are among the most widely prescribed drugs in neurologic practice. It is estimated that more than 1.25 million people in the United States have chronic epilepsy. Approximately 4% of the population who live to age 80 may be given a diagnosis of epilepsy at some time in their lives, and 10% may experience at least one seizure.[22] The overall age-adjusted incidence of epilepsy in the United States is estimated to be 56.7/100,000.[22] The figure is the average of two peaks of incidence in the perinatal period and in the years past age 65, when the incidence is about 1/1000, with a period of lower incidence in midlife. Although most patients are able to live full lives with good seizure control, epilepsy remains one of the most disruptive and distressing human diseases.

Fundamental information about the pathogenesis and pathophysiology of epilepsy in humans is relatively sparse. Anticonvulsant drugs were discovered serendipitously, and their spectrum of activity in human epilepsy has been defined by careful clinical observation and clinical experience. Although treatment of epilepsy with drugs remains largely empirical, research during the past decade has provided new insights into how the drugs work at a molecular level. Understanding these mechanisms may clarify basic features of epileptogenicity and help to identify new drugs. At a practical level, a mechanistic classification of anticonvulsant drugs provides a more rational framework for prescribing them and monitoring their use. This section presents information about anticonvulsant drug mechanisms in a clinical context. The chapter presents three mechanisms of action of current anticonvulsant drugs and a fourth mechanism that is likely to be used by future drugs. Drugs in current use are placed into three groups according to their major mechanism of action, and this classification is related to their clinical spectrum of activity. The relationship of this information to clinical use for chronic epilepsy and status epilepticus is discussed in the final sections.

CLASSIFICATION OF SEIZURES AND THE EPILEPSIES

Seizures are the clinical manifestations of synchronous, episodic, paroxysmal, abnormal electrical discharge of groups of neurons in the central nervous system (CNS). Seizures produce many different types of behavioral manifestations ranging from brief episodes of staring to complex automatic behaviors.[22] Seizures are usually described as either having a local or focal onset in a specific region in the nervous system, or having a generalized onset (Table 3–1). Partial seizures are those in which the first behavioral or electroencephalographic change can be localized to a portion of one cerebral hemisphere. Partial seizures are further classified into those during which consciousness is impaired (a complex partial seizure) or into those during which consciousness is not impaired (a simple partial seizure). Simple partial seizures may evolve to complex partial seizures,

and simple and complex partial seizures may evolve to generalized tonic-clonic seizures. Generalized tonic-clonic seizures are then described as secondarily generalized. Primary generalized seizures are those in which the first clinical changes indicate involvement of both cerebral hemispheres. Major forms of generalized seizures are absence seizures, myoclonic seizures, tonic seizures, tonic-clonic seizures, and atonic seizures.

Epilepsy may be defined as the condition of chronic recurring seizures. Two classifications of the epilepsies continue to be used. In the first classification, the epilepsies are divided into (1) the localization-related (focal, local, partial) epilepsies; (2) the generalized epilepsies; (3) the epilepsies and syndromes that have undetermined origin; and (4) the special epilepsy syndromes (Table 3–2). In the second classification, the epilepsies are divided into (1) primary (idiopathic); (2) secondary (symptomatic); or (3) cryptogenic forms. The idiopathic epilepsies are those for

---

Table 3–1 INTERNATIONAL CLASSIFICATION OF SEIZURES

I. Partial (focal, local) seizures
   A. Simple partial seizures (consciousness not impaired)
     1. With motor symptoms
     2. With somatosensory or special sensory symptoms
     3. With autonomic symptoms
     4. With psychic symptoms
   B. Complex partial seizures (with impairment of consciousness)
     1. Beginning as simple partial seizures and progressing to impairment of consciousness
     2. With impairment of consciousness at onset
   C. Partial seizures evolving to secondarily generalized seizures
     1. Simple partial seizures evolving to generalized seizures
     2. Complex partial seizures evolving to generalized seizures
     3. Simple partial seizures evolving to complex partial seizures to generalized seizures
II. Generalized seizures (convulsive or nonconvulsive)
   A. Absence seizures
     1. Typical absences
     2. Atypical absences
   B. Myoclonic seizures
   C. Clonic seizures
   D. Tonic seizures
   E. Tonic-clonic seizures
   F. Atonic seizures (astatic seizures)
III. Unclassified epileptic seizures
   Includes all seizures that cannot be classified because of inadequate or incomplete data and some that defy classification in hitherto-described categories. This includes some neonatal seizures such as rhythmic eye movements, chewing, and swimming movements.

Source: Proposal for revised clinical and electroencephalographic classification of epileptic seizures. Epilepsia 22:489–501, 1981.

Table 3-2 INTERNATIONAL CLASSIFICATION OF EPILEPSIES AND EPILEPTIC SYNDROMES

I. Localization-related (focal, local, partial) epilepsies and syndromes
   A. Idiopathic (with age-related onset): At present, two syndromes are established:
      1. Benign childhood epilepsy with centrotemporal spike
      2. Childhood epilepsy with occipital paroxysms
   B. Symptomatic: This category comprises syndromes of great individual variability.
II. Generalized epilepsies and syndromes
   A. Idiopathic (with age-related onset, in order of age appearance)
      1. Benign neonatal familial convulsions
      2. Benign neontal convulsions
      3. Benign myoclonic epilepsy in infancy
      4. Childhood absence epilepsy (pyknolepsy, petit mal)
      5. Juvenile absence epilepsy
      6. Juvenile myoclonic epilepsy (impulsive petit mal)
      7. Epilepsy with grand mal seizures (generalized tonic-clonic seizures) on awakening
   B. Idiopathic and/or symptomatic (in order of age of appearance)
      1. West's syndrome (infantile spasms, Blitz-Nick-Salaam Krampfe)
      2. Lennox-Gastaut syndrome
      3. Epilepsy with myoclonic-astatic seizures
      4. Epilsepsy with myoclonic absences
   C. Symptomatic
      1. Nonspecific etiology
      2. Specific syndromes: Epileptic seizures may complicate many disease states. Under this heading are included those diseases in which seizures are presenting or predominant feature.
III. Epilepsies and syndromes undetermined as to whether they are focal or generalized
   A. With both generalized and focal seizures
      1. Neonatal seizures
      2. Severe myoclonic epilepsy in infancy
      3. Epilepsy with continuous spikes and waves during slow-wave sleep
      4. Acquired epileptic aphasia (Landau-Kleffner syndrome)
   B. Without unequivocal generalized or focal features
IV. Special syndromes
   A. Situation-related seizures (Gelegenheitsanfalle)
      1. Febrile convulsions
      2. Seizures related to other identifiable situations, such as stress, hormones, drugs, alcohol, or sleep deprivation
   B. Isolated, apparently unprovoked epileptic events
   C. Epilepsies characterized by specific modes of seizures precipitated
   D. Chronic progressive epilepsia partialis continua of childhood

Source: Proposal for the classification of the epilepsies and epileptic syndromes. Epilepsia 26:268–278, 1985.

which no cause other than a possible hereditary predisposition can be found from history, physical examination, electroencephalogram (EEG), imaging studies, and routine laboratory testing. The symptomatic epilepsies and syndromes include those that are secondary to an underlying abnormality of the nervous system produced by such causes as tumor, vascular disease, trauma, infections, or toxic-metabolic disturbances. The cryptogenic epilepsies are presumed to be symptomatic, but the cause of the epilepsy is unknown. The significance of this scheme is that the symptomatic epilepsies may be subject to therapeutic intervention such as treating an infection or removing a tumor, whereas the idiopathic epilepsies are produced by fixed or structural abnormalities that are not currently subject to intervention. This is a somewhat artificial distinction as all of the epilepsies presumably are due to a CNS abnormality that may or may not eventually be subject to treatment. Nonetheless, the major first approach to therapy in the epilepsies is to identify correctly the seizure type, the form of epilepsy that is represented, and whether the epilepsy is idiopathic, cryptogenic, or symptomatic. Diagnosis is based primarily on historical information obtained from the patient, family members and seizures witnesses, family history, and a detailed neurologic examination. At a minimum, an EEG and a brain imaging study, either computed tomography or magnetic resonance imaging, is obtained. For complex cases when the seizure type is unclear from the description or when seizures fail to respond as expected to therapy, additional detailed electrodiagnostic testing including video EEG or telemetry may be needed. An excellent description of seizure diagnosis can be found in another book in the *Contemporary Neurology Series* by Engel.[22] Some forms of epilepsy and isolated symptomatic seizures can be abolished simply by removing the underlying etiology (e.g., cerebral tumor, abscess, or fever). A small percentage of patients with intractable, usually partial, seizures can be successfully treated with surgical removal of the damaged area of the nervous system that gave rise to their seizures. A large percentage of children with epilepsy become seizure-free. Anticonvulsant drugs, however, remain the principal treatment for the vast majority of patients with epilepsy.

CLINICAL CLASSIFICATION OF ANTICONVULSANT DRUGS

Despite substantial interest in developing new, safer, and more efficacious anticonvulsant drugs, six classes of anticonvulsant drugs, which have been in use for 15 to 75 years, continue to be the primary drugs used to treat patients with epilepsy. The anticonvulsant drugs classes include hydantoins (phenytoin); iminostilbenes (carbamazepine); barbiturates (phenobarbital, primidone); fatty acids (sodium valproate); benzodiazepines (clonazepam, diazepam, nitrazepam, lorazepam); and succinimides (ethosuximide). Multiple anticonvulsant drugs are available because they often have somewhat different clinical spectra of action, can be administered with different dosing regimens, evoke different idiopathic allergic reactions, have different dose-dependent toxicities, and have variations in their absorption and metabolism (Table 3–3). Once a correct diagnosis has been made, a relatively selective anticonvulsant drug may be chosen.

Because selection of an anticonvulsant drug is usually dictated by the specific seizure diagnosis in individual pa-

Table 3–3 PHARMACOKINETIC PROPERTIES OF ANTICONVULSANT DRUGS

Drug Use	Daily Dosage (mg/kg)	Rx Plasma Concentration (µg/mL)	Plasma Half-life (h)	Peak Time (h)	Time to Steady-State (d)	Protein Bound (%)
Carbamazepine GTCS; CPS; SPS	10–20	4–12	12 ± 3	2–6	2–4	80
Phenytoin GTCS; CPS; SPS	5–7	10–20	24 ± 12	4–8	5–10	90
Na Valproate absence; GTCS; CPS; MCS	20–60	50–100	12 ± 6	1–4	2–4	90
Primidone GTCS; CPS; SPS	10–15	5–15	12 ± 6	2–4	4–7	0–20
Phenobarbital GTCS; CPS; SPS	2–3	10–30	96 ± 12	4–8	14–21	40–50
Ethosuximide absence	15–40	40–100	60 ± 6	2–4	5–8	0
Clonazepam absence; MCS; CPS; SPS	0.1–0.2	0.02–0.08	12–40	1–4	6	87

Key: GTCS = Generalized tonic-clonic seizures, CPS = Complex partial seizures; SPS = Simple partial seizures; MCS = Myoclonic seizures.

**Table 3-4 CLINICAL SPECTRUM OF ACTIVITY OF
ANTICONVULSANT DRUGS**

Drug	Tonic-Clonic and Partial Seizures	Generalized Absence	Myoclonic
Phenytoin	++	0	0
Carbamazepine	++	0	0
Primidone	++	0	0
Valproate	++	++	++
Phenobarbital	+	0	+
Clonazepam	+	+	++
Ethosuximide	0	++	0

Key: ++ = Very effective; + = May be helpful; 0 = Ineffective or harmful.

tients, anticonvulsant drugs have often been classified in terms of their therapeutic efficacy against specific seizures types in man (Table 3-4).[21,100] Phenytoin, carbamazepine, and primidone are effective against primary and secondarily generalized tonic-clonic seizures and partial seizures, but are ineffective against myoclonic and generalized absence seizures. From the perspective of their mechanism of action, they are referred to later in this text as type I anticonvulsant drugs. Sodium valproate, barbiturates, and benzodiazepines have a broader range of action, but use of drugs from the last two drug classes is limited by sedation and development of tolerance. These drugs also have common mechanistic features and are referred to here as type II anticonvulsant drugs. Phenobarbital is considered to be less efficacious than the aforementioned drugs for generalized tonic-clonic and partial seizures and is effective against myoclonic seizures, but has no role in the therapy of generalized absence seizures. In contrast, valproate has been demonstrated to have efficacy in the treatment of generalized tonic-clonic, myoclonic, and absence seizures. Benzodiazepines such as diazepam and clonazepam have been used primarily against generalized absence and myoclonic seizures, and diazepam and lorazepam have been used in the treatment of status epilepticus. Some benzodiazepines have been shown also to have efficacy against generalized tonic-clonic seizures. Finally,

ethosuximide remains the drug of choice for generalized absence seizures, but has no significant efficacy against generalized tonic-clonic, partial, or myoclonic seizures. Ethosuximide and similar drugs trimethadione and dimethadione are grouped as type III anticonvulsant drugs from the standpoint of their mechanism. Therefore, anticonvulsant drugs can be classified as those that are effective against tonic-clonic and partial seizures but not against myoclonic or absence seizures, those with mixed efficacy, and those that are selective for generalized absence seizures. Although this classification of anticonvulsant drugs has therapeutic usefulness, it does not provide information concerning the mechanisms of action of the drugs. It does, however, suggest that anticonvulsant drugs may have different mechanisms of action.

MECHANISMS OF ACTION OF ANTICONVULSANT DRUGS

At the present time, there are three major actions of anticonvulsant drugs that are likely to underlie their anticonvulsant action (Table 3-5). These actions are reduction of sodium current, enhancement of GABAergic (gamma-aminobutyric acid) inhibition, and reduction of a transient (T) calcium current. In addition, some experimental anticonvulsant drugs under develop-

Table 3-5 MAJOR CELLULAR MECHANISMS OF ANTICONVULSANT DRUGS

Reduction of sodium current
Enhancement of GABAergic inhibition
Reduction of transient calcium current
Reduction of excitatory amino acid
  neurotransmission

ment reduce the action of the excitatory amino acid, glutamic acid on specific receptors called N-methyl-D-aspartic acid (NMDA) receptors.

Effects of Anticonvulsant Drugs on Sodium Channels

All anticonvulsant drugs have been shown to alter some membrane property of neurons and axons.[23,34,52,78] However, to be potential anticonvulsant drug mechanisms, the membrane effects must be produced at concentrations achieved in the cerebrospinal fluid (CSF) and in plasma free of protein binding in ambulatory patients. A direct membrane effect produced only at toxic free-plasma concentrations is unlikely to be a relevant anticonvulsant drug mechanism of action.

Most seizures are accompanied by excessive high frequency discharge of action potentials, either at the focus of the seizure or in propagation pathways. High-frequency discharge of action potentials permits massive excitatory input to be delivered to neurons in projection pathways and thus allows propagation of seizure activity. Phenytoin, carbamazepine, and sodium valproate all are able to block the ability of central neurons to fire action potentials at high frequency. It is likely that this blockade of high-frequency repetitive firing underlies their anticonvulsant action, as these effects of the anticonvulsant drugs are produced at free serum concentrations of the drugs present during clinical administration. In addition, phenobarbital and the benzodiazepines (diazepam, clonazepam, nitrazepam, and lorazepam) all block sustained,

high-frequency repetitive firing (SRF) of action potentials at concentrations that are higher than those achieved in ambulatory patients but that are equivalent to those achieved during the treatment of generalized tonic-clonic status epilepticus. Thus, it is likely that any anticonvulsant drug that is effective against generalized tonic-clonic seizures, partial seizures, and generalized tonic-clonic status epilepticus has a primary action to block SRF.

Phenytoin, carbamazepine, sodium valproate, anticonvulsant benzodiazepines (diazepam, nitrazepam, clonazepam, and lorazepam), phenobarbital, and primidone block SRF of action potentials in vertebrate cortical and spinal cord neurons in cell culture.[52,58] However, only phenytoin, carbamazepine, and sodium valproate reduce SRF (Fig. 3-1) at therapeutic free-plasma concentrations.

The anticonvulsant drug-induced block of SRF has several important properties. First, the block is *voltage-dependent*. When neurons are held at large negative potentials, membrane depolarization can produce SRF. Following membrane depolarization, however, SRF is limited to a few action potentials. Second, the effect of the anticonvulsant drugs is *use-dependent*. Under normal circumstances following membrane depolarization, neurons fire a train of action potentials with varying degrees of spike frequency adaptation. In the presence of an anticonvulsant drug, however, there is a progressive alteration of action potentials within the train. The initial action potential is unaffected but each subsequent action potential has a smaller amplitude and a lower rate of rise. Eventually, firing of action potentials fails during the depolarization. Third, the effect of the anticonvulsant drugs is *time-dependent*. Under normal circumstances, a train of action potentials can be elicited in neurons; following membrane repolarization, a depolarization can evoke an action potential that is unaffected. In the presence of an anticonvulsant drug, however, a train can be evoked with

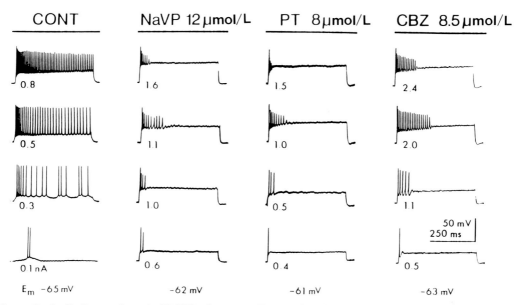

Figure 3–1. Sodium valproate (NaVP), phenytoin (PT), and carbamazepine (CBZ) limited SRF of action potentials. Intracellular recordings were made from spinal cord neurons in cell culture as increasing depolarizing current pulses were applied. Current pulse magnitude in nanoamps is shown below each of the traces. The membrane potentials from which the depolarizing pulses were applied are shown below each column. In control medium (CONT), SRF was obtained for all depolarizations. With NaVP, PT, and CBZ, limitation of SRF was seen at each of the membrane potentials. (Adapted from McLean and Macdonald.[58–60])

limitation of repetitive firing. For several hundred milliseconds following membrane repolarization, an evoked action potential will still be of reduced amplitude and rate of rise; that is, once the effect of the anticonvulsant drug has been produced, it takes several hundred milliseconds to be removed.

Phenytoin and carbamazepine reduce the amplitude of sodium-dependent action potentials by increasing the voltage dependency of steady-state inactivation and by reducing the rate of recovery of sodium channels from inactivation.[12,55,58,60,97] Phenytoin, carbamazepine, phenobarbital, and diazepam all inhibit the binding of [H³] batrachotoxinin A 20-α-benzoate (BTX-B), a toxin that binds to sodium channels at a site related to activation of sodium channel ion flux[96] and reduces batrachotoxin-stimulated ²⁴Na influx in brain synaptic terminals.[98]

The effects of the anticonvulsant drugs on sodium channels are similar to those of local anesthetic drugs.[13,35,43,88] The action of these drugs has been interpreted using the modulated-receptor hypothesis.[12,35] The sodium channel exists in three main conformations: a resting or activatable state, an open or conducting state, and an inactive or nonactivatable state. Under normal circumstances, when membrane potential is large and negative, most of the sodium channels open in proportion to the level of membrane depolarization. With progressive depolarization, some channels are converted to the inactive state, and membrane depolarization now will produce opening of fewer channels. If the membrane is depolarized, all channels may be in the inactive state and no channels will open. To remove channel inactivation, the membrane must be again hyperpolarized to a large negative voltage. In the modulated-receptor hypothesis, it has been postulated that drugs bind to the different forms of these channels with different affinity.

In the case of the anticonvulsant drugs, it is likely that they bind to the inactive form of the channel. Therefore, when a neuron has a large negative membrane potential, all of the channels are in the closed conformation and are not bound with high affinity by the anticonvulsant drugs. In contrast, when the cell is depolarized, a fraction of the channels are in an inactive state, allowing equilibrium to shift toward the bound, inactive conformation of the channel. In such a model, anticonvulsant drugs can produce time-, voltage-, and use-dependent block of sodium-dependent action potentials because the fraction of inactive channels is increased by membrane depolarization and by repetitive firing. Because the drug that is bound to the inactive channels takes time to dissociate, there is time dependence of the block. Therefore, it is likely that anticonvulsant drugs block SRF of sodium action potentials by selectively binding to the inactive form of the sodium channel.

The effect of the anticonvulsant drug, however, will be highly voltage-dependent. If the neuron is at a very large negative membrane potential or is hyperpolarized, then very few of the channels will be in the inactive state, and therefore very little of the anticonvulsant drug will be bound. If, however, the neuron is in a depolarized state, then many of the channels will be bound and the effect of the anticonvulsant drug will be profound. Thus, the anticonvulsant drug will be most effective in neurons that have their membrane potential reduced and their firing at high frequency. This is the characteristic phenomenon seen in neurons that are undergoing epileptic discharge, and therefore it is likely that this is an effective mechanism of action for these anticonvulsant drugs.

Although the apparent mechanism of action of sodium valproate is similar to that of phenytoin and carbamazepine, sodium valproate has not been shown to bind to the BTX-B binding site on sodium channels[96] or to block batrachotoxin-stimulated ^{24}Na influx in brain synaptic terminals.[98] Thus, it is likely

that blockade of SRF may be responsible, at least in part, for preventing generalized tonic-clonic and partial seizures but not for generalized absence seizures.

Effects of Anticonvulsant Drugs on Calcium Channels

In addition to effects on sodium channels, the clinically used anticonvulsant drugs have been demonstrated to have effects on calcium channels.[52] Calcium entry into neurons has been shown to be through three different voltage-dependent calcium channels.[71] These channels have been called the L channel, the N channel, and the T channel. These calcium channels differ in their voltage dependency for activation and inactivation, rate of inactivation, and individual channel conductance. In addition, they have different agonist and antagonist pharmacology. L-channel conductance is large, and L current is long-lasting and slowly inactivating. T-channel conductance is small, and T currents are transient and inactivate rapidly. N-channel conductance is intermediate in magnitude, and N current inactivates at a rate between that of the T and L currents. Phenytoin, barbiturates, and benzodiazepines have been demonstrated to reduce calcium influx into synaptic terminals[3,25,44,75] and to block presynaptic release of neurotransmitter[41,66,79, 97] at concentrations that are supertherapeutic. Barbiturates block both L and N currents without affecting T current at anesthetic but not free serum anticonvulsant drug concentrations (Figure 3–2).[28,29] Similarly, phenytoin[61] and diazepam[85] have been demonstrated to block calcium current at supratherapeutic concentrations.

In contrast, ethosuximide and the trimethadione metabolite dimethadione have been demonstrated to affect T current in thalamic neurons[11] and in primary afferent neurons[30] at therapeutically relevant concentrations (Fig. 3–3). It has been proposed that T calcium currents are important pacemaker cur-

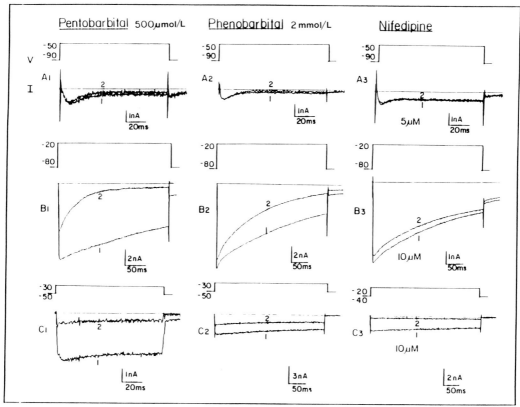

Figure 3-2. Pentobarbital and phenobarbital reduced N- and L- but not T-calcium currents, whereas nifedipine selectively reduced L-calcium current. T-, L- and N/L-calcium currents were evoked from different membrane potentials with varying depolarizing commands. A control current was obtained (line 1 on each graph) and the effects of pentobarbital (A_1, B_1, C_1), phenobarbital (A_2, B_2, C_2), and nifedipine (A_3, B_3, C_3) were determined by applying the drugs to the neuron. The current was evoked again (line 2) and superimposed on the control current. (A) None of the drugs altered T-calcium current. (B) Pentobarbital and phenobarbital, but not nifedipine, increased the rate of inactivation primarily of the N component of the N/L-calcium current. (C) Pentobarbital, phenobarbital, and nifedipine decreased L-calcium current. Recordings were made from mouse dorsal root ganglion neurons grown in cell culture. (From Gross and Macdonald,[29] p 447, with permission.)

rents in thalamic neurons and that these currents may be responsible, in part, for the 3-Hz rhythm seen in the EEG of patients with generalized absence seizures.[11] Blockade of T calcium current by ethosuximide or trimethadione, then, would disrupt the slow rhythmic firing of thalamic neurons and disrupt the spike-and-wave discharge. However, sodium valproate, but not clonazepam, may alter T calcium currents.[42]

Enhancement of GABAergic Inhibition

Synaptic inhibition is an important mechanism for regulation of CNS excitability. Enhancement of inhibition, therefore, would be an effective means for decreasing abnormal excitability. Inhibition in the nervous system is mediated by a number of neurotransmitters and their corresponding receptors. Rapid inhibition is mediated primarily

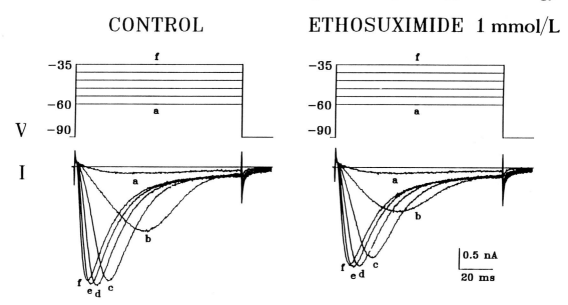

Figure 3–3. Ethosuximide reduced T-calcium current. Voltage clamp recordings were obtained from acutely dissociated rat nodose ganglion neurons using the whole-cell recording technique. Neurons were held at −90 mV, and depolarizing commands were applied in 5-mV increments to −60 to −35 mV. This voltage clamp sequence evoked a series of T-calcium currents. In the presence of ethosuximide, currents at each command were reduced in amplitude from those produced under control conditions.

by amino-acid neurotransmitters, including GABA and glycine acting on postsynaptic GABA$_A$ receptors and glycine receptors, respectively. Additional postsynaptic inhibition that has a slower time course may be mediated by GABA acting at GABA$_B$ receptors,[5,67] norepinephrine action at α-2 receptors,[95] and opioid peptides acting at μ-opioid and δ-opioid receptors.[69] Inhibition can also be produced presynaptically by reducing the release of neurotransmitter. It is likely that a number of amino-acid and neuropeptide transmitters interact with presynaptic receptors to reduce calcium entry and therefore, to block synaptic transmitter release.[19] These neurotransmitters include GABA,[20] adenosine,[52] neuropeptide Y,[24] dynorphin A,[8] and norepinephrine.[94] Rapid forms of inhibition mediated by glycine and GABA$_A$ receptors are produced by activation of neurotransmitter receptors where the proteins forming the receptor also form the channel.[27,80] The slower forms of inhibition and the presynaptic regulation of

calcium entry are likely mediated by receptors that bind transmitter and then bind guanosine 5′-triphosphate- (GTP) binding proteins (G-proteins). The G-proteins are heterotrimers which, upon interaction with a neurotransmitter-bound receptor, dissociate into a GTP-bound α-subunit and a $\beta\gamma$ dimer.[26] It is likely that the α-subunit of the G-protein interacts with calcium channels to reduce presynaptic calcium entry.[24,37,82] It has also been demonstrated that the postsynaptic GABA$_B$,[2] α-2-adrenergic,[1] and μ-opioid[1] receptors are coupled to potassium channels via G-proteins.

Of the many forms of inhibition, the only form that has been shown clearly to be regulated by anticonvulsant drugs is GABAergic inhibition. GABA is a neutral amino acid that is synthesized from glutamic acid by the enzyme glutamic acid decarboxylase. It is metabolized in neurons and glia by the enzyme GABA transaminase. When GABA is released, it binds to postsynaptic GABA$_A$ receptors. The GABA$_A$ receptor has been shown to be an oligomeric complex consisting of at least two binding sites for GABA, allosteric regulatory binding sites for benzodiazepines and β-carbolines, picrotoxin-like convulsant drugs and barbiturates, and a chloride channel (Fig. 3–4).[74,76,87] The receptor appears to be formed from three peptide subunits, α, β, and γ chains with an unknown stoichiometry,[77,80] and there are multiple forms of α, β, and γ chains.[46,77] Each peptide chain spans the membrane at least four times, having four membrane, or M, regions. The juxtaposition of portions of the M regions is thought to form the chloride ion channel, which is opened by GABA binding. There are series of positive charges around the extracellular portion of the M proteins which presumably are involved in regulating neg-

atively charged chloride ion entry. The channel is closed when GABA is not bound to the receptor but opens following GABA binding. Thus, the $GABA_A$ receptor forms the chloride ion channel.

Benzodiazepines have been shown to enhance the binding of GABA to its receptor[63,86] and to enhance $GABA_A$ receptor current (Fig. 3–5).[9,50] Phenobarbital, however, has been demonstrated not to enhance the binding of GABA to its receptor,[73] but to enhance $GABA_A$ receptor current (see Fig. 3–5).[51] The benzodiazepines (diazepam, clonazepam, nitrazepam, and lorazepam) have all been shown to enhance $GABA_A$ receptor chloride current at low nanomolar concentrations which are achieved in CSF and in plasma unbound to plasma proteins.[84] Similarly, phenobarbital has been demonstrated to en-

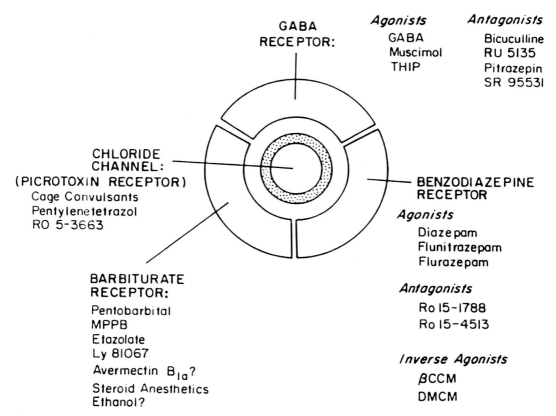

Figure 3–4. GABA receptor channels have multiple binding sites for drugs to regulate GABA-evoked current flow. The portions of the receptor that surround the channel do not represent individual GABA receptor channel subunits. (From Olsen et al,[72] p 2, with permission.)

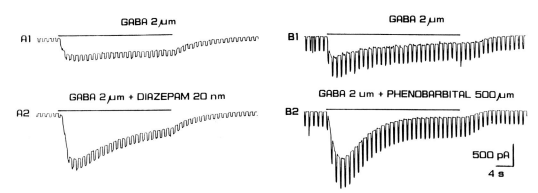

Figure 3–5. GABA receptor chloride currents were enhanced by diazepam and phenobarbital. Mouse spinal cord neurons in cell culture were voltage clamped at −75 mV using the whole-cell recording technique. GABA (2 μm) was applied by pressure ejection from blunt-tipped micropipettes positioned adjacent to the neuron. GABA receptor current (A1) was enhanced when diazepam was applied with GABA (A2). GABA receptor current (B1) was also enhanced when GABA was applied with phenobarbital (B2). The equilibrium potential for chloride ions was 0 mV, and therefore the GABA receptor currents were inward (downgoing). (From Twyman et al,[92] p 215, with permission.)

hance GABA$_A$ receptor current at a concentration achieved in ambulatory patients in CSF and in plasma unbound to plasma proteins.[81]

Although both benzodiazepines and barbiturates enhance GABA$_A$ receptor current, they do so by different mechanisms.[89,92] When GABA binds to its receptor and gates open the chloride ion channel, the channel opens and closes rapidly, forming bursts of openings interrupted by brief closures (Fig. 3–6 A and B).[31,54] This bursting behavior of GABA$_A$ receptor channels appears to be a general property of neurotransmitter-gated receptor channels.[10] Benzodiazepines have been demonstrated to increase the frequency of occurrence of these bursting GABA$_A$ receptor currents (Fig.3–6C).[4,86,92] Barbiturates, however, do not modify the frequency of occurrence of bursting GABA$_A$ receptor currents, but instead appear to modify the stability of individual openings (Fig. 3–6D).[53,92] The GABA$_A$ receptor channel bursts are still present, but the openings within the bursts are prolonged and there is more current flow per burst. Thus, benzodiazepines and barbiturates enhance GABA$_A$ receptor currents by binding to different binding sites and by regulating different properties of the GABA$_A$ receptor channel

(Fig. 3–7). This chloride current results in membrane hyperpolarization and, therefore, neuronal inhibition. In many areas of the nervous system, abnormal GABAergic inhibition may underlie the development of seizures, and blockade of inhibition may result in more effective propagation of the seizure discharge to the rest of the nervous system.

Sodium valproate does not bind to GABA$_A$ receptors and does not appear to enhance GABA$_A$ receptor chloride current by a postsynaptic mechanism. Nevertheless, sodium valproate has been demonstrated to increase brain GABA levels. The elevation in brain GABA concentrations may be due to an effect of sodium valproate on enzymes involved in the synthesis and degradation of GABA. Sodium valproate is a weak inhibitor of GABA transaminase and a stronger inhibitor of succinic semialdehyde dehydrogenase. Furthermore, sodium valproate has been shown to activate the major synthetic enzyme glutamic acid decarboxylase. It is thought that this combined action of sodium valproate to enhance GABA synthesis and to block GABA degradation may account for the increase in brain GABA concentrations. Furthermore, this effect of sodium valproate appears to be selective in that the in-

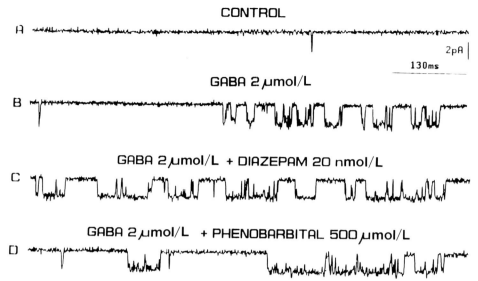

Figure 3–6. Single channel GABA receptor currents were enhanced by diazepam and phenobarbital. Patches of mouse spinal cord neurons in cell culture were removed using the "outside-out" configuration for patch clamp recording. GABA was applied to the excised patches by local pressure ejection. (*A*) Before application of GABA, only rare, brief spontaneous currents were recorded. When channel opening occurred, it produced a downward current deflection. (*B*) Following application of GABA (2 μm), single-channel currents increased in frequency and occurred as single openings or in bursts of openings. (*C*) In the presence of diazepam, GABA evoked increased single channel activity. (*D*) In the presence of phenobarbital, GABA again increased GABA receptor channel activity. Patches were voltage clamped at −75 mV, and chloride equilibrium potential was 0 mV. Diazepam increased the frequency of channel opening without altering the duration of openings, whereas phenobarbital did not increase the frequency of channel openings but evoked longer openings. (From Twyman et al,[92] p 216, with permission.)

crease in GABA levels may occur in GABAergic neuronal terminals rather than in glial cells. Thus, it has been proposed, but not conclusively demonstrated, that sodium valproate may enhance GABAergic transmission by increasing presynaptic GABA stores and by facilitating the release of GABA. This presynaptic mechanism may result in increased GABAergic inhibition.

Effects of Anticonvulsant Drugs on Excitatory Mechanisms

Excitation in the nervous system is produced primarily by the excitatory amino acid glutamate and possibly by aspartate and small depeptide acidic amino acids.[56] (Excitatory amino acid neurotransmission is discussed in Chapter 1.) Glutamate binds to three different receptors, named for agonists that are selective for those receptors: the NMDA receptor, the quisqualate receptor, and the kainate receptor.[16,39,62,93] These three receptors are most probably different proteins with different physiologic and pharmacologic properties. The NMDA receptor operates a channel permeable to Na^+ and Ca^{2+} but showing a voltage-dependent block by Mg^{2+}.[70] The NMDA channel is effectively closed or blocked at large negative potentials by magnesium ions but the block by magnesium ion is relieved when the membrane potential is reduced. The net effect of this is that with strong synaptic depolarization of neurons by excitatory amino acids or by other excitatory neurotransmitters or membrane voltage-dependent conductances, synaptically released excitatory amino acids can now strongly produce further depolarization by opening

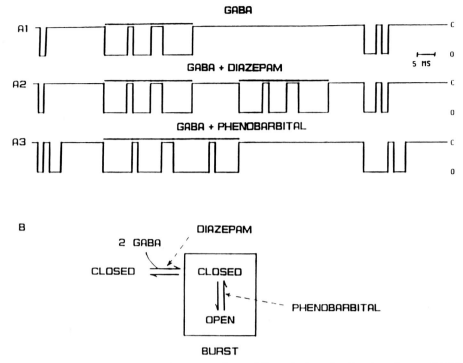

Figure 3 – 7. Barbiturates and benzodiazepines have different sites of action to enhance GABA receptor current. GABA (A_1) evoked frequent channel openings in bursts of one or more openings. Prolonged bursts are overscored. With diazepam (A_2), bursts with long openings were of the same duration but were more frequent, resulting in more GABA receptor current. In the presence of phenobarbital (A_3), bursts were prolonged and consisted of longer single channel openings. In a simplified burst kinetic model for the GABA receptor channel complex (B), two molecules of GABA bind to the receptor to gate open the channel in bursts. Diazepam enhanced GABA binding affinity to increase burst frequency without altering individual GABA receptor bursts. Phenobarbital altered the GABA receptor bursts by prolonging the time spent in the open state. This site of action may be at or near the channel to modify the properties of channel gating. (From Twyman et al,[92] p 219, with permission.)

NMDA receptor channels that are unblocked by magnesium due to the membrane depolarization. NMDA receptors have been strongly implicated in paroxysmal discharge of neurons in hippocampus. It is likely that they are involved in abnormal paroxysmal activity in other areas of the nervous system as well.

The quisqualate and kainate receptors (see Chapter 1) also allow cations to enter cells and do not have the property of voltage dependency produced by magnesium blockade.

None of the conventionally used anticonvulsant drugs appear to affect glutamate receptors at therapeutic concentrations.[52] The only exception to this is

phenobarbital, which has been shown to block glutamate responses in high magnesium solution, an effect probably mediated at the quisqualate receptor.[51,68] Barbiturates do not, however, modify the binding of quisqualate to its receptor at therapeutic plasma concentrations.[38] Sodium valproate does not modify synaptic acidic amino acid responses but has been shown to decrease release of aspartic acid from brain synaptic terminals. It has been suggested, therefore, that sodium valproate may act presynaptically to reduce release of excitatory amino acids. Despite the absence of an action of clinically used anticonvulsant drugs on glutamate receptors, a number of experimental drugs that act on glutamate receptors have an anticonvulsant action in experimental animals. Initially it was shown that competitive NMDA receptor antagonists such as 2-amino phosphonohepano and 2-amino-6-phosphonovalerate[15,64,65] are potent anticonvulsant drugs in rodent and primate models of epilepsy. Similarly, the NMDA channel antagonist MK-801[99] has been shown to be an effective anticonvulsant drug in experimental animals. Whether these anticonvulsant drugs will be of clinical use depends on their effects on NMDA receptors involved in the normal functioning of the brain. NMDA receptors are involved in synaptic plasticity and learning; thus, it is possible that NMDA antagonists will have significant cognitive side effects. It remains an open question whether these anticonvulsant drugs will be of clinical use.

MECHANISTIC CLASSIFICATION OF ANTICONVULSANT DRUGS

The foregoing review suggests that anticonvulsant drugs can be divided on a mechanistic basis into at least three classes, based on their ability to block SRF by enhancing sodium channel inactivation; to enhance GABAergic inhibition; and to block slow, pacemaker-driven repetitive firing by blocking T calcium current (Table 3–6). Type I anticonvulsant drugs such as phenytoin and carbamazepine limit SRF but do not modify GABAergic synaptic transmission or T calcium current. Type II

drugs such as phenobarbital, valproate, and the benzodiazepines have dual actions to enhance GABAergic synaptic transmission and to block SRF, but may or may not alter T calcium current. Type III drugs such as ethosuximide and dimethadione, on the other hand, have no effect on either postsynaptic GABA responses or SRF, but block T calcium currents.

These results further suggest that the ability of a Type I anticonvulsant drug to block generalized tonic-clonic seizures and some forms of partial seizures and to block maximal electroshock seizures in experimental animals may correlate with the ability of the drug to block SRF. On the other hand, the ability of a type II drug to enhance GABAergic synaptic transmission may be one mechanism to block myoclonic seizures and pentylenetetrazol seizures in experimental animals. Whether or not generalized absence seizures are blocked by enhancement of GABAergic inhibition is uncertain but remains a possibility. Type III anticonvulsant drugs may be effective against generalized absence seizures in humans and PTZ seizures in experimental animals due to their effect on T calcium current.

This mechanistic classification of anticonvulsant drugs must remain tentative at the present time as the actions described have not been directly demonstrated to be anticonvulsant in experimental animals. Nonetheless, it is likely that cellular mechanisms such as those demonstrated in in vitro models are important for anticonvulsant efficacy. Further investigation may lead to a classification of these drugs on mechanistic rather than empiric bases.

Table 3–6 ANTICONVULSANT DRUG CLASSIFICATION

Type	Action	Drugs
I	Reduce sodium current	Phenytoin, carbamazepine, primidone
II	Enhance GABA current, reduce sodium current and/or reduce T calcium current	Phenobarbital, sodium valproate, diazepam, clonazepam, lorazepam
III	Reduce T calcium current	Ethosuximide, trimethadione (dimethadione)

CLINICAL USE OF ANTICONVULSANT DRUGS FOR CHRONIC THERAPY

Decision to Initiate and Discontinue Therapy

The relative risks and benefits of anticonvulsant drug therapy should be considered before initiating therapy.[21] Many of the risks of therapy, especially the effects on learning and memory, may be more harmful to the patient than the underlying risk of seizure recurrence (see Chapter 1). Recent epidemiologic studies have defined certain groups of patients with a rather low risk of seizure recurrence after a single unprovoked episode.[33] In these patients, it is prudent to withhold anticonvulsant therapy until additional seizures occur. Similarly, simple febrile convulsions in young children are generally harmless, and chronic anticonvulsant therapy is generally withheld except in unusual circumstances. Follow-up studies have also demonstrated that many children who are seizure-free for several years while on medication remain so after its discontinuation.[36,83] Therefore, most pediatric seizure patients are withdrawn from medication after a seizure-free interval of 2 to 4 years.

Initiating Chronic Anticonvulsant Therapy

Prior to initiation of anticonvulsant drug therapy, routine evaluation of blood elements and liver function should be obtained. A follow-up laboratory evaluation should occur within the first 2 weeks of drug administration and then at increasing intervals during maintenance therapy. The total daily dose and dosing schedule are determined on a milligram-per-kilogram basis to achieve a therapeutic plasma concentration (see Table 3–3). Published therapeutic plasma levels should be considered guidelines and should not be adhered to slavishly. Adequacy of plasma level is primarily determined by therapeutic response in the presence of acceptable or no toxicity. The dosing interval ideally should be one half the plasma half-life (see Chapter 1). Phe-

nytoin can be administered at a higher dose to achieve a more rapid attainment of therapeutic plasma level, but loading should not be attempted with sodium valproate or primidone. Loading with carbamazepine can sometimes be achieved, although vomiting is a frequent side effect. Loading of phenobarbital or clonazepam will be limited by sedative side effects.

In a newly presenting patient, the major goal is to manage the patient with a single appropriate anticonvulsant drug. The patient should be asked to keep a seizure diary so that the number of seizures can be compared to the dosing schedule and plasma levels of the anticonvulsant drug. If the patient cannot be controlled with the selected anticonvulsant drug, it should be increased until mild toxicity is encountered (high-dose monotherapy). If the anticonvulsant drug fails, consideration should be given to the initial diagnosis. Was it a correct diagnosis, does the patient have functional seizures, and is the patient compliant in taking his or her medications? If the answers to these question indicate that the anticonvulsant drug is a failure, a crossover to another anticonvulsant drug should be attempted. The second anticonvulsant drug should be added to the first, and a therapeutic plasma level obtained. The initial anticonvulsant drug should be withdrawn slowly, and high-dose monotherapy with the second anticonvulsant drug should be attempted. If the patient cannot be maintained on a single appropriate anticonvulsant drug, then referral to an epilepsy specialist is warranted for further work-up. Use of more than one anticonvulsant drug simultaneously greatly increases the risk of drug interactions and toxic side effects (Table 3–7).

Therapy for Pregnant Women with Epilepsy

The problems and management of pregnant women with epilepsy has been the subject of considerable discussion and controversy (for review see Yerby[102]). It is clear, however, that mother and fetus are subject to addi-

Table 3–7 SOME ANTICONVULSANT DRUG INTERACTIONS

Anticonvulsant Drugs	Drugs That Raise Its Level	Drugs That Lower Its Level	Raises Levels of	Lowers Level of	Unusual Interactions
Carbamazepine	Erythromycin, cimetidine, calcium channel blockers, isoniazid, propoxyphene	Phenobarbital, phenytoin, primidone	Isoniazid	Phenytoin, warfarin, doxycycline, haloperidol, theophylline	May alter effectiveness of oral contraceptives. May increase neurotoxicity of lithium.
Phenytoin	Choramphenicol, dicumarol, disulfiram, tolbutamide, isoniazid, phenothiazines, diazepam, ethosuximide, phenobarbital, valproate, ethanol, methylphenidate, salicylates, cimetidine, propoxyphene	Carbamazepine, chronic alcohol, reserpine, clonazepam, phenobarbital, valproate		Digoxin, dicumarol, corticosteroids, 50H-chole-calciferol, thyroxine, quinidine	Oral calcium solutions reduce absorption.
Valproate	Salicylates, carbamazepine, dicumarol, ethosuximide	Ethosuximide	Phenobarbital, ethosuximide	Phenytoin, ethosuximide	May produce status with clonazepam and coma with barbiturates.
Primidone, phenobarbital	Valproate, MAO inhibitors, chloramphenicol		Phenytoin	Oral anticoagulants, digoxin, antidepressants, contraceptives, quinidine, griseofulvin, corticosteroids, doxycycline	Enhances effect of alcohol.
Ethosuximide	Valproate	Phenytoin		Griseofulvin	

Source: Adapted from McEvoy[57] and Anon., Neurofax. Ciba-Geigy, 1989, pp 34–35.

tional risks if the mother has epilepsy.[102] Many of these increased risks are due to the administration of anticonvulsant drugs. The general risks of pregnancy to mother and infant include:

1. Seizure frequency during pregnancy is increased 33%.
2. Vaginal bleeding during pregnancy and in the postpartum period is increased 10%.
3. The infant has a 3% risk of developing epilepsy.
4. If no prophylactic vitamin K is given to the mother, there is a 10% risk of perinatal hemorrhage in the infant.

There is a 4% to 6% risk of fetal congenital malformation if anticonvulsant drugs are taken during pregnancy.[102] Most of the commonly used anticonvulsant drugs, including phenytoin,[32] carbamazepine,[40] and valproate[18] have been associated with minor congenital malformations such as dysmorphic facies and distal hypoplasia. Trimethadione[103] has been associated with more severe congenital abnormalities, and therefore should not be given to women of childbearing age.

Valproate in pregnancy has been associated with a teratogenic syndrome described in Chapter 1. Pregnant women taking the drug should be followed using methods to detect spinal dysraphism (e.g., α-fetoprotein and ultrasound).

Primidone may share the potential for teratogenicity of other anticonvulsant drugs, although a strong relationship has not been established. Primidone is distributed into breast milk of nursing mothers, and this may produce a significant plasma level in the infant. There is little evidence that this transfer is harmful under most circumstances, but the infants should be observed for somnolence.

The similarity of the fetal syndromes produced by phenytoin and carbamazepine has led to the suggestion that their mechanism of teratogenicity may be similar. Both drugs are metabolized through the arene oxide pathway to an epoxide intermediate prior to excretion.[47] The severity of the fetal hydantoin syndrome correlates with the activity of epoxide hydrolase, an enzyme used to metabolize epoxides.[7] Because both phenytoin and carbamazepine are metabolized through this common pathway, it is possible that the epoxide intermediate is responsible for the fetal malformations. This suggestion is further supported by the observation that the combination of carbamazepine, phenobarbital, and valproate is particularly teratogenic and is associated with accumulation of carbamazepine epoxide due to inhibition of epoxide hydrolase by valproate acid.[47] Use of multiple anticonvulsant drugs during pregnancy markedly increases the risk for congenital malformations possibly due to combined actions of the drugs to increase epoxide metabolites.

The management of women of childbearing age with epilepsy includes patient education and use of monotherapy prior to conception. The need for the anticonvulsant drug should be confirmed. If the diagnosis is incorrect, then the anticonvulsant drug should be discontinued with an appropriate taper. If the diagnosis is correct, the woman should be acquainted with the risks to the fetus of having generalized seizures during pregnancy and of the risks of taking anticonvulsant drugs. She should be adequately treated with a single appropriate anticonvulsant drug and should take multivitamins. Monitoring of anticonvulsant drug levels should begin prior to conception and should continue during pregnancy because of the tendency of drug levels to fall due to a larger volume of distribution. It should be emphasized that with proper care the majority of women deliver healthy, normal infants.

Therapy for Partial and Generalized Tonic-Clonic Seizures

The drugs that are most useful for simple, partial complex, and generalized tonic-clonic seizures are carbamazepine, phenytoin, and sodium valproate (see Table 3–3). Primidone, though very effective, produces more cognitive side effects than the aforementioned drugs. Phenobarbital and clonazepam are less effective than the other drugs and produce more cognitive side effects, but they are useful in certain complicated patients.

CARBAMAZEPINE

Carbamazepine has become a popular drug for treatment of seizures because of its effectiveness and relative freedom from cognitive side effects.[22,57] In addition to seizures, it is approved for treatment of trigeminal neuralgia. It is also prescribed for a number of other conditions not approved in the labeling, including neuropathic pain, movement disorders, and affective disorders (see Chapters 2, 7, and 9).

Pharmacokinetics and Administration. Carbamazepine (Tegretol) is available in a chewable tablet, a larger tablet for adults, and a suspension. It is slowly but reliably absorbed from the gastrointestinal tract in 2 to 8 hours.[57] The suspension may be absorbed more rapidly than the tablets, and steady-state concentrations are reportedly comparable when the suspension is administered three times a day and tablets are administered twice a day.

The plasma half-life is usually longer at the initiation of therapy (25 to 65 hours) than several weeks later (12 ± 3 hours) because of a tendency for the drug to induce its own metabolism. Metabolism is through oxidation by the liver to form hydroxylated metabolites. Although plasma levels remain fairly steady after initiation of therapy, there is a wide variation in the dose needed to produce a specific plasma concentration. Often the doses needed to produce a therapeutic plasma concentration seem higher in adults (1 to 2 g) than for other anticonvulsant drugs.

Therapy should be initiated with a low dose to avoid side effects including vomiting, diplopia, and ataxia. In children, 10 to 15 mg/kg is a good starting dose, divided two to three times per day.

Individuals older than 12 years of age can be started on 200 mg twice daily. The therapeutic range of plasma concentration is 4 to 12 μg/mL. Dosing with the suspension should be divided into smaller doses than used for tablets. The dose is gradually increased during the first 3 to 4 weeks of therapy to achieve a therapeutic response. As the drug induces its own metabolism over the first weeks of usage, some upward adjustment of dose is usually required to maintain a therapeutic level.

Side Effects and Interactions. Carbamazepine can produce a variety of neurologic side effects at toxic levels. Dizziness, diplopia, and agitation are among the most common. Children with a spike-wave EEG pattern are predisposed to develop exacerbation of atypical absence or generalized convulsive seizures. The most common systemic effects are nausea, vomiting, and abdominal pain, which may be dose related. Leukopenia is fairly common but usually transient and harmless. The risk of aplastic anemia in patients on the drug appears to be five to eight times greater than in general population. A skin rash is a prominent allergic manifestation. Prominent drug interactions (see Table 3–7) occur with calcium channel blockers and erythromycin. Initiation of both verapamil and erythromycin therapy may raise carbamazepine levels into the toxic range within a few days.

PHENYTOIN

Phenytoin is one of the oldest anticonvulsant drugs and is as effective as carbamazepine for most patients.[22,57] A choice between the two drugs is often based on the individual clinician's preferences and/or patient susceptibility to cognitive and cosmetic side effects. Phenytoin has also been used to treat cardiac arrhythmias and trigeminal neuralgia.[57]

Pharmacokinetics and Administration. Phenytoin is available as a capsule, a sustained-release capsule, a chewable tablet, and a suspension for oral administration.[57] Parenteral use is discussed in the section on status epilepticus (see p 109). Although the drug is generally completely and rapidly absorbed, there is great variability in absorption from different preparations and from the same form by different manufacturers. Care should be taken when changing from one preparation to another. Gastrointestinal absorption is erratic in infants younger than 1 year of age, and the drug is very difficult to administer orally at this age.

Phenytoin is metabolized by hydroxylation in the liver, and this process is saturable, as described in Chapter 1. This type of metabolism may cause considerable variation in the blood level achieved by a given dose of drug. Generally a blood level between 10 to 20 μg/mL is effective for reducing seizures. Typically, the dose per kilogram needed to increase the plasma concentration from 10 to 20 μg/mL is lower than the dose needed to achieve a level of 10 μg/mL, especially in children. The half-life of the drug in adults in the midtherapeutic range is approximately 24 hours. In infants and children, however, the half-life is often much shorter, so that once-daily administration is adequate for many adults but children typically maintain a more stable plasma level if the daily dose is divided.

Phenytoin therapy is usually initiated at a dose of 5 to 7 mg/kg per day in adults. In children, the average starting dose is 5 mg/kg per day divided two to three times per day. A therapeutic concentration is generally achieved in a week. In situations in which rapid loading is needed, a loading dose of 20 mg/kg may be given orally, divided during a 4- to 8-hour period. Intravenous loading is described below. Patients being loaded with phenytoin would be monitored for cardiovascular and neurologic condition. After initiation of therapy, the patient's response and plasma drug concentration are used as a guide to dose titration.

Side Effects and Interactions. Phenytoin can cause a wide range of side effects, some of which are dose related (e.g., ataxia, cognitive dulling), and others which probably are not (e.g., hypertrichosis, gingival hyperplasia, lymphadenopathy, rashes). A rare form of liver toxicity may be related to a genetic inability to detoxify metabolites of phenytoin (see Chapter 1). This disorder is a model for other types of genetically determined drug side effects. Phenytoin has a number of interactions with metabolism of drugs, outlined in Table 3–7.

VALPROATE

Valproic acid and its sodium salt, valproate, are the anticonvulsant drugs with the widest spectrum of activity against generalized tonic-clonic and absence seizures. Valproate is valued for its broad activity and relative freedom from cognitive side effects, but gastrointestinal and hepatic toxicity have limited its use.[22,57]

Pharmacokinetics and Administration. Liquid valproic acid, valproate sodium capsules, and enteric-coated divalproex sodium (Depakote) tablets are available. The enteric-coated form is a complex of sodium valproate and valproic acid, which are absorbed in the small intestine. Sodium valproate is converted to valproic acid before it is absorbed (about 4 hours). Absorption of the enteric-coated tablets takes about 2 hours longer. The half-life of valproate is approximately 8 to 12 hours, and the drug is metabolized by first-order kinetics. Doses of 10 to 30 mg/kg generally produce plasma levels in the therapeutic range of 50 to 100 μg/mL. Valproate is generally started at a dose of 10 to 15 mg/kg per day, and the dose is increased at 1- to 2-week intervals in increments of 5 to 10 mg/kg to achieve a therapeutic effect. The top dose is generally 60 mg/kg per day, but higher doses have been used safely.

Side Effects and Interactions. The most frequent side effects are nausea, vomiting, and gastroesophageal reflux. This can be minimized by slowly increasing the dose, administering with meals, and by using the enteric-coated preparation.[57] Severe CNS depression has been reported when valproate is combined with other depressants, but cognitive function is usually preserved when the drug is used alone. The most malignant side effect is hepatic necrosis, discussed in Chapter 1. This rare effect may be related to production of toxic metabolites in susceptible individuals, especially children. Minor elevation in amino transferases and serum ammonia are relatively common, with little clinical significance. Decreased platelet adhesiveness and prolonged bleeding time have been described, and at high doses, peripheral edema and tremor may occur.

Administration of valproate together with phenobarbital routinely leads to an increase in the plasma concentration of phenobarbital. Valproate generally causes a reduction in plasma levels of phenytoin (see Table 3–7). An interaction between clonazepam and valproate to cause absence status epilepticus has been described, but often the drugs have been used safely together.

PRIMIDONE

Primidone (Mysoline) is an effective barbiturate-type anticonvulsant drug, but its use is limited by its cognitive and motor side effects. Its primary use is as an additional drug in complex patients such as those with severe partial complex seizures.[22,57]

Pharmacokinetics and Administration. Primidone is absorbed in about 4 hours and is metabolized by the liver into two metabolites, phenylethylmalonamide (PEMA) and phenobarbital.[57] The approximate half-life of primidone is 10 to 20 hours, and the half-life of PEMA is 10 to 24 hours. The half-life of phenobarbital is from 2 to 4 days. PEMA has relatively weak anticonvulsant activity so that the primary anticonvulsant effect is mediated by primidone and phenobarbital. In newborn infants, little of the primidone is metabolized to phenobarbital, and the drug is an effective anticonvulsant with relatively few

side effects. Phenobarbital may be administered to supplement the phenobarbital metabolized from primidone in certain situations. To avoid phenobarbital toxicity, however, this combination usually should not be used.

Primidone should be started cautiously because of the high incidence of side effects in patients who have not received the drug. A typical starting dose in children is 2 to 5 mg/kg in divided doses, advancing to a maintenance dose of 10 to 25 mg/kg. A target effective plasma concentration of 12 mg/mL is generally aimed for. A typical adult dose is 100 mg at bedtime for 3 days, followed by 100 mg twice a day for a week and 100 mg three times daily for another week, and a maintenance dose of 10 to 15 mg/kg per day administered daily in three divided doses.

Side Effects and Interaction. The most common side effects are drowsiness, ataxia, lethargy, nausea, and vomiting. Ataxia and vertigo are particularly likely to occur with administration of this drug, but they tend to diminish with continued use. Other side effects may include skin rashes and hematologic reactions. Interactions with other drugs are similar to those produced by phenobarbital.

PHENOBARBITAL

Phenobarbital and related compounds such as mephobarbital and primidone are among the oldest and safest anticonvulsant drugs. Phenobarbital is especially useful for controlling seizures in infants because other anticonvulsant drugs are more difficult to use at this age. The popularity of barbiturate anticonvulsant drugs has waned, however, because of their propensity to produce cognitive dulling and depression in susceptible individuals.

Pharmacokinetics and Administration. Phenobarbital is completely absorbed, and peak blood concentrations are reached within 8 to 12 hours. The half-life is among the longest of the anticonvulsant drugs, ranging from 2 to 3 days in children to 3 to 4 days in adults. The dosage is linearly related to the blood level throughout a broad range of plasma concentrations. The usual oral dose of phenobarbital is 3 to 5 mg/kg in young children. In adults, the general starting dose is approximately 1 mg/kg with the maintenance dose being about 2 to 3 mg/kg per day administered in a single daily dose. Children require more on a milligram per kilogram basis than adults. A plasma phenobarbital concentration of 10 to 20 μg/mL or higher is generally therapeutic, and the drug may be safely used up to a plasma concentration of approximately 40 μg/mL. Even blood levels of 60 μg/mL or higher may be used in acutely ill patients with careful monitoring of the cardiorespiratory system.[14] In these cases, the drug may be administered intramuscularly and intravenously, as described in the section below on status epilepticus.

Side Effects and Interactions. The principal adverse effect of phenobarbital is to diminish memory and learning. School performance of children taking phenobarbital should be monitored carefully. Older patients who take phenobarbital may be susceptible to confusion and depression. High doses of phenobarbital used to control status epilepticus may produce cardiorespiratory depression. In addition, the drug may produce a variety of rashes and allergic phenomena including the Stevens-Johnson syndrome. Valproate routinely increases the plasma concentration of phenobarbital by approximately 50%. Barbiturates tend to decrease the blood levels of oral anticoagulants, digoxin, and a variety of other drugs by activating the mixed-function oxidase drug-metabolizing enzymes (see Table 3–7).

Therapy for Absence Seizures

Absence seizures produce brief lapses in consciousness, which may recur many times throughout the day. The primary drugs use to treat absence seizures are ethosuximide and valproate.[22] Ethosuximide remains the primary drug, especially in children, because of the higher risk of hepatotoxicity and other side effects during therapy with valproate. Valproate is especially valuable for patients with both generalized tonic-clonic and absence seizures, however.

ETHOSUXIMIDE

Pharmacokinetics and Administration. Ethosuximide is available in capsules and oral solution.[57] The drug is generally absorbed from the gastrointestinal tract in about 4 hours, and the drug is metabolized with a half-life of about 30 hours in children and 60 hours in adults. Because of its long half-life, it can be administered once a day, and a typical dose for a child 3 to 6 years of age is 250 mg at bedtime. The dose is usually titrated to eliminate the absence seizures, which are usually quite obvious. The starting dose in adults should be 20 mg/kg per day. A typical maintenance dose is about 15 to 40 mg/kg per day, and a target plasma concentration is in the range of 40 to 100 μg/mL; however, levels up to 150 μg/mL may be required. When beginning the medication, the dose should be adjusted cautiously because some patients experience nausea and vomiting at the initiation of therapy.

Side Effects and Interaction. Ethosuximide is relatively benign. The most common side effects are gastrointestinal symptoms of anorexia, weight loss, gastric upset, cramps, and abdominal pain, especially at the initiation of therapy. The drug may produce a number of other hematologic and immune-mediated side effects.

VALPROATE

The use of valproate for absence seizure is similar to its use for other seizures described previously.

Therapy for
Myoclonic Seizures

Myoclonic seizure disorders comprise a varied combination of problems. Drugs that are particularly effective for myoclonic seizures include clonazepam, valproate, phenobarbital (to some extent), and other less commonly used anticonvulsant drugs such as adrenocorticotropic hormone (ACTH).[22] The mechanism of action of ACTH in myoclonic seizure disorders is not well understood. Valproate has already been described and only clonazepam will be considered here. Children with myoclonic seizure disorders have an unusually high incidence of underlying metabolic disorders, and this group tends to be more refractory than those with other forms of epilepsy.

CLONAZEPAM

Pharmacokinetics and Administration. Clonazepam is generally well absorbed from the gastrointestinal tract and is generally metabolized with an apparent half-life of 12 to 40 hours.[57] The drug is converted by the liver to several metabolites, some of which have anticonvulsant activity. Although therapeutic blood levels for clonazepam and other benzodiazepines have been published, there is little reliable evidence of a good relationship between blood level and therapeutic effect. Titration of clonazepam is usually performed by increasing the dose and monitoring the clinical effect rather than by using blood levels.

The drug is available in tablets. A typical initial dose for infants and children is 0.01 to 0.03 mg/kg administered two to three divided doses. The dosage is generally increased by 0.25 to 0.5 mg every 3 to 4 days until seizure control or side effects are observed. Children typically tolerate up to 0.2 mg/kg. The adult dosage typically is between 1 to 1.5 mg daily, and the dose is titrated upward every few days to a maximum of approximately 20 mg or until a therapeutic effect is noted.

Side Effects and Interactions. The primary side effects of clonazepam are sedation, drowsiness, hypotonia, and ataxia. In children, it is rather common to see increased aggressiveness and irritability. In addition, the drug may have several other side effects such as drooling and hypersecretion in the upper respiratory tract. The drooling may be related to reduced activity of the swallowing mechanism. A variety of other hematologic and skin manifestations have been reported. The drug has been reported to produce absence status epilepticus when used with valproate in certain patients, but clinical experience suggests that this effect may be infrequent. The possibility of toxic overdose needs to be considered with this drug as well as with the barbiturate drugs, because of its potential to depress the cardiorespiratory system.

THERAPY FOR
STATUS EPILEPTICUS

Status epilepticus has been defined as a condition characterized by "epileptic seizures that are so frequently repeated or so prolonged as to create a fixed and lasting condition".[45] The actual definition of the point at which sequential seizures become status epilepticus is often unclear, but seizures lasting longer than 30 minutes are typically put in this category.[17] The most serious form is generalized tonic-clonic status epilepticus, but absence status, partial complex, and simple partial status epilepticus and epilepsia partialis continua are frequently observed. Status epilepticus, especially when it is prolonged for more than 1 hour, is associated with significant medical and neurologic morbidity. This morbidity may be related to (1) primary damage to the CNS by excessive excitation, (2) brain injury from systemic metabolic alterations from status epilepticus, and (3) the damage produced by the underlying process producing status epilepticus.[49] Generally, the morbidity of status epilepticus is closely associated with the seriousness of the underlying condition. For example, status epilepticus in the setting of hypoxic ischemic encephalopathy or herpes encephalitis generally has a poorer outcome than status epilepticus associated with fever in children or with drug withdrawal.

In the treatment of status epilepticus, it is important to provide adequate but not overzealous therapy.[17,45] In particular, it is important to guard cardiorespiratory functioning during the period when potentially depressing drugs are being administered. A suggested protocol for treatment of status epilepticus in adults is shown in Table 3–8. The major components of successful therapy include attention to the airway, cardiorespiratory function, and metabolic factors such as adequate serum glucose, along with adequate anticonvulsant therapy. The primary drugs used in adults are intravenous phenytoin and a benzodiazepine, either lorazepam or diazepam. In children, especially infants, phenobarbital is used more commonly as a primary drug for status epilepticus. For both adults and children, pentobarbital coma is used to terminate seizures that have been refractory to other therapies. Several other drugs have been used for status epilepticus

but are not considered here in detail. For example, paraldehyde infused as a 4% solution in the dose of 0.12 to 3.0 mL/kg over 15 to 30 minutes has been used but is limited by cardiovascular side effects. Similarly, lidocaine given as a 50- to 100-mg intravenous bolus followed by an infusion of 1 to 2 mg/kg has been used, but its tendency to produce toxic CNS side effects has limited its popularity. Valproate has also been given rectally for status epilepticus but has a rather slow onset of action.

Phenytoin

Phenytoin is an excellent drug for treatment of status epilepticus because of its relative lack of sedative effects. It is generally administered in a loading dose of 18 to 20 mg/kg intravenously. The drug is not absorbed reliably after intramuscular injection. Phenytoin should be diluted to 5 mg/mL or less in normal saline solution and infused at a rate of not greater than 50 mg/min. Cardiovascular monitoring should be performed because the diluent, propylene glycol, is cardiotoxic. This loading dose results in a peak plasma concentration of approximately 25 μg/mL at the end of

Table 3–8 PROTOCOL FOR EMERGENCY TREATMENT OF STATUS EPILEPTICUS IN ADULTS

0–5 min	Assessment	
	Airway management	
	Blood draw:	Drug levels
		Glucose
		Toxic screen
		BUN, electrolytes
5–10 min	Start IV infusion	
	Administer:	Glucose (25 g)
		B vitamins
10–30 min	Lorazepam:	4–8 mg IV
		or
	Diazepam:	10–20 mg IV
		and
	Phenytoin:	20 mg/kg IV in <5 mg/mL solution in normal saline; rate of 50 mg/min with cardiac and blood pressure monitoring.
30–60 min	If seizures persist:	Phenobarbital 10 mg/kg IV at 100 mg/min. May repeat 2–3 times if airway is secure.
>1 h	Consider pentobarbital coma, general anesthesia	

Source: Adapted from Davies et al[16] and Kalant and Grose.[41]

the infusion and a half-life in range from 12 to 24 hours.[6] In children, the half-life tends to be shorter after intravenous administration than after oral administration, and the maintenance dose (approximately 5 mg/kg per day) should be started at approximately 12 hours. A phenytoin prodrug (ACC-9653) is being developed to overcome some of the problems with parenteral phenytoin.[45] This drug can be injected intramuscularly and is rapidly converted into phenytoin in the body. It also can be injected intravenously with fewer reactions at the injection site than phenytoin. In children, phenytoin is generally well tolerated, although the half-life can be much shorter than the typical 24-hour half life in adults.

Benzodiazepines

The primary benzodiazepines used for status epilepticus are diazepam and lorazepam.[91] Both drugs are quite active in abolishing status epilepticus, although their effects may be short-lived. They are quite sedating and may produce respiratory depression, especially when combined with barbiturate anticonvulsant drugs. In adults, a dose of 10 to 20 mg of diazepam or 4 to 8 mg of lorazepam is used.[6,45] In children, doses of diazepam of 0.3 mg/kg and of lorazepam of 0.03 to 0.05 mg/kg may be used.[48] Repeated higher doses of benzodiazepines may be used to stop seizures if careful monitoring and respiratory support are provided. Although human studies suggest little difference between the two drugs with respect to their ability to stop status epilepticus, lorazepam's more prolonged duration in the plasma may be an advantage.[91] The drug is less lipid soluble than diazepam, so that the fall in plasma level due to redistribution after administration is less than for diazepam.[6] The use of either drug should be followed by the infusion of an anticonvulsant drug with prolonged action, such as phenytoin or phenobarbital.

Phenobarbital

Phenobarbital has been used intramuscularly and intravenously for status epilepticus and is effective and relatively safe when adequate monitoring is performed.[6,45,58] The major drawback is prolonged sedation after high doses. It is the primary drug used for treatment of infants. The initial dose is usually 10 mg/kg and additional boluses may be given, to a total of approximately 40 mg/kg. This dose leads to a plasma concentration of approximately 40 μg/mL in most patients. Even higher doses may be used to control status epilepticus, although in infants, levels approaching 60 μg/mL are associated with cardiac depression.[14] In the suggested protocol for treatment of status epilepticus in adults (see Table 3–8), phenobarbital is a secondary drug after the patient has been given phenytoin and a benzodiazepine. The maintenance dose of phenobarbital is dependent on the desired blood level.

Pentobarbital Coma

Pentobarbital coma effectively produces cortical suppression for refractory status epilepticus.[45,48] Generally this therapy is reserved for patients who continue in status epilepticus after receiving maximal tolerated doses of benzodiazepines, phenytoin, and phenobarbital. Patients with seizures that have continued for more than 1 hour are thought to be at greater risk for brain injury and are potential candidates for this therapy. Induction of pentobarbital coma should be performed only by individuals trained in critical-care neurology and/or anesthesia in an intensive-care setting. A suggested protocol for pentobarbital coma is shown in Table 3–9.[45] Generally, the pentobarbital loading is titrated to cause a burst suppression pattern on the EEG. In children, a loading dose of 8 mg/kg of pentobarbital as a bolus has been used, followed by a continuous pentobarbital infusion of 3 mg/kg per hour.[48] EEG is

Table 3–9 PROTOCOL FOR PENTOBARBITAL COMA IN REFRACTORY STATUS EPILEPTICUS

Preparation:	Intubate and mechanically ventilate in intensive care unit
	Cardiovascular and EEG monitoring
Loading dose:	5–8 mg/kg IV bolus
	Supplement with 25–50 mg every 5 min to produce EEG burst suppression
Maintenance:	3–5 mg/kg per h
Plasma therapeutic concentrations:	25–50 μg/mL

used to monitor patients as they emerge from coma. This therapy is associated with several potential adverse effects, especially if the patient has other organ system dysfunction such as renal failure. Although this therapy is in common use, its efficacy for altering the outcome of status epilepticus has not definitely been proved.

CONCLUSION

Most anticonvulsant drugs were discovered serendipitously and their clinical role has been defined empirically. Recent evidence reviewed in this chapter indicates that there are four major mechanisms whereby these drugs exert their anticonvulsant effects. Three of these mechanisms are used by current anticonvulsant drugs and the fourth, modulation of excitatory neurotransmission, is a potential mechanism for future anticonvulsant drugs. The antiepileptic drugs in current use appear to exert their effect by (1) reduction of sodium currents across neuronal membranes, (2) reduction of transient T calcium currents, and (3) enhancement of GABAergic inhibition. The anticonvulsant drugs can be grouped according to their mechanism of action. Drugs that are effective for partial and generalized tonic-clonic seizures (carbamazepine, phenytoin, and primidone) preferentially and selectively reduce sodium currents. In contrast, drugs that preferentially reduce transient T calcium currents, such as ethosuximide, are selectively effective for absence seizures. Drugs such as sodium valproate, which

is active against both generalized tonic-clonic seizures and absence seizures, the benzodiazepines, and phenobarbital have a mixed spectrum of activity. They are also active against myoclonic seizures. These drugs act by a combination of several mechanisms of action including enhancement of GABAergic currents, reduction in sodium currents, and reduction in transient T calcium currents. The correlations between mechanisms of action and clinical activity provide a basis for thinking about therapy with current drugs and planning new therapeutic strategies.

Current principles for the use of anticonvulsant drugs minimize the use of any drugs unless absolutely necessary and restrict the number of patients placed on two or more anticonvulsant drugs. Recent research has also suggested guidelines for discontinuation of anticonvulsant drugs in patients who are at low risk for seizure recurrence. A persistent and troubling side effect of anticonvulsant drugs is their effect on learning and memory. This problem is especially important in children, and future work is needed to overcome it. Progress is also needed in therapy for refractory partial complex epilepsy and status epilepticus.

REFERENCES

1. Aghajanian, GK and Wang, YY: Pertussis toxin blocks the outward currents evoked by opiate and α_2-agonists in locus coeruleus neurons. Brain Res 371:390–394, 1986.
2. Andrade, R, Malenka, RC, and Nicoll,

RA: A G protein couples serotonin and GABA$_B$ receptors to the same channels in hippocampus. Science 234:1261–1265, 1986.

3. Blaustein, MP and Ector, AC: Barbiturate inhibition of calcium uptake by depolarized nerve terminals in vitro. Mol Pharmacol 11:369–378, 1975.

4. Bormann, J: Electrophysiology of GABA$_A$ and GABA$_B$ receptor subtypes. Trends in Neuroscience 11:112–116, 1988.

5. Bowery, NG, Doble, A, Hill, DR, Hudson, AL, Middlemiss, DN, Shaw, J, and Turnball, MJ: (−)-baclofen decreases neurotransmitter release in the mammalian CNS by an action at a novel GABA receptor. Nature 283:92–94, 1980.

6. Browne, TR: The pharmacokinetics of agents used to treat status epilepticus. Neurology 40(Suppl 2):28–32, 1990.

7. Buehler, BA: Epoxide hydrolase activity in fibroblasts: Correlation with clinical features of the fetal hydantoin syndrome. Proceedings of the Greenwood Genetic Center 6:117, 1987.

8. Chavkin, C, James, IF, and Goldstein, A: Dynorphin is a specific endogenous ligand of the κ opioid receptor. Science 215:413–415, 1982.

9. Choi, DW, Farb, DH, and Fischbach, GD: Chlordiazepoxide selectively augments GABA action in spinal cord cell cultures. Nature 269:342–344, 1977.

10. Colquhoun, D and Sakmann, B: Fast events in single-channel currents activated by acetylcholine and its analogues at the frog muscle endplate. J Physiol (Lond) 369:501–557, 1985.

11. Coulter, DA, Hugenard, JR, and Prince, DA: Anticonvulsants depress calcium spikes and calcium currents of mammalian thalamic neurons in vitro. Society of Neuroscience Abstracts 14:262, 1988.

12. Courtney, KR and Etter, EF: Modulated anticonvulsant block of sodium channels in nerve and muscle. Eur J Pharmacol 88:1–9, 1983.

13. Courtney, KR: Mechanism of frequency-dependent inhibition of sodium currents in myelinated nerve by the lidocaine derivative GEA 968. J Pharmacol Exp Ther 195:225–236, 1975.

14. Crawford, TO, Mitchell, WG, Fishman, LS, and Snodgrass, SR: Very high dose phenobarbital for refractory status epilepticus in children. Neurology 38:1035–1050, 1988.

15. Croucher, MJ, Collins, JF, and Meldrum, BS: Anticonvulsant action of excitatory amino acid antagonists. Science 216:899–901, 1982.

16. Davies, JD, Evens, RH, Francis, AA, et al: Conformational aspects of the actions of some piperidine dicarboxylic acids at excitatory amino acid receptors in the mammalian and amphibian spinal cord. Neurochem Res 7:1119–1133, 1982.

17. Delgado-Escueta, AV, Wasterlain, C, Treiman, DM, and Porter, RJ: Management of status epilepticus. N Engl J Med 306:1337–1340, 1982.

18. DiLiberti, JH, Farndon, PA, Dennis, NR, and Curry, CJ: The fetal valproate syndrome. Am J Med Genet 19:473–481, 1984.

19. Dunlap, K and Fischbach, GD: Neurotransmitters decrease the calcium component of sensory neurone action potentials. Nature 276:837–839, 1978.

20. Dunlap, K: Two types of γ-aminobutyric acid receptor on embryonic sensory neurones. Br J Pharmacol 74:579–585, 1981.

21. Eadie, MJ and Tyrer, JH: Anticonvulsant Therapy: Pharmacological Basis and Practice. Churchill Livingstone, New York, 1980.

22. Engel, J: Seizures and Epilepsy. FA Davis, Philadelphia, 1989.

23. Esplin, D: Effect of diphenylhydantoin on synaptic transmission in the cat spinal cord and stellate ganglion. J Pharmacol Exp Ther 120:301–323, 1957.

24. Ewald, DA, Sternweis, PC, and Miller, RJ: Guanine nucleotide-binding protein Go-induced coupling of neuropeptide Y receptors to Ca2$^+$ channels in sensory neurons. Proc Natl Acad Sci USA 85:3633–3637, 1988.

25. Ferrendelli, JA and Daniels McQueen, S: Comparative actions of phenytoin and other anticonvulsant drugs on potassium- and veratridine-stimulated calcium uptake in synaptosomes. J Pharmacol Exp Ther 220:29–34, 1982.

26. Gilman, AG: G proteins and dual con-

trol of adenylate cyclase. Cell 36:577–579, 1986.

27. Grenningloh, G, Rienitz, A, Schmitt, B, Methfessel, C, Zensen, M, Beyreuther, K, Gundelfinger, ED, and Betz, H: The strychnine-binding subunit of the glycine receptor shows homology with nicotinic acetylcholine receptors. Nature 328:215–220, 1987.

28. Gross, RA and Macdonald, RL: Barbiturates and nifedipine have different and selective effects on calcium currents of mouse DRG neurons in culture: A possible basis for differing clinical actions. Neurology 18:443–451, 1987.

29. Gross, RA and Macdonald, RL: Differential actions of pentobarbitone on calcium current components of mouse sensory neurones in culture. J Physiol (Lond) 405:187–203, 1988.

30. Gross, RA, Kelly, KM, and Macdonald, RL: Ethosuximide and dimethidione selectively reduce calcium currents in cultured sensory neurons by different mechanisms. Neurology 39:(Suppl 1), 412, 1989.

31. Hamill, OP, Bormann, J, and Sakmann, B: Activation of multiple-conductance state chloride channels in spinal neurons by glycine and GABA. Nature 305:805–808, 1983.

32. Hanson, JW, Myrianthopoulos, NC, Harvey, MA, and Smith, DW: Risks to the offspring of women treated with hydantoin anticonvulsants, with emphasis on the fetal hydantoin syndrome. J Pediatr 89:662–668, 1976.

33. Hauser, WA: Should people be treated after a first seizure? Arch Neurol 43:1287–1288, 1986.

34. Hershkowitz, N and Raines, A: Effects of carbamazepine on muscle spindle discharges. J Pharmacol Exp Ther 204:581–591, 1978.

35. Hille, B: Hydrophilic and hydrophobic pathways for the drug-receptor reaction. J Gen Physiol 69:497–515, 1977.

36. Holowach Thurston, J, Thurston, DL, Hixon, BB, and Keller, A: Prognosis in childhood epilepsy. Additional followup of 148 children 15–23 years after withdrawal of anticonvulsant therapy. N Engl J Med 306:831–836, 1982.

37. Holz, GG, Rane, SG, and Dunlap, K:

GTP binding proteins mediate transmitter inhibition of voltage-dependent calcium channels. Nature 319:670–672, 1986.

38. Honore, T, Davies, SN, Drejer, J, Fletcher, EJ, Jacobsen, P, Lodge, D, and Nielsen, FE: Quinoxalinediones: Potent competitive non-NMDA glutamate receptor antagonists. Science 241:701–703, 1988.

39. Jones, AW, Smith, DAS, and Watkins, JC: Structure-activity relations of dipeptide antagonists of excitatory amino acids. Neuroscience 13:573–581, 1984.

40. Jones, KL, Lacro, RV, Johnson, KA, and Adams, J: Pattern of malformations in the children of women treated with carbamazepine during pregnancy. N Engl J Med 320:1661–1666, 1989.

41. Kalant, H and Grose, W: Effects of ethanol and pentobarbital on release of acetylcholine and from cerebral cortex slices. J Pharmacol Exp Ther 158:386–393, 1967.

42. Kelly, K, Gross, RA, and Macdonald, RL: Valproic acid and its 22-en metabolite selectively reduce the T calcium current component in sensory neurons. Neurology 40(Suppl): 329, 1990.

43. Khodorov, BI: Sodium inactivation and drug-induced immobilization of the gating charge in nerve membrane. Prog Biophys Mol Biol 37:49–89, 1981.

44. Leslie, SW, Friedman, MB, and Coleman, RR: Effects of chlordiazepoxide on depolarization-induced calcium influx into synaptosomes. Biochem Pharmacol 29:2439–2443, 1980.

45. Leppik, I: Status epilepticus: The next decade. Neurology 40(Suppl 2):4–8, 1990.

46. Levitan, ES, Schofield, PR, Burt, DR, Rhee, LM, Wisden, W, Kohler, M, Norihisa, J, Rodriguez, HF, Stephenson, A, Darlison, MG, Barnard, EA, and Seeburg, PH: Structural and functional basis for GABA$_A$ receptor heterogeneity. Nature 335:76–79, 1988.

47. Lindhout, D, Hoppener, RJ, and Meinardi, H: Teratogenicity of antiepileptic drug combinations with special emphasis on epoxidation (of carbamazepine). Epilepsia 25:77–83, 1984.

48. Lockman, LA: Treatment of status epilepticus in children. Neurology 40 (Suppl 2):43–46, 1990.

49. Lothman, E: The biochemical basis and pathophysiology of status epilepticus. Neurology 40(Suppl 2):13–23, 1990.

50. Macdonald, RL and Barker, JL: Benzodiazepines specifically modulate GABA-mediated postsynaptic inhibition in cultured mammalian neurones. Nature 271:563–564, 1978.

51. Macdonald, RL and Barker, JL: Different actions of anticonvulsant and anesthetic barbiturates revealed by use of cultured mammalian neurons. Science 200:775–777, 1978.

52. Macdonald, RL and McLean, MJ: Anticonvulsant drugs: Mechanisms of action. In Delgado-Escueta, AV, Ward, AA, Jr, Woodbury, DM, and Porter, RJ, (eds): Advances in Neurology, Vol 44. Raven Press, New York, 1986, pp 713–736.

53. Macdonald, RL, Rogers, CJ, and Twyman, RE: Kinetic properties of the GABA$_A$ receptor main conductance state of mouse spinal cord neurones in culture. J Physiol (Lond) 410:479–499, 1989.

54. Macdonald, RL, Rogers, CJ, and Twyman, RE: Barbiturate regulation of kinetic properties of the main conductance state of the GABA$_A$ receptor channel of mouse spinal cord neurones in culture. J Physiol (Lond) 417:483–500, 1989.

55. Matsuki, N, Quandt, FN, Ten Eick, RE, and Yeh, JZ: Characterization of the block of sodium channels by phenytoin in mouse neuroblastoma cells. J Pharmacol Exp Ther 228:523–530, 1984.

56. Mayer, ML and Westbrook, GL: The physiology of excitatory amino acids in the vertebrate central nervous system. Prog Neurobiol 28:197–276, 1987.

57. McEvoy, GK: AHFS Drug Information. American Society of Hospital Pharmacists, Bethesda, MD, 1989, pp 1076–1106.

58. McLean, MJ and Macdonald, RL: Multiple actions of phenytoin on mouse spinal cord neurons cell culture. J Pharmacol Exp Ther 227:779–789, 1983.

59. McLean, MJ and Macdonald, RL: Sodium valproate, but not ethosuximide, produces use- and voltage-dependent limitation of high frequency repetitive firing of action potentials of mouse central neurons in cell culture. J Pharmacol Exp Ther 237:1001–1011, 1986.

60. McLean, MJ and Macdonald, RL: Carbamazepine and 10,11-epoxycarbamazepine produce use- and voltage-dependent limitation of rapidly firing action potentials of mouse central neurons in cell culture. J Pharmacol Exp Ther 238:727–738, 1986.

61. McLean, MJ and Macdonald, RL: Benzodiazepines, but not beta carbolines, limit high frequency repetitive firing of action potentials of spinal cord neurons in cell culture. J Pharmacol Exp Ther 244:789–795, 1988.

62. McLennan, J: Receptors for excitatory amino acids in the mammalian central nervous system. Prog Neurobiol 20: 251–271, 1983.

63. Meiners, BA and Salama, AI: Enhancement of benzodiazepine and GABA binding by the novel anxiolytic, tracazolate. Eur J Pharmacol 78:315–322, 1982.

64. Meldrum, BS, Croucher, MJ, Czuczwar, SJ, Collins, JF, Curry, K, Joseph, M, and Stone, TW: A comparison of the anticonvulsant potency of +2-amino-5-phosphonopentanoic acid and +2-amino-7-phosphonohepatanoic acid. Neuroscience 9:925–930, 1983.

65. Meldrum, BS, Croucher, MJ, Badman, G, and Collins, JF: Anticonvulsant action of excitatory amino acid antagonists in the photosensitive baboon, Papio Papio. Neurosci Lett 39:101–104, 1983.

66. Mitchell, PR and Martin, IL: The effects of benzodiazepines on K$^+$-stimulated release of GABA. Neuropharmacology 17:317–320, 1978.

67. Newberry, NR and Nicoll, RA: Comparison of the action of baclofen with γ-aminobutyric acid on rat hippocampal pyramidal cells in vitro. J Physiol (Lond) 265:465–488, 1985.

68. Nicoll, RA: Pentobarbital: Action on frog montoneurons. Brain Res 96:119–123, 1975.

69. North, RA: Receptors on individual neurones. Neuroscience 17:899–907, 1986.

70. Nowak, L, Bregostovski, P, Ascher, P, Herbert, A, and Prochiantz, A: Magnesium gates glutamate-activated channels in mouse central neurones. Nature 307:462–465, 1984.

71. Nowycky, MC, Fox, AP, and Tsien, RW: Three types of neural calcium channels with different calcium agonist sensitivity. Nature 316:440–443, 1985.

72. Olsen, RW, Bureau, M, Ransom, RW, Deng, L, Dilber, A, Smith, G, Krestchatisky, M, and Tobin, AJ: The GABA receptor-chloride ion channel protein complex. In Kito, S, et al (eds): Neuroreceptors and Signal Transduction. Plenum Press, New York, 1988, pp 1–14.

73. Olsen, RW and Snowman, AM: Chloride-dependent enhancement by barbiturates of γ-aminobutyric acid receptor binding. J Neurosci 2:1812–1823, 1982.

74. Olsen, RW and Venter, JC (eds): Benzodiazepine/GABA receptors and chloride channels: Structure and functional properties. In Receptor Biochemistry and Methodology, Vol 5. Alan R Liss, New York, 1986, p 15.

75. Ondrusek, MG, Belknap, JK, and Leslie, SW: Effects of acute and chronic barbiturate administration on synaptosomal calcium accumulation. Mol Pharmacol 15:386–395, 1979.

76. Polc, P, Bonetti, EP, Shaffner, R, and Haefely, W: A three-state model of the benzodiazepine receptor explains the interactions between the benzodiazepine antagonist Ro 15-1788, benzodiazepine tranquilizers, β-carbolines and phenobarbitone. Naunyn-Schmiedeberg's Archives of Pharmacology 321:260–264, 1982.

77. Pritchett, DB, Sontheimer, H, Shivers, BD, Ymer, S, Kettenmann, H, Schofield, PR, and Seeburg, PH: Importance of a novel GABA$_A$ receptor subunit for benzodiazepine pharmacology. Nature 338:582–585, 1989.

78. Raines, A and Standaert, FG: Pre- and post-junctional effects of DPH at the cat soleus neuromuscular junction. J Pharmacol Exp Ther 153:361–366, 1966.

79. Richter, JA and Waller, MB: Effects of pentobarbital on the regulation of acetylcholine content and release in different regions of rat brain. Biochem Pharmacol 26:609–615, 1977.

80. Schofield, PR, Darlison, MG, Fujita, N, Burt, DR, Stephenson, FA, Rodriguez, H, Rhee, LM, Ramachandran, J, Reale, V, Glencorse, TA, Seeburg, PH, and Barnard, EA: Sequence and functional expression of the GABA$_A$ receptor shows a ligand-gated receptor super-family. Nature 328:221–227, 1987.

81. Schulz, DW and Macdonald, RL: Barbiturate enhancement of GABA-mediated inhibition and activation of chloride ion conductance: Correlation with anticonvulsant and anesthetic actions. Brain Res 209:177–188, 1981.

82. Scott, RH and Dolphin, AC: Regulation of calcium currents by a GTP analogue: Potentiation of baclofen-mediated inhibition. Neurosci Lett 69:59–64, 1986.

83. Shinnar, S, Vining, SPG, Mellits, ED, DiSouza, BJ, Holden, K, Baumgardner, RA, and Freeman, JM: Discontinuing anticonvulsant medication in children with epilepsy after two years without seizures: A prospective study. N Engl J Med 313:976–980, 1985.

84. Skerritt, JH and Macdonald, RL: Benzodiazepine receptor ligand actions on GABA responses. Benzodiazepines, CL 218872, Zopiclone. Eur J Pharmacol 101:127–134, 1984.

85. Skerritt, JH, Werz, MA, McLean, MJ, and Macdonald, RL: Diazepam and its anomalous p-chloro-derivative Ro 5-4864: Comparative effects on mouse neurons in cell culture. Brain Res 310:99–105, 1984.

86. Skerritt, JH, Willow, M, and Johnston, GAR: Diazepam enhancement of low affinity GABA binding to rat brain membranes. Neurosci Lett 29:63–66, 1982.

87. Somjen, GG: Effects of ether and thiopental on spinal presynaptic terminals. J Pharmacol Exp Ther 140:393–401, 1963.

88. Strichartz, GR: The inhibition of sodium currents in myelinated nerve by

quaternary derivatives of lidocaine. J Gen Physiol 62:37–57, 1973.

89. Study, RA and Barker, JL: Diazepam and (−)- pentobarbital: Fluctuation analysis reveals different mechanisms for potentiation of γ-aminobutyric acid responses in cultured central neurons. Proc Natl Acad Sci USA 78:7180–7184, 1981.

90. Tallman, J and Gallager, D: The GABAergic system: A locus of benzodiazepine action. Annu Rev Neurosci 8:21–44, 1985.

91. Treiman, DM: The role of benzodiazepines in the management of status epilepticus. Neurology 40(Suppl 2):32–42.

92. Twyman, RE, Rogers, CJ, and Macdonald, RL: Differential regulation of $GABA_A$ receptor channels by diazepam and phenobarbital. Ann Neurol 25: 213–220, 1989.

93. Watkins, JC and Evans, RH: Excitatory amino acid transmitters. Annu Rev Pharmacol Toxicol 21:165–204, 1981.

94. Werz, MA and Macdonald, RL: Dynorphin reduces calcium-dependent action potential duration by decreasing voltage-dependent calcium conductance. Neurosci Lett 46:185–190, 1984.

95. Williams, JT, Henderson, G, and North, RA: Characterization of α_2-adrenoceptors which increase potassium conductance in rat locus coeruleus neurones. Neuroscience 14:95–101, 1985.

96. Willow, M and Catterall, WA: Inhibition of binding of [^{3}H] Batrachotoxinin A 20-a-benzoate to sodium channels by the anticonvulsant drugs diphenylhydantoin and carbamazepine. Mol Pharmacol 22:627–635, 1982.

97. Willow, M, Gonoi, T, and Catterall, WA: Voltage clamp analysis of the inhibitory actions of diphenylhydantoin and carbamazepine on voltage-sensitive sodium channels in neuroblastoma cells. Mol Pharmacol 27:549–558, 1985.

98. Willow, M, Kuenzel, EA, and Catterall, WA: Inhibition of voltage-sensitive sodium channels in neuroblastoma cells and synaptosomes by the anticonvulsant drugs diphenylhydantoin and carbamazepine. Mol Pharmacol 25:228–234, 1984.

99. Wong, EHF, Kemp, JA, Priestley, T, Knight, AR, Woodruff, GN, and Iversen, LL: The anticonvulsant MK-801 is a potent N-methyl-D-aspartate antagonist. Proc Natl Acad Sci USA 83:7104–7108, 1986.

100. Woodbury, DM, Penry, JK, and Pippenger, CE: Anticonvulsant Drugs, ed 2. Raven Press, New York, 1982.

101. Yaari, Y, Pincus, JH, and Argov, Z: Depression of synaptic transmission by diphenylhydantoin. Ann Neurol 1:334–338, 1977.

102. Yerby, MS: Problems and management of the pregnant woman with epilepsy. Epilepsia 28(Suppl 3):S29–S36, 1987.

103. Zackai, EH, Mellman, WJ, Neiderer, B, and Hanson, JW: The fetal valproate syndrome. J Pediatr 87:280–284, 1975.

Chapter 4

STROKE AND HYPOXIC-ISCHEMIC DISORDERS

William A. Pulsinelli, M.D., Ph.D.,
Michael Jacewicz, M.D., and
Alastair M. Buchan, M.D., M.R.C.P.

The number of new and recurrent cases of cerebrovascular disease (stroke) exceeds 400,000 yearly in the United States.[166] With a mortality rate of approximately 25% to 30%,[211] the 100,000 plus who die each year make stroke the third leading cause of death in this country. Adding the number of people who suffer persistent neurologic deficits after cardiopulmonary resuscitation,[118] more than 500,000 patients annually suffer the effects of hypoxic-ischemic brain damage in the United States alone.

This chapter reviews current clinical and experimental pharmacotherapies for acute stroke and its prevention. Therapies intended for the prophylaxis of atherosclerosis (e.g., antihypertensive and cholesterol-lowering drugs) and hemorrhagic stroke are not discussed. A brief review of normal cerebral metabolism, thrombus formation, and the pathogenesis of ischemic brain damage caused by focal or global ischemia is presented as background. Reviews by Siesjö[180] and Plum and Pulsinelli[158] provide a more detailed description of the molecular mechanisms of cerebral ischemia.

NORMAL CEREBRAL BLOOD FLOW AND METABOLISM

The mechanisms governing cerebrovascular smooth muscle tone and thereby blood flow to the brain are complex, interdependent, and incompletely understood. Conceptually, at least five levels of vasoregulation can be distinguished:

1. *Autoregulation*, a process whereby small arteries and arterioles dilate or constrict to maintain a constant cerebral blood flow (CBF) over a range of systemic blood pressure changes[104,110]

2. *Metabolic coupling*, an undefined mechanism that allows regional CBF to increase or decrease in proportion to local metabolism[114]
3. *Regulation through extrinsic nerves*, which includes innervation of vascular smooth muscle via the sympathetic (vasoconstrictor) network arising from the superior cervical ganglia, the trigeminovascular system,[139a] and the cholinergic (vasodilator) network putatively arising from cranial nerve VII[119]
4. *Regulation by intrinsic neural pathways*, for example, cerebral vasodilation mediated by projections from the fastigial nucleus and ascending cholinergic fibers of the basal forebrain[165]
5. *Regulation by the endothelium*, which degrades blood-borne vasoactive substances such as norepinephrine, serotonin, and kinins and secretes vasoactive substances such as prostacyclin, endothelium-derived relaxing factor, and endothelin, a powerful vasoconstricting peptide[208,220]

These several regulatory mechanisms interact to maintain blood flow to the normal resting human brain at approximately 55 mL/100g per minute.

Normally, the energy needed to perform the brain's work—that is, to maintain cell membrane potentials; to synthesize, package, and release neurotransmitters; and to maintain cell structure—is derived primarily from the oxidation of glucose to CO_2 and water.[186] The brain possesses the requisite enzymes to oxidize fatty acids and ketone bodies, but in the absence of glucose, these fuels can only partially support normal energy needs.[93] Glucose enters the brain via a carrier-mediated transport process with a K_m (7 to 8 mmol/L) for transport close to the concentration of glucose in blood. Accordingly, glucose concentrations in the brain closely reflect small changes in the blood-glucose concentration greater and less than 7 to 8 mmol. The brain normally extracts and metabolizes approximately 10% (30 μmol/100 g per minute) of glucose available from blood

in a single pass. In contrast, approximately 50% (156 μmol/100 g per minute) of the O_2 delivered to the brain is extracted in a single pass. The approximate fivefold difference in the metabolic rate for oxygen versus the metabolic rate for glucose indicates that the great majority of glucose is metabolized via oxidative pathways, with the net production of approximately 30 moles of adenosine triphosphate (ATP) per mole of glucose. The small excess of glucose not metabolized aerobically goes toward the formation of lactate and the synthesis of other carbon constituents of the brain.[186]

CEREBRAL ISCHEMIA: THRESHOLDS FOR INJURY

The progressive decline of CBF is signaled at specific blood flow thresholds by the acceleration of glycolysis, the loss of electroencephalographic activity, the depolarization of membrane potentials, and the alteration of ion fluxes (Table 4–1). The earliest measurable change as blood flow falls lower than 30 to 35 mL/100 g per minute is an increase in the extracellular[86] (and presumably intracellular) hydrogen ion concentration. At flows between 15 to 25 mL/100 g per minute, sensory evoked potentials disappear and the electroencephalogram (EEG) becomes isoelectric.[8] At flows less than 15 mL/100 g per minute, extracellular potassium rises, and shortly thereafter the extracellular calcium concentration

Table 4–1 EFFECTS OF REDUCED CEREBRAL BLOOD FLOW ON PRIMATE BRAIN METABOLISM

Blood Flow (mL/100 g per min)	Effect
55	Normal resting flow
<30–35	Increased H+ ion concentration
15–25	EEG isoelectric Sensory evoked potentials disappear
<15	Extracellular potassium rises and calcium falls
<10–18	Irreversible brain injury

falls[8,87] as the cell membrane depolarizes. Although the threshold values mentioned previously were measured in primates,[14,196] they are remarkably similar for a variety of species including humans, whose EEG begins to slow at blood flow values of 15 to 18 mL/100 per minute.[193]

Estimates of the CBF values below which irreversible brain injury results vary from approximately 10 mL/100 g per minute[196] to 18 mL/100 g per minute.[14] The variability in thresholds for cellular injury stems partly from the dynamic nature of brain cell vulnerability but more importantly from the *degree* and *duration* of ischemia.[14] Certain neuron populations succumb to relatively brief periods of ischemia, whereas others are more resistant.[162,163] The combined variable of *degree* and *duration* of ischemia is particularly important when defining the therapeutic relevance of the so-called ischemic penumbra, that is, regions of the brain lying at the edge of an area of ischemia, where the lack of oxygen is sufficiently severe to cause electric silence but not to depolarize membranes. Initially, it was thought that such regions would recover upon cerebral reperfusion; more recent data, however, suggest that the penumbra may itself die if too long deprived of oxygen and substrate.[14]

The description of CBF thresholds for ischemic injury is further complicated by the distinctly different patterns of brain damage that evolve after *global* cerebral ischemia (e.g., with cardiac arrest) versus *focal* ischemia (e.g., with thromboembolic arterial occlusion).[162] In addition to the intensity and duration of ischemia, hypotension, hypoxia, hyperglycemia, fever, and other metabolic factors can modify the distribution and extent of ischemic damage. Given the complex metabolic environment, ischemia-induced changes in vascular reactivity may alternatively temper (i.e., vasodilate) or aggravate (i.e., vasoconstrict) the ischemic insult such that the hemodynamic and pathologic consequences become difficult to predict.

Transient, global ischemia of the brain triggers a remarkable swing in CBF between an initial brief period of high CBF and a later, more prolonged period of low CBF. Upon cerebral recirculation, blood flow to the brain recovers immediately to values greater than normal. This hyperemic response is transient, lasting only minutes. Cerebral blood flow then falls to approximately 50% of normal values and remains reduced for at least several hours. Some researchers argue that this late or "delayed" cerebral hypoperfusion further jeopardizes already compromised brain cells. Experimental studies, however, demonstrate that delayed cerebral hypoperfusion does not prevent the recovery of normal high-energy metabolite levels even in brain tissue destined to develop irreversible damage.[162]

Occlusion of an extracranial or intracranial blood vessel supplying the brain (focal ischemia) induces a variable and dynamic response in the vascular smooth muscle of blood vessels lying in the ischemic core and in the boundary zones of ischemia. Regions of dense ischemia may show a gradual or steep topographic transition between areas with severely reduced CBF and areas of normal blood flow. In other instances, blood flow to the rim of brain tissue surrounding the ischemic zone may be greater than normal. Reversal of focal vascular occlusion frequently causes a pattern of blood flow change in the ischemic regions similar to that described for recirculation after global ischemia. An initial brief hyperemia is followed by a more prolonged hypoperfusion of the previously ischemic zone. How and whether such changes in CBF affect focal cerebral infarction remain the topics of vigorous research.

The phenomenon of "no-reflow," defined as the absence of CBF after reversal of cerebrovascular occlusion, was initially described for complete (zero CBF) global ischemia. In fact, "no-reflow" proved to be an artifact of abnormally low cerebral perfusion pressure. Accordingly, it has little relevance to acute focal ischemia of the brain, especially since CBF in focal ischemia is rarely, if ever, reduced to zero.

MOLECULAR CHANGES DURING ISCHEMIA

Energy Metabolism

When CBF falls lower than 10 to 15 mL/100 g per minute, the supply of oxygen and glucose fall so low that the brain depletes its high-energy organic phosphates (phosphocreatine, ATP) and its carbohydrate (glucose, glycogen) stores within seconds to minutes. (Table 4–2).[120] The glycolytic rate increases in an attempt to maintain ATP levels, and lactic acid accumulates in the tissue in proportion to the preischemic stores of tissue glucose and glycogen.[158,180] In the absence of oxygen, mitochondrial respiration ceases and the nicotinamide adenine dinucleotide (NADH) level rapidly rises in mitochondria and cytoplasm. To maintain the cytoplasmic NAD^+ necessary for glycolysis, cytoplasmic NADH is oxidized via the conversion of pyruvate to lactate. Eventually, even this pathway fails due to either substrate (glucose) depletion or feedback inhibition by hydrogen ions at the phosphofructokinase step. At this

point, all energy-requiring systems cease to operate. Importantly, however, the complete shutdown of oxidative and glycolytic pathways does not necessarily signal irreversible brain damage, since all brain cells can recover from a few minutes of absent energy stores.

Lipid Metabolism

The depletion of high-energy organic phosphates produces a rapid reversal in the energy-dependent glycerophospholipid synthetic pathway, thereby causing an accumulation of diglycerides.[9,97] The diglycerides are further hydrolyzed by several lipolytic enzymes to cause a 10-fold to 20-fold rise of free fatty acids and glycerol.[62] The polyunsaturated fatty acid, arachidonate, is released in greatest concentration, and this is accompanied by comparatively large rises in the concentrations of palmitic and stearic acid.[9,97] This accumulation of free fatty acids may initiate irreversible cellular injury through several mechanisms. High concentrations of fatty acids in partially ischemic tissue can uncouple oxidative phosphorylation and retard recovery of normal energy metabolism after ischemia is reversed. Moreover, the metabolism of arachidonic acid through cyclo-oxygenase- and lipoxygenase-catalyzed reactions forms products that greatly affect platelet aggregation and vascular smooth-muscle contractility. Furthermore, mono-oxygenase products of arachidonic acid can initiate potentially damaging free-radical intermediates.[221]

Free Radicals

Highly reactive molecules or ions called *free radicals*, with an unpaired electron, are formed normally as a consequence of both the enzymatic peroxidation of lipids and mitochondrial respiration. Cellular defense mechanisms against normally generated free radicals include the enzymes superoxide dismutase, catalase, and peroxidase. The reducing agents, glutathione and vitamins E and C, also protect against

Table 4–2 MAJOR MOLECULAR CHANGES DURING ISCHEMIA

ENERGY METABOLISM
Fall in tissue oxygen, glucose, and high-energy phosphates
Early increase in glycolytic rate
Increased production of organic acids

LIPID METABOLISM
Accumulation of diglycerides
Increased free fatty acids: Arachidonic, palmitic, and stearic acids
Generation of free radicals

NEUROTRANSMITTERS
Reduced production of monoamine neurotransmitters
Enhanced release of catecholamines and EAAs

ION HOMEOSTASIS
Movement of potassium out of and sodium into neurons
Increased levels of intracellular calcium

free radicals by acting as radical scavengers. Free-radical accumulation is unlikely in the totally ischemic brain since oxygen, which is important for their formation, is absent. In focal stroke where some blood flow is usually present , however, and in instances of cerebral recirculation, the conditions are ideal for free-radical generation.[181a] Despite such opportunistic conditions, the evidence that free-radical mechanisms participate in ischemic brain injury is indirect. Reports of conjugated dienes in the brains of animals subjected to global brain ischemia[213] and the ability of some antiradical agents to reduce ischemic brain damage[84a,118a] are at present the most convincing evidence for the participation of enhanced formation of free radicals in the pathophysiology of brain ischemia. Nevertheless, it remains unclear whether free-radical mechanisms participate in vascular (blood flow) mediated process or if they contribute directly to brain cell injury.

Neurotransmitter Chemistry

Cerebral hypoxia-ischemia induces many changes in the synthesis of neurotransmitters and in their release and reuptake by neurons and glia. Which of these changes, if any, are directly relevant to cerebral dysfunction or cell death from stroke is currently the focus of much research.

The synthesis and degradative metabolism of dopamine, norepinephrine, and serotonin require oxygen in approximately 12-μmol/L concentrations.[71] Since the oxygen tension of normal brain lies close to this level, mild hypoxia or reduction of cerebral circulation potentially can alter brain monoamine neurotransmitter levels. Similarly, cerebral hypoxia-ischemia alters the brain concentrates of the excitatory amino acid (EAA) neurotransmitters aspartate and glutamate, and the inhibitory transmitters, gamma-aminobutyric acid (GABA) and glycine. Glycine, which also facilitates activation of excitatory amino acid receptors, is derived from glycolytic intermediates, whereas GABA, aspartate, and glutamate are synthesized from intermediates of the citric acid cycle. Ischemia-induced changes in the concentrations of glycolytic and the citric acid cycle intermediates therefore can alter the concentrations of the amino acid neurotransmitters. In addition, ischemia-induced changes in the formation of the acetyl moiety from glucose and pyruvate impairs the formation of acetylcholine.

Intense research has focused on the relationship between EAA neurotransmitters and brain damage accompanying stroke. High concentrations of glutamate and aspartate, and their analogues such as kainic acid or ibotenic acid, are toxic to central nervous system (CNS) neurons. Olney,[145,146] having noted that their neurotoxic properties paralleled their ability to cause neuron excitation, formulated the "excitotoxic hypothesis" of neuronal injury. This hypothesis has been invoked to explain cell damage for a variety of neurodegenerative diseases and for brain damage from epilepsy; it is also used to explain the pathogenesis of neuronal death from stroke.[170] Ischemia of sufficient intensity to deplete high-energy organic phosphates causes synaptic depolarization and the release of many neurotransmitters, including glutamate, aspartate, and glycine.[15,19] Activation of postsynaptic receptors for the EAAS, and in particular the N-methyl-D-aspartate (NMDA) and amino-3-hydroxy-5-methyl-4-isoxozale proprionate (AMPA) receptor, opens monovalent and divalent cation channels. The influx of sodium and, more importantly, calcium[91,180] may then trigger a cascade of biochemical changes that lead to irreversible cell injury.

Ion Homeostasis

At CBF values less than 10 to 15 mL/100 g per minute, ischemia-induced neuronal depolarization leads to movement of potassium out of and sodium into brain cells. In cell cultures, hypoxia-induced influx of sodium and chloride ions is associated with the influx of water, cell swelling, and rupture of neurons.[168,169] A similar mechanism of ischemic cell death *in vivo* seems unlikely, however, since the vast majority of brain cells can tolerate many minutes of ischemic depolarization with only minimal cell swelling. Moreover, upon cerebral reperfusion, the neurons that are destined to die shrink and involute rather than swell.

Calcium, one of several second messengers, modulates many important cellular enzymes. For this reason, the intracellular calcium concentration is tightly regulated between 10^{-6} to 10^{-8} mol/L in the face of extracellular calcium levels of 10^{-3} mol/L. Calcium gains entry to the cell largely via volt-

age-dependent and ligand-(neurotransmitter) sensitive cation channels (Fig. 4–1) present in the plasma membrane. Energy-dependent and ion co-transport mechanisms of the plasma membrane, as well as storage by the endoplasmic reticulum and mitochondria, further regulate the intracellular calcium concentration. Ischemia-induced membrane depolarization and release of neurotransmitters allow calcium to enter neurons and attain abnormally high intracellular concentrations. Intracellular calcium levels may also increase during ischemia through stimulation of the phosphatidylinositol system, which through the formation of inositol triphosphate, triggers the release of calcium from the endoplasmic reticulum.[78] Calcium-activated enzymes that may participate in cell in-

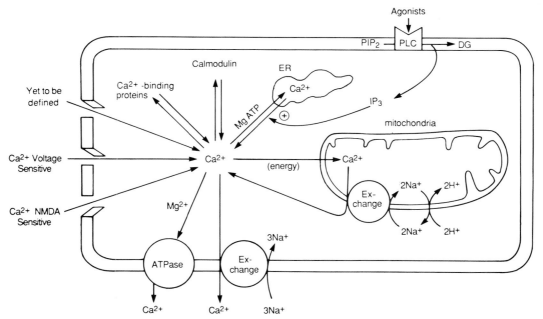

Figure 4–1. A neuron showing the mechanisms of calcium homeostasis. Calcium enters neurons via NMDA-sensitive or voltage-sensitive channels in the plasma membrane. Intracellular free calcium can also be increased via agonist stimulation of membrane phospholipase C (PLC) and the formation of inositol triphosphate (IP3). Inosital triphosphate stimulates calcium release from endoplasmic reticulum (ER). Intracellular calcium is buffered by binding to proteins and energy-dependent translocation into ER and mitochondria. Calcium is pumped from the cell via an Mg^{2+} dependent ATPase and by a Na^+/Ca^{2+} ion exchanger. Calcium bound to calmodulin exerts its regulatory control over multiple cell functions. (Modified from Swanson PD, et al: Calcium buffering systems in brain. In Rodnight R, et al [eds]: Chemisms of Brain. Churchill Livingstone, London, 1981).

jury include calcium-dependent phospholipases, which cause breakdown of membrane glycerophospholipids,[97] and calcium-dependent proteases, which degrade neurofilaments and disassemble microtubules.[123]

HISTOLOGIC PATTERNS OF ISCHEMIC BRAIN DAMAGE

Ischemic injury to the brain can be conveniently subdivided into two broad categories based on the histologic pattern and the type of ischemic insult (Table 4–3). Cerebral infarction, defined as an area of brain in which all tissue components including neurons, glial cells, and at least some endothelial cells are irreversibly injured,[158] is most frequently caused by focal ischemia. In contrast to focal infarction, brain damage from global ischemia affects specific populations of highly vulnerable neurons. This "selective neuronal necrosis" is usually caused by temporary cardiac asystole but also accompanies prolonged hypoxemia or carbon monoxide poisoning. If global ischemia is sufficiently long and co-exists with other conditions such as hyperglycemia, multifocal cerebral infarcts may develop. The neurons known to be most vulnerable to hypoxia-ischemia are the pyramidal neurons in the CA1 zone of the hippocampus and in layers 3, 5, and 6 of the neocortex; the cerebellar Purkinje cells; and the small- and medium-sized neurons in the striatum.[24,162]

Table 4–3 HISTOLOGIC PATTERNS OF ISCHEMIC INJURY

CEREBRAL INFARCTION
Irreversible injury of all tissue components
Time course: Complete in 4–8 hours

SELECTIVE NEURONAL NECROSIS
Hippocampus CA1 zone
Neocortex layers 3, 5, and 6
Cerebellar Purkinje's cells
Small- and medium-sized striatal neurons
Time course: Varies from a few hours in the striatum to 48–72 hours in the hippocampus

Infarction and selective neuronal necrosis differ from each other not only in the severity and distribution of the ischemic insult, but also in the time for maturation of the injury. Cerebral infarction proceeds rapidly to maximal damage and is usually complete within 4 to 8 hours of ischemia onset.[44a] In contrast, selective ischemic necrosis of neurons in experimental animals,[163] and probably in humans as well,[155] evolves during several hours in some cells (e.g., striatal neurons) while damage to the pyramidal neurons in the CA1 zone of the hippocampus requires 48 to 72 hours to mature. Differences in the severity and duration of ischemia as well as the different maturation times for infarction versus selective neuronal necrosis have important implications for the pathogenesis and pharmacologic intervention of stroke. To reduce cerebral infarction, therapy should be initiated quickly after the onset of ischemia. Efforts to reduce selective neuronal necrosis, however, especially in the hippocampus, might still be effective even if begun several hours after the onset of ischemia.

THERAPIES TO ENHANCE BRAIN OXYGEN AND SUBSTRATE SUPPLY

Antithrombotic Therapy

Most strokes, whether caused by cerebral atherosclerosis or by emboli from the heart or the carotid arteries, involve the process of thrombosis at some stage. Antithrombotic therapies for cerebral and myocardial ischemia have stimulated vigorous research and debate for the past three decades. Despite many clinical trials, however, considerable uncertainty remains about the effectiveness of such measures in stroke. Accordingly, this section presents certain guidelines, derived from "consensus opinion," for antithrombotic therapy of selected types of cerebral ischemia.

THROMBUS FORMATION

The heart and the carotid and intracranial arteries represent the most important origins for stroke-related thrombosis. Although the mechanism for initiating a thrombus is similar at each site, the rate of clot propagation and its composition differs as a function of the local hemodynamics and other rheologic factors. "White" thrombi, composed principally of platelets and fibrin, form in areas where blood flow velocity is high and shearing forces near the vascular endothelium are maximum. In areas of low blood flow or blood stasis, such as in the recesses of an enlarged atrial appendage, large numbers of red blood cells are trapped by fibrin to form a "red" thrombus. Turbulent blood flow with an admixture of high and low velocities favors the formation of thrombi composed of mixtures of platelets, red blood cells, and fibrin.

Thrombi undergo constant change regardless of their initial composition. Proteolytic enzymes from white blood cells, plasma, and the endothelium can remodel the clot and in the process cause embolism, ulceration of an atherothrombotic plaque, or complete clot lysis. Alternatively, the clot may be incorporated into an atherosclerotic plaque and/or continue to enlarge until it occludes the lumen of the blood vessel.

PLATELETS AND THROMBOSIS

Arterial thrombus formation occurs almost exclusively at sites of atherosclerosis or injured endothelium.[96] Endothelial damage caused by direct mechanical trauma, hemodynamic stress, infection-inflammation, or immunologic processes exposes collagen of the vessel basal membrane. The collagen, in turn, causes platelets to adhere, aggregate (Fig. 4–2), and form a nidus from which either a red or white thrombus can evolve. An endothelium-derived protein, von Willebrand's factor, binds to glycoprotein receptors on the platelet membrane[12] and fosters the "adhesion" reaction of platelets to basal membrane collagen.

Collagen, circulating epinephrine, thrombin, and a platelet-derived prostaglandin called thromboxane A_2 (TXA_2) stimulate platelets to release into the circulation[121] the contents of their various cytoplasmic granules (Fig. 4–3). The intensity of this response determines whether the platelets release a few or many substances including adenosine diphosphate (ADP), serotonin, platelet factors 3 and 4, coagulation factor 5, fibrinogen, β-thromboglobulin, and TXA_2.

The release-promoting agents, collagen, epinephrine, and TXA_2, stimulate two lipolytic enzymes, phospholipase A_2 and phospholipase C in platelet membranes (see Fig. 4–3). It is unclear whether these enzymes are activated directly or through a specific G-activated protein and/or calcium ions. In either case, activation of phospholipase A_2 releases arachidonic acid from membrane-bound glycerophospholipids. The enzymes cyclo-oxygenase and thromboxane synthetase then metabolize arachidonic acid to form TXA_2.[96]

The activation of phospholipase C causes the formation of inositol triphosphate and diacylglycerol (see Fig. 4–3). Inositol triphosphate stimulates release of Ca^{2+} ions from microsomes, a step that triggers myosin phosphorylation and contraction of the platelet. Diacylglycerol activates protein kinase C, which in turn phosphorylates a 47 KD protein. The resulting phosphoprotein, in conjunction with the contraction of the platelet, leads to the secretion of serotonin, ADP, and the other substances mentioned previously.[76]

COAGULATION PROTEINS

The coagulation of blood involves a series of reactions in which more than 12 coagulating factors (proteases) are activated through an orderly sequence of proteolytic reactions (see Fig. 4–2). This proteolytic cascade produces soluble fibrin monomers that polymerize to

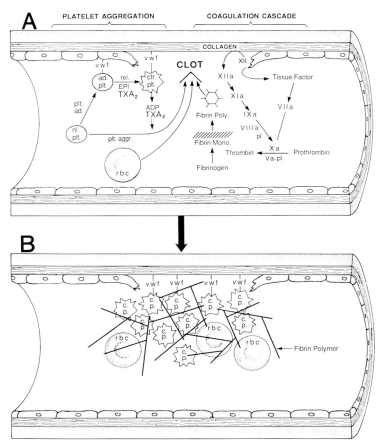

Figure 4–2. Cutaway view of a blood vessel showing interaction between platelet aggregation and the coagulation cascade (*A*) to form a thrombus (*B*) at the site of a vascular wall injury. Abbreviations: ADP = adenosine diphosphate; ad. plt. = adhered platelets; ctr. plt. and c.p. = contracted platelets; EPI = epinephrine; mono = monomer; nl. plt. = normal platelets; pl = platelet membrane; poly = polymer; rbc = red blood cell; TXA$_2$ = thromboxane A$_2$; Va-XIIa = activated clotting proteases; vwf = von Willebrand factor.

form insoluble fibrin with cross-links of sufficient strength to stabilize the clot.[30] The sequential nature of the coagulation cascade amplifies what initially may be a weak clotting signal; the system also contains multiple control points allowing its fine regulation.

Activation of the intrinsic system, so-called because all components are contained in plasma, occurs when factor XII contacts a nonendothelialized vascular surface. Activation of factor XII, in turn, activates factors XI, IX, and, with the cooperation of factor VIII, factor X. Factor X represents the crossover point between the intrinsic and extrinsic coagulation systems; the latter being so named because in the test tube, extrinsic tissue thromboplastin (usually derived from human or rabbit brain) is used to initiate coagulation. Both systems probably participate in thrombus formation in vivo, but current knowledge cannot fully explain the precise activation of the extrinsic system. The latter involves activation of factor VII through the release of tissue factor from the injured endothelium. The distinction between the two systems has practical applications in that the two most frequently used measures of hemostasis, the partial thromboplastin time

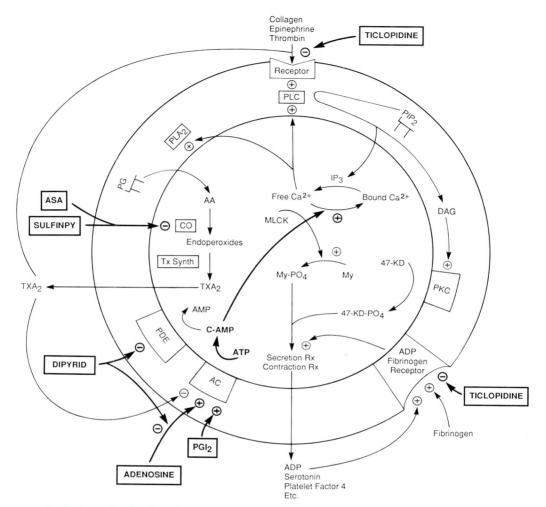

Figure 4-3. A single platelet showing important membrane receptors and cellular enzyme mechanisms of secretion, contraction and aggregation. Thin arrows represent mechanisms that facilitate platelet aggregation; thick arrows represent pathways that inhibit platelet aggregation. Thin-walled boxes indicate enzymes that promote platelet activation, and thick-walled boxes signify agents that inhibit platelet aggregation. Platelet aggregation is triggered by collagen, thrombin, or epinephrine membrane receptors that activate PLC and then the sequential release of intracellular IP_3 and calcium, activation of phospholipase A_2 and thromboxane production, stimulation of regulatory protein phosphorylation; and finally, contraction/secretion of ADP and so on by the platelet. The + signs signify stimulation or facilitation of a particular receptor or enzyme and the − signs indicate inhibition at this site. Abbreviations: AA = arachidonic acid; AC = adenylate cyclase; ASA = aspirin; C-AMP = cyclic AMP; CO = cyclooxygenase; DAG = diacylclycerol; DIPYRID = dipyridamole; 47-KD = 47 kilodalton protein; IP_3 = inositol triphosphate; MLCK = myosin light chain kinase; My = myosin; PDE = phosphodiesterase; PG = glycerophospholipids; PGI_2 = prostacyclin; PIP_2 = phosphotidylinositol biphosphate; PKC = protein kinase C; PLA_2 = phospholipase A_2; PLC = phospholipase C; SULFINPY = Sulfinpyrazine; Tx Synth = thromboxane synthetase; TXA_2 = thromboxane A_2.

(PTT) and the prothrombin time (PT), reflect the activity of the intrinsic and extrinsic systems respectively.[30]

Activation of factor X through either the intrinsic or extrinsic system converts prothrombin to thrombin, which in turn splits off soluble fibrin monomers from fibrinogen. Through the action of factor XIII, the soluble fibrin monomers are converted to insoluble fibrin polymers, completing the clotting cascade.

Circulating platelets normally possess little procoagulant activity until they are exposed to collagen. Activation of the platelet-aggregating and release reactions causes several events that lead to platelet procoagulant activity. Contraction of the platelets exposes membrane phospholipids that bind factors V and X, thereby markedly enhancing the rate of prothrombin conversion to thrombin. In addition, platelet phospholipids may enhance the activation of factor X by providing a surface for the reaction of factors VII and IX.[55]

PHYSIOLOGIC
ANTITHROMBOTIC
MECHANISMS

Left unchecked, the active mechanisms leading to platelet aggregation and thrombus formation would rapidly clot the body's entire circulation. Several physiologic processes prevent such uncontrolled thrombogenesis. The neg-

atively charged endothelial cells repel like-charged platelets. In addition, rapidly flowing blood clears activated coagulation factors from areas of endothelial injury, and the liver removes these activated proteases from the circulation.[96]

Normal endothelial cells suppress platelet aggregation through the synthesis and release of prostacyclin (PGI$_2$), a prostaglandin metabolite of arachidonic acid (Fig. 4–4). Platelet adenylate cyclase activity is enhanced by PGI$_2$ and the resulting accumulation of intracytoplasmic cyclic adenosine monophosphate (AMP) (Fig. 4–3) stimulates the sequestration of free calcium by normal intracellular storage sites and facilitates the inhibition of phospholipase C activity. The latter changes act in concert to suppress platelet aggregation. In addition to its potent platelet antiaggregatory properties, prostacyclin also dilates cerebral blood vessels.

Endothelial cells synthesize two agents with anticoagulant activity. The first, heparan sulfate, is a glycosoaminoglycan attached to specific plasma membrane proteins[23,167] on the luminal

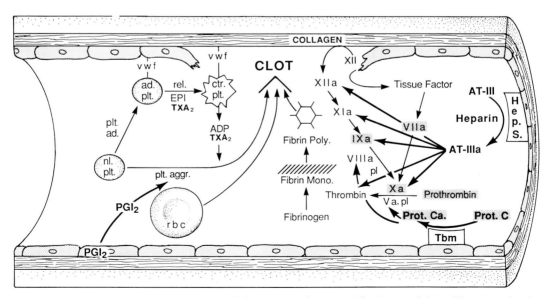

Figure 4–4. Cutaway view of a blood vessel showing mechanisms of anticoagulation. Heparin activates antithrombin III (AT-III), which inhibits multiple components of the coagulation cascade. Shaded factors represent vitamin-K-dependent proteases and the site of coumadin action. Activated protein C (Prot. Ca) inhibits factors VIII and V. Prostacyclin (PGI$_2$) inhibits platelet activation. Abbreviations: Hep. S. = heparan sulfate; Prot. C. = protein C; Tbm = thrombomodulin; for other abbreviations see Figure 4–2 legend.

surface of endothelial cells (see Fig. 4–4). In this position, heparan sulfate stimulates the activity of antithrombin III, a circulating protease capable of slowly inhibiting the coagulation factors II, IX, X, XI, and XII. Naturally occurring heparan sulfate or administered heparin markedly enhance the activity of antithrombin III. Thrombomodulin, the second endothelial-derived factor with anticoagulant properties, is a receptor lying on the luminal surface of endothelial cells that binds thrombin. The thrombin so bound is unable to split fibrin monomers from fibrinogen. In addition, the binding of thrombin to thrombomodulin, in conjunction with factor V, stimulates the activation of protein C. Activated protein C is a potent anticoagulant which, in the presence of calcium ions, phospholipids, and protein S, inactivates factors V and VIII by cleaving their polypeptide chains.[39]

Equally important, activated protein C triggers the fibrinolytic system (Fig. 4–5). Protein C is thought to neutralize a circulating inhibitor of tissue plas-minogen activator (tPA), thereby increasing the concentration of active tPA in the circulation.[39] Plasminogen binds to fibrin polymer as the thrombus is formed.[40] Activated tPA binds strongly to the plasminogen-fibrin polymer complex within the clot, converting plasminogen into plasmin. Plasmin in turn degrades fibrin into soluble fragments (fibrin degradation products) causing clot dissolution. Active plasmin, which may escape into the circulation, is quickly neutralized by α-2-macroglobulin and α-2-antiplasmin.

Anticoagulants

PHARMACOLOGY

Heparin. Commercially available heparin contains a heterogeneous group of mucopolysaccharides composed of repeating disaccharide units of different lengths. Heparin markedly accelerates the binding of circulating antithrombin III to activated coagulation factors II (prothrombin), IX, X, XI, and

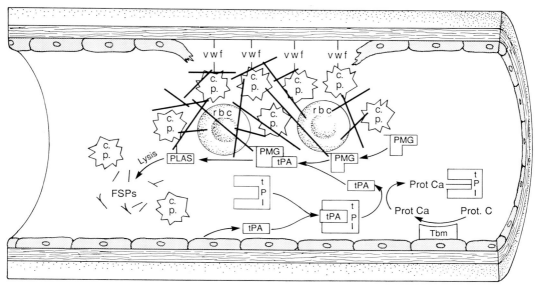

Figure 4–5. Mechanism of clot lysis by tissue plasminogen activator. Tissue plasminogen activator (tPA) is released from endothelial cells and bound to a circulatory inhibitor (tPI). Activated protein C (Prot Ca) releases tPA from the inhibitor, enabling tPA to bind to plasminogen already present in the clot. Plasminogen (PMG) is converted to plasmin (PLAs), which lyses clot into fibrin split products (FSPs). Abbreviations: c.p. = contracted platelets; Tbm = thrombomodulin.

Table 4–4 RISK OF MAJOR HEMORRHAGE* FROM ANTICOAGULATION

Drug	Indication	Average Risk
Heparin (acute)	TIA	4%[†][134]
	Acute, progressing stroke	3%[†][134]
	Cardiogenic emboli	4%[†][134]
Warfarin sodium (chronic)	MI, CVA	5%–7%[‡][118]

*Defined as requiring transfusion and/or hospitalization, intracranial or fatal.
†Per event
‡Per year
Abbreviations: TIA = transient cerebral ischemic attack; MI = myocardial infarction; CVA = any ischemic cerebrovascular accident.

XII, with the predominant effect on factor X (see Fig. 4–4). The binding of antithrombin III to the activated coagulation factors irreversibly inhibits their procoagulant activity.[23,167]

Heparin is poorly absorbed from the gastrointestinal tract, and must be administered either by deep injection into body fat or intravenously. Heparin produces immediate anticoagulation with a dose-dependent half-life ranging up to 5 hours after an intravenous dose.

Continuous intravenous infusion is the method of choice for administering heparin to patients with acute stroke. An initial bolus of 5000 U is followed by a maintenance infusion adjusted to a level (approximately 1000 to 2000 U/h) that will maintain the activated PTT in the range of 1.5 to 2 times the patient's preheparin control value.

The principal complication of heparin therapy is hemorrhage from preexisting sites of vascular damage or bleeding (Table 4–4). In addition, heparin administered for 1 week or longer can produce thrombocytopenia in as many as 25% of patients, either by increasing platelet aggregation or by inducing antiplatelet antibodies. The latter condition is more frequently encountered with heparin derived from bovine lungs than from porcine intestines. Paradoxically, heparin may promote coagulation by reducing antithrombin III levels, and also by stimulating platelet aggregation. Purified, low-molecular-weight heparins (heparinoids), currently under active clinical study, may avoid the proaggregatory effect of heparin on platelets.[16]

Hydroxycoumarins. Several orally active anticoagulants, which share the 4-hydroxycoumarin structure, modify coagulation through a post-translational inhibition of vitamin K–dependent proteins synthesized in the liver. The clotting proteases, that is, factors II (prothrombin), VII, IX, and X, and the naturally occurring anticoagulant, protein C, require carboxylation of several amino terminal glutamate residues for their activity.[23] The hydroxycoumarins block the cyclic oxidation-reduction of vitamin K necessary for the carboxylation of these proteins.

Bioavailability, predictable absorption, and duration of action make racemic sodium warfarin (Coumadin) the drug of choice for chronic anticoagulation.[96] Sodium warfarin is rapidly absorbed from the gastrointestinal tract, reaching peak concentrations within 1 hour after ingestion. Therapeutic effects, however, do not begin for 6 to 8 hours and reach peak anticoagulant activity only 72 to 96 hours after ingestion. Differences in the half-lives of the vitamin K-dependent proteins, and the fact that warfarin sodium inhibits an anticoagulant protein (protein C), account for this complex and delayed therapeutic efficacy. Because protein C and factor VII possess similar half-lives (i.e., 6 hours), a combination of procoagulant and anticoagulant activity occurs during the first 6 to 12 hours after the initial warfarin dose. With longer administration of sodium warfarin, the anticoagulant activity predominates as the half-life for prothrombin (i.e., 60 hours) is exceeded.

Many factors can alter the anticoagulant response to hydroxycoumarinlike drugs. Disease processes that alter hepatic function, the availability of vitamin K in the diet, and many drugs modify the anticoagulation response to sodium warfarin by altering its absorption, its binding to albumin, or its metabolism or excretion. The *Physicians' Desk Reference* (Medical Economics Books, Nadell, NJ) provides a complete list of these interacting agents.

The one-stage PT is a sensitive index of the activities of factors II, VII, and X, and accordingly is used most frequently to monitor warfarin therapy. The optimal therapeutic range, however, remains controversial. Prothrombin times beyond 2.5 control values are associated with a greater risk of hemorrhage (see Table 4–4), as shown by the Dutch study on long-term oral anticoagulation following myocardial infarction (MI) in the elderly.[184] The matter is further complicated because protimes measured in Europe, where the assay employs human thromboplastin, differ from measurements in North America, where rabbit brain thromboplastin is used. The method in North America yields values that are one half to one third of those obtained by the European method. Accordingly, PTs reported simply as 1.5 to 2 times the control value in North America versus Europe actually reflect markedly different degrees of anticoagulation. Based on results from the Dutch study,[184] protimes measured using rabbit-brain thromboplastin should be prolonged to approximately 1.3 to 1.7 times control values.[159]

CLINICAL EXPERIENCE AND GUIDELINES

Most studies employing oral anticoagulants and heparin to treat or prevent stroke were conducted without the scientifically rigorous methods now demanded of clinical trials, nor in most cases were patients treated sufficiently early after the onset of symptoms. Moreover, most therapeutic trials classified stroke types on the basis of temporal patterns, such as transient ischemic attack (TIA) or progressing stroke, rather than by their vascular or hematologic pathogenesis. Such classification schemes may obscure detection of otherwise effective therapies for a particular subpopulation of patients.[56] Despite the less-than-desirable nature of this classification system, however, we are bound to it in the following description of therapeutic trials for stroke.

Early studies performed on patients with TIAs or stroke failed to demonstrate a reduction of subsequent stroke for those taking sodium warfarin as opposed to placebo. Sodium warfarin failed not only to reduce the risk of stroke preceded by a TIA or a minor stroke, but also increased mortality from cerebral hemorrhage. Similar trials have not been repeated in the modern era, leaving largely unknown the effects of anticoagulants on stroke morbidity and mortality.

TIA. In five randomized trials performed between 1961 to 1985,[28] a total of 117 patients with TIA were treated with sodium warfarin and compared with 110 control patients. Treatment with sodium warfarin reduced the incidence of TIA to 21% from 30% in the control population, but no differences emerged for the endpoints of stroke and death. Although anecdotal observations suggest that patients with crescendo TIA suffer a high risk of stroke, no prospective study exists on this point, nor do any data describe the effect of anticoagulation in this group. If aspirin fails to prevent recurrent or crescendo TIA in patients with carotid lesions, and no contraindications exist, our practice is to administer heparin and to prescribe warfarin sodium for a brief period (1 to 3 months), with precise PT regulation.

Progressing Stroke. Approximately two thirds of patients with acute anterior circulation ischemia experience fluctuations of neurologic signs and symptoms during the first 24 to 48 hours.[104a] In patients with vertebrobasilar ischemia, an unstable course occurs in an equal or slightly greater proportion of the patients for periods lasting as long as 96 hours.[104b,104c] Approximately 40% of the patients with an unstable course will show progressive worsening of their neurologic deficits.[104a]

The pathophysiologic basis for progressive deterioration over days of patients with acute stroke remains a mystery but is likely to involve several related but independent processes. Increasing brain edema, the dynamic interaction of multiple vasoactive and metabolic factors, and progressive thrombus extension are only some of the possible causes for stroke progression. Importantly, these factors, which vary greatly in their impact from patient to patient, may explain why anticoagulation therapy aimed at preventing the extension of thrombosis helps a limited number of patients and then only partially.

Anticoagulation of patients with acute progressing stroke is based on "suggestive but not conclusive" studies.[67] Of the four studies performed during the 1960s, only two were randomized and both suffered from weaknesses in design and the lack of computed tomography (CT) scanning. Nevertheless, all four showed a trend toward improved outcome in patients treated acutely with heparin versus controls. A recent double-blind, placebo-controlled trial[52] demonstrated no significant difference between heparin-treated and placebo-treated patients whose therapy was initiated within 48 hours of symptoms. Since a sizeable but unreported number of patients was entered into the study between 24 and 48 hours, however, a time when the greater proportion of such patients would have already completed their stroke, firm conclusions are hardly possible.

On the basis of these data, no prevalent opinion has evolved for the use of anticoagulants in acute stroke when the pathogenesis is uncertain.[56,179] Our own practice is to anticoagulate with heparin all partial-stroke patients who present within 12 hours of anterior circulation ischemia or 24 hours of vertebrobasilar ischemia, who have no other contraindications, and whose CT scan is free of hemorrhage. Patients admitted after these time limits are anticoagulated if they show clinical signs of deterioration.

Patients who have no cardiogenic source of emboli are treated chronically with aspirin after discontinuing heparin. Patients with a demonstrable source of emboli from the heart are switched to sodium warfarin for a few months or chronically, depending upon the nature of the heart lesion.

Completed Stroke. Anticoagulation is without benefit and potentially dangerous following a completed stroke[67] except when indicated as prophylaxis against recurrent cardioembolic stroke. Large infarcts in particular may undergo hemorrhagic conversion with catastrophic consequences. In nine trials during the early sixties, a total of 956 patients with completed stroke were randomly assigned to either sodium warfarin or placebo therapy. Recurrent stroke developed in 18% of the sodium warfarin–treated patients and in 16% of controls; of those treated with sodium warfarin, 25% died, compared to 20% of controls.[28]

Cardiogenic Stroke. Cardiogenic emboli may account for up to one third of all ischemic strokes.[191] Intracardiac thrombi form in the presence of structural abnormalities of the heart chambers and valves, and also as a consequence of arrhythmias, which promote blood stasis. Patients with atrial fibrillation and mitral stenosis from rheumatic heart disease have a 17-fold increase in the risk of thromboembolism.[44,215] Anticoagulants are recommended as a prophylaxis against stroke in patients with rheumatic heart disease, (Table 4–5) especially in

Table 4-5 PROPHYLAXIS AGAINST CARDIOEMBOLIC STROKE: INDICATIONS FOR ANTICOAGULATION*

Rheumatic heart disease	Mitral valve plus embolism or atrial fibrillation
	Mitral valve plus left atrium >5.5 cm
	Aortic valve plus embolism or atrial fibrillation
Nonvalvular atrial fibrillation	Embolism
	Left atrial thrombus—2D echo
	Prior to DC conversion
	Dilated/Hypertrophic cardiomyopathy
	Thyrotoxic heart disease
	Age >60—Individual basis
Myocardial infarction	Anterior or septal infarct
	Massive infarct
	Intramural thrombus—2D echo
	Akinetic wall
Prosthetic valves	Mitral or aortic valve
Other valvular disease	Mitral valve prolapse plus embolism
	Mitral annular calcification plus embolism
	Nonbacterial thrombotic endocarditis
Congenital heart disease	Paradoxic embolism

*Indications summarized largely from references 53, 54, 117, 179, and 191.

those who experience a cardioembolic event.[117]

The incidence of stroke in nonrheumatic atrial fibrillation (AF) is increased sixfold,[215] but the decision to initiate long-term anticoagulation (see Table 4–5) is not generally made unless an embolic event has been documented.[53] Data from a recent, randomized but unblinded trial of warfarin versus aspirin (75 mg) or placebo therapy in patients with nonvalvular AF showed that careful anticoagulation significantly reduced the incidence of thromboembolism.[154] A preliminary report of a similar study of chronic anticoagulation for nonvalvular AF in the United States indicated that treatment with warfarin or aspirin (325 mg) reduced the risk of an embolic event by 81%.[191] Aspirin caused a 49% risk reduction, but a direct comparison with warfarin therapy is still under study.

The risk of cardiogenic emboli in the aftermath of MI is lower than with rheumatic heart disease. Nevertheless, the comparatively large population with myocardial ischemia results in a substantial number of patients with MI-related stroke. This is particularly true if the myocardial ischemia has caused a large infarct, anterior-wall or septal involvement, atrial fibrillation, or conges-tive heart failure (see Table 4–5). Two-dimensional echocardiography makes possible the visualization of intracardiac thrombi. Two studies using this technique in conjunction with anticoagulation have shown that 32% and 34% of anterior wall MIs are associated with thrombi. No anticoagulated patient suffered an embolic event, whereas six of seven nonanticoagulated patients in one study,[108] and 7 of 18 in the other[214] suffered an embolic complication. It is clear that cerebral embolism can complicate MI and reasonable to recommend that the echocardiographic demonstration of a mural thrombus or an akinetic wall segment should warrant acute anticoagulation (see Table 4–5) with high-dose heparin.

Anticoagulation is indicated for those patients who already have suffered a cardiogenic embolism, since 10% to 20% of such patients re-embolize within the first 2 to 4 weeks if untreated.[34,35] Exactly when to anticoagulate requires balancing the risk of hemorrhagic conversion of the infarct (see Table 4–4) against reducing the risk of early re-embolization.[34,35] In the absence of anticoagulants, hemorrhagic conversion of a bland infarct occurs in most instances by 48 hours and is more likely to complicate large infarcts. It is prudent to delay anticoagulation for cardioembolic stroke for 24 to 48 hours and to wait even longer (approximately 7 days) for those with massive cardioembolic strokes or hemorrhagic conversion.

Heparin should be given as a continuous intravenous infusion of 1000 U/h without an initial bolus, with the PTT carefully maintained at 1.5 to 2 times control (50 to 70 seconds). Rapid anticoagulation is not necessary after cardiogenic emboli so that an initial bolus is unnecessary.[134] As shown in Table 4–4, the risk of brain hemorrhage for short-term anticoagulation with heparin is 4% for cardioembolic stroke.[134] Alternatively, heparin can be completely avoided and oral administration of sodium warfarin can begin, since the prolongation of the PT does not occur for 36 to 48 hours. As explained previously, however, sodium warfarin therapy without prior heparinization may be accompanied by a hypercoaguable state during the first 6 to 12 hours.

Cerebral Venous Thrombosis. Anticoagulant therapy in cerebral venous thrombosis (CVT) has been controversial because the associated cerebral infarction is frequently hemorrhagic.[11,29] In the pre-CT-scan era, Gettelfinger and Kokmen[70] underscored the potential danger when two of their three heparinized patients (including one who also received a thrombolytic drug urokinase) developed fatal cerebral hemorrhage; their four nonheparinized patients made good recoveries. In contrast, Krayenbuhl[113] did not observe brain hemorrhage in 73 patients when anticoagulation was "well-controlled"; he reported a 7% mortality in patients treated with antibiotics and anticoagulation, whereas 37% of those treated with antibiotics alone and 70% of untreated patients died. Most recent studies, especially those using the CT scan to screen for hemorrhages, have reported results favoring the use of anticoagulants in CVT. Di Rocco and associates[50] treated five patients with heparin and urokinase early after

symptom onset with excellent recovery, despite evidence of parenchymal injury (i.e., hemiparesis, seizures) in four patients. Bousser's group[20] emphasized that heparin for CVT was at the very least not harmful, as none of their 23 heparinized patients died and 19 made full recoveries. In a preliminary report, Villringer and colleagues[209] found that 4 of 10 nonheparinized patients either died or suffered severe neurologic deficits, while their 10 heparinized patients made excellent recoveries or had "slight neurologic deficits." Overall, current evidence[101a,126a] supports the early use of heparin, or at the very least, antiplatelet agents, to treat CVT; the development of hemiparesis, seizures, and other evidence of tissue injury does not contraindicate anticoagulant therapy, provided that cerebral hemorrhage has been excluded by CT or magnetic resonance imaging.

Antiplatelet Agents

PHARMACOLOGY

Aspirin. Aspirin (acetylsalicylic acid), a nonsteroidal anti-inflammatory agent, is well absorbed in the stomach and small intestine within 4 to 10 minutes of oral administration. It is hydrolyzed in the liver with a half-life of 15 to 20 minutes, producing salicylic acid, which is inactive and excreted by the kidney. Although usually well tolerated, aspirin prolongs the bleeding time and can cause gastric erosion and gastrointestinal bleeding.

At low doses (<150 mg) aspirin acts by irreversibly acetylating *platelet cyclo-oxygenase*, thereby blocking TXA_2 synthesis (see Fig. 4–3). The loss of TXA_2 decreases platelet phospholipase C and increases adenylate cyclase activities. The resulting fall in platelet inositol triphosphate and diacylglycerol levels, plus the enhanced platelet cyclic AMP levels, lead to inhibition of platelet aggregation. At higher doses, aspirin transiently inhibits *endothelial cell cyclo-oxygenase*, and the salicylate moiety inhibits endothelial cell lipoxygenase as well, both being effects that can lessen the beneficial effect of TXA_2 suppression. These considerations make uncertain the optimal dose of aspirin for stroke therapy. Very low doses of aspirin (30 to 50 mg/d) might be optimal for inhibiting platelet aggregation,[151] but clinical trials have used higher doses ranging from 325 to 1500 mg/d. A large trial conducted in the United Kingdom of patients with TIAs[204] found no difference between those treated with 325 mg as compared to 1350 mg, but neither of the two groups in that trial showed a substantial risk reduction.

Dipyridamole. Dipyridamole (Persantine) is an orally active vasodilator with antiplatelet properties. It is excreted in the bile as the glucuronide metabolite. Its half-life is approximately 12 hours. Side effects are rare and include gastrointestinal irritation, headache, and dizziness. Dipyridamole directly inhibits platelet cyclic AMP phosphodiesterase and indirectly stimulates adenylate cyclase by blocking the reuptake of adenosine; both actions enhance platelet cyclic AMP levels and thereby potentiate the antiaggregatory action of PGI_2 (see Fig. 4–3) Theoretically, dipyridamole may act synergistically when combined with aspirin, since both agents act at different sites. The dose is 75 to 100 mg given four times daily.

Sulfinpyrazone. This phenylbutazone derivative competitively inhibits platelet cyclo-oxygenase (see Fig. 4–3), thereby inhibiting platelet aggregation. It is orally absorbed, reaches peak plasma concentrations at 1 to 2 hours, and has a half-life of 2 to 3 hours. Sulfinpyrazone is protein bound and largely excreted via the kidneys, where it acts as a uricosuric agent. Like aspirin, it too tends to promote gastrointestinal bleeding. The usual dose is 200 mg given four times a day.

Ticlopidine. This compound is chemically unrelated to other platelet antiaggregants. Orally administered in a dose of 500 mg/d, its activity persists for approximately 1 week. Its mechanism of action is not well defined but may involve alteration of the platelet membrane binding sites for thrombin, fibrinogen, ADP, and platelet activating factor (see Fig. 4–3).[92] Ticlopidine neither inhibits platelet thromboxane synthetase, nor blocks prostacyclin synthesis in the arterial wall. Nevertheless, it does interfere with aggregation induced by TXA_2, giving it a theoretic advantage over aspirin.

Principal side effects noted in two large trials of ticlopidine for TIA[92] or stroke[65] included a 20% to 24% incidence of diarrhea, a 14% to 17% incidence of skin rash, and 1% to 2% incidence of neutropenia.

Suloctidil. Suloctidil is a peripheral vasodilator without a well-defined antithrombotic mechanism.

Pentoxifylline. This methylxanthine derivative is a recently introduced agent that improves microcirculatory flow by increasing erythrocyte deformability, reducing plasma fibrinogen concentrations, and inhibiting platelet aggregation. It also possesses mild CNS stimulatory properties.

CLINICAL EXPERIENCE AND GUIDELINES

Many randomized clinical trials of various platelet antiaggregants have been conducted. Since treatment is neither expensive nor necessarily toxic, even a moderate risk reduction would be advantageous for the individuals with cerebrovascular disease.

TIA. Antiplatelet trials for stroke prevention in patients with TIA have yielded mixed results; some studies showed remarkable risk reduction and others none (Table 4–6). To reconcile this dilemma, an Antiplatelet Trialists' Collaboration overview was published[5] in which all original data from 25 separate studies (13 for stroke, 10 for MI, 2 for unstable angina) were subjected to a "meta-analysis," allowing a valid sta-

Table 4-6 RESULTS OF ASPIRIN THERAPY
FOR TIA/MINOR STROKE

Study	Number of Patients		Outcome: Stroke and/or Death	
	Aspirin	Control	Aspirin	Control
Canadian[31]	290	294	46 (16%)	68 (23%)
French Study[21]	400	204	53 (13%)	38 (19%)
US Study[58]	153	150	21 (14%)	27 (18%)
German Study[171]	29	29	0 (0%)	4 (14%)
Danish Study[187]	101	102	21 (21%)	17 (17%)
UK TIA Trial[204]	1621*	814	312 (19%)	178 (21%)
European SPS[200]	1250	1250	200 (16%)	296 (23%)
TOTALS	3844	2844	653 (17%)	628 (22%)

*815 at 1300 mg/d and 806 at 325 mg/d.

tistic evaluation of data compiled from separate trials that have inherent differences. This analysis of "all published, intention-to-treat" cerebral vascular trials examined the effects of treatment on nonfatal stroke, that is, stroke with survival to the end of the scheduled treatment period, on nonfatal MI, and on vascular death. For patients who entered the analysis because of a cerebrovascular event (i.e., TIA or minor stroke) and who were treated with antiplatelet agents, the overall reduction in any vascular event was 22%; for vascular death, 15%; and for nonfatal stroke, 22%. The risk reduction for patients entered with myocardial disease was similar for the endpoints of any vascular event (26%) or vascular death (14%), but was higher for nonfatal stroke (40%). Calculations estimated that antiplatelet treatment for 100 people with TIA or minor stroke would prevent, during 2 years, one death and three nonfatal events. Although an earlier study[31] suggested that the benefit was limited to men, two[21,204] out of three subsequent larger trials found benefits for antiplatelet therapy in women as well.

Aspirin represents the mainstay of antiplatelet therapy for preventing stroke; the addition of other antiplatelet agents provides no significant additional benefit. Sulfinpyrazone did not improve the outcome when added to aspirin and had no beneficial effect when used alone.[31] Suloctidil has been found in one carefully controlled trial to be of no benefit.[66] Dipyridamole did not increase the protective effect of aspirin in two trials,[3,21] but dipyridamole alone may be useful for those with prosthetic heart valves or those intolerant to aspirin. Ticlopidine has recently been shown to provide a small (12%) but significant ($P = 0.048$) risk reduction compared to ASA for the prevention of stroke and death in patients with TIA.[92] In a separate study,[65] ticlopidine reduced the risk of recurrent stroke, MI, or vascular death by 30% compared to placebo ($P = 0.006$) in patients with recent thromboembolic stroke. Ticlopidine was equally effective in men and women in both studies.

Two studies[61,147] comparing aspirin versus sodium warfarin in patients with TIAs showed no difference in either stroke or TIA incidence between the two therapies.

Progressing Stroke. No published data describe whether the acute administration of aspirin to patients with progressing stroke has an effect. Hsu and colleagues[99] have given pentoxifylline (PTX) in a randomized, placebo-controlled trial for acute stroke. The investigators started treatment within 12 hours of stroke onset; of the patients studied, 139 received pentoxifylline and 131 received placebo. Of the PTX-treated patients, 15 (11%) died, as did 14 (11%) of the control group. Treatment was associated with modest improvement in the neurologic status during the first few days of intravenous pentoxifylline infusions, but this was not maintained after patients were switched to oral medication. No significant side effects were noted.

Completed Stroke. In contrast to most antiplatelet trials, which have examined TIA patients, a large French study evaluated patients who presented with a stroke. Results suggested that aspirin reduced the risk of stroke both for those with TIA and those who had already suffered a minor stroke.[21] Attempting to confirm this, the Swedish Cooperative Study[195] assigned 253 stroke patients to 1.5 g of aspirin and 252 patients to a placebo group within 3 weeks of the event. During a follow-up period of 2 years, they failed to detect a difference in either the stroke rate (12% in the aspirin group and 13% in the placebo group) or death rate (13% in both groups). Unpublished results from the Canadian-American Ticlopidine Study,[65] however, demonstrated that ticlopidine therapy in patients presenting with a minor stroke significantly reduced death and the recurrence of stroke compared to placebo therapy.

Cardiogenic Stroke. The use of aspirin as prophylaxis in patients with asymptomatic nonvalvular AF is now well established.[191] Some researchers also recommend the use of aspirin for those at an increased risk of cardioembolic stroke due to endothelial damage caused by mitral valve prolapse. The use of dipyridamole in conjunction with sodium warfarin in patients with prosthetic heart valves is considered standard therapy.[188]

Cerebral Venous Thrombosis. Data on the effectiveness of antiplatelet therapy in CVT are limited. In one study of 16 women treated with aspirin and dipyridamole for CVT,[55] none developed cerebral hemorrhage and all but 2 recovered normal neurologic function.

Primary Prevention. Given information from the Antiplatelet Trialists' Study,[5] there appears to be little benefit of prophylactic aspirin therapy for healthy individuals or those with asymptomatic carotid stenosis. Antiplatelet therapy is relatively innocuous, however, and the desire to prevent cardiovascular events is strong. Nevertheless, this rationale must be tempered by the results from a recent American trial[189] for the primary prevention of MI, which although suggesting a dramatic reduction in the expected number of myocardial infarcts, failed to alter the incidence of stroke. In fact, an increase in the number of hemorrhagic strokes was recorded. Results from a similar British study[156] did not confirm the reduction of MI, and also failed to show a reduction in the incidence of stroke, though the latter study did not demonstrate an increase of cerebral hemorrhage. At this time, giving healthy people aspirin as a prophylaxis against stroke seems unwarranted. Whether individuals with asymptomatic carotid artery bruits or stenosis would benefit from long-term prophylactic aspirin remains to be tested.

Thrombolytic Therapy

The recent success with thrombolytic therapy in the management of acute myocardial ischemia has rekindled interest in its use for the treatment of acute stroke. During the era prior to brain imaging, fear of accentuating or inducing intracerebral hemorrhage with fibrinolytic drugs all but precluded their use for acute stroke. Nevertheless, the advent of fibrin-specific thrombolytic agents such as tPA and anisoylated plasminogen-streptokinase complex (APSAC), plus a clearer appreciation of the timing and pathogenesis of hemorrhagic infarction, have generated new enthusiasm for these agents.

PHARMACOLOGY

tPA. Tissue plasminogen activator is a naturally occurring protein that preferentially binds and activates plasminogen bound to fibrin (see Fig. 4–5).

It has recently been synthesized using recombinant techniques, and a single- and double-chain variety are available. The half-lives of these two molecules are approximately 8 and 5 minutes respectively.[40]

Streptokinase. Streptokinase, a protein derived from beta-hemolytic streptococci, binds in a 1:1 stoichiometric ratio to circulating plasminogen, thereby opening an active site on the plasminogen molecule. The plasminogen-streptokinase complex converts other circulating plasminogen molecules to plasmin. Plasmin in turn lyses fibrin within thrombi, as well as circulating fibrinogen and coagulation factors II (prothrombin), V, and VIII. A newer form of streptokinase, APSAC has the advantage over streptokinase of a longer half-life, a greater degree of fibrin versus fibrinogen selectivity, and a lower incidence of hypotensive side effects.[139] Streptokinase and, to a somewhat lesser degree, APSAC result in a systemic fibrinolytic state with decreased levels of circulating plasminogen and fibrinogen as well as factors V and VIII. The concomitant increase in lysis fragments of fibrinogen and fibrin inhibits thrombus extension. The circulating half-lives for streptokinase and APSAC are approximately 20 and 90 minutes, respectively. Both agents are capable of initiating allergic reaction, but recent experience indicates that the frequency of anaphylaxis may be less for APSAC than for streptokinase therapy.[40]

Urokinase. Urokinase is a naturally occurring proteolytic enzyme that directly converts circulating plasminogen to plasmin. Single-chain urokinase-plasminogen activator complex synthesized with recombinant techniques has greater fibrin specificity than does urokinase because of the former's greater affinity for fibrin-bound plasminogen. The half-life of urokinase is approximately 15 minutes; the half-life of single-chain urokinase-plasminogen activator is approximately half that of urokinase.[40]

Comparative Properties of Thrombolytic Agents. Although the three agents just discussed differ in their proteolytic efficacy on a per-milligram-weight basis, the efficacy of thrombolysis and coronary artery reperfusion are essentially equal for all three classes of drugs when given in therapeutically effective doses. The different classes of fibrinolytic drugs variably affect circulating fibrinogen, with streptokinase and APSAC producing the greatest, urokinase producing an intermediate, and single-chain r-tPA producing the least degree of the fibrinolytic state. Although theoretically the less severe systemic fibrinolysis caused by tPA compared to streptokinase should provide a lower frequency of bleeding complications, clinical experience with all three fibrinolytic agents indicates a similar frequency and severity of hemorrhagic events.[40,153a]

CLINICAL EXPERIENCE
AND GUIDELINES

Acute or Progressing Stroke. A recent review[46] revealed that up until the early 1980s, a total of 261 patients were treated in seven separate thrombolytic studies, of which only three included control patients. Of the treated patients, 50% improved, but approximately 10% sustained intracerebral hemorrhage and 14% died. Unfortunately, methodologic weaknesses that included the late entry of patients and the unavailability of CT scans led to the premature and possibly erroneous conclusion that fibrinolytic therapy was unsafe and of little benefit.

A new study,[47] which used either streptokinase or urokinase, was remarkable in that there was a mean onset-to-treatment interval of 7.6 hours. Recanalization of cerebral vessels in 15 of 20 patients with carotid territory stroke was proven by selective angiography. Of the 15 patients who demonstrated recanalization, 10 exhibited some clinical improvement. Of the 20 patients with carotid territory stroke, 4 developed hemorrhagic transformation on CT scan, although these were not associated with clinical deterioration.

Several new tPA safety studies, which require prompt administration of the drug, are underway. One[25] relies solely on the clinical status as an end-point and administers r-tPA within 90 or 180 minutes; others[46a,153a,201] seek angiographic evidence of recanalization and allow 4 to 8 hours for patient entry. Preliminary data from these studies are encouraging, with evidence of clinical improvement and partial recanalization. Hemorrhagic transformations have not exceeded the expected frequency in either study. The hope is that these trials will lead to a randomized, blinded, and placebo-controlled study in the near future. Until such trials are completed, however, and despite encouraging anecdotal reports, thrombolytic therapy should only be used by experienced physicians in the setting of an experimental study with stringent inclusion/exclusion criteria.

Hemodilution and Viscosity Reduction

Hemodilution as a treatment for ischemic stroke takes its rationale from a number of rheologic properties closely associated with stroke.[83,202] Cerebral ischemia can reduce deformability of red blood cells, increase their aggregation, and impede local microcirculation. Factors that enhance blood viscosity (e.g., polycythemia, paraproteinemia, and high hematocrit levels) increase the risk and extent of cerebral infarction.[90,106,149] In particular, rheologic factors may be critically important in the pathogenesis of focal perfusion defects observed during recirculation after *complete* cerebral ischemia.[74,105] In contrast, a reduction in blood viscosity with agents such as dextran 40 may lower cerebrovascular resistance and improve perfusion even in regions of relatively low blood flow.[79,217,218] A potentially limiting consequence of hemodilution, however, is that it lowers the

blood's oxygen-carrying capacity[60,98] an effect that of itself might explain the observed blood flow alterations.

PHARMACOLOGY

Dextran 40 contains a mixture of branched polysaccharides (molecular weight of approximately 40,000), so that a small percentage of patients show allergic responses without previous exposure. Itching, skin rash, joint pains, and other mild symptoms can develop, but serious reactions are unusual. After hapten-dextran (20 mL) is administered to block potential antibodies, dextran 40 is infused intravenously either alone or in combination with venesection (250 to 500 mL over 2 to 4 hours daily). The dosage is adjusted to the desired hematocrit level and the patient's cardiovascular status. After a single dose, over 24 hours the kidneys excrete up to 50% of dextran 40, consisting mostly of components of lower molecular weight. The body slowly oxidizes the remainder over several weeks, during which time it can still contribute to plasma expansion.

CLINICAL EXPERIENCE AND GUIDELINES

Intravascular volume expansion and induced arterial hypertension are reported to reverse ischemic deficits caused by vasospasm in subarachnoid hemorrhage, provided that treatment is started before brain infarction develops.[107] The efficacy of hemodilution therapy is uncertain for other types of ischemic stroke. Since stroke patients are often volume depleted when they arrive at the hospital, hemodilution with a volume expander (e.g., dextran 40 or other synthetic starch) has been advocated to improve cardiovascular output as well as to reduce blood viscosity.[80] To avoid pulmonary edema in patients with cardiac disease, however, invasive cardiac output monitoring may be necessary.[80] Alternatively, isovolemic hemodilution can be achieved by combining venesection with dextran or albumin infusion.[101,190] Although early studies suggested an improved outcome,[101,217] two major randomized studies of hemodilution have subsequently shown no benefit. In one study,[174,175] hemodilution was started within 12 to 48 hours of stroke onset, and in the second,[190] within 12 hours, including a large subgroup that began treatment within 6 hours. The mean reduction of hematocrit level from 43% to 40% during the 6 to 12 hours after stroke onset[190] could still represent too little treatment too late. A preliminary report from the Hemodilution in Stroke Study Group[95] suggests possible benefit for subgroups of patients treated within 12 hours and for whom treatment goals (a 15% decrease in hematocrit level or a 10% increase in cardiac output) were effectively achieved. Subgroup analysis by the Scandinavian Stroke Study Group,[175] however, failed to demonstrate clinical benefit in patients whose treatment was started within 12 hours of stroke onset.

Another strategy to decrease blood viscosity is to increase red blood cell deformability with agents such as the methylxanthine, pentoxifylline. Some experimental studies using this agent[102,111] have suggested improved blood flow to the normal and ischemic brain, but others[103,188] have not supported these observations. A recent double-blind, multicentered study[99] demonstrated a small clinical improvement that was not sustained for more than a few days.

Perfluorochemicals

The *perfluorochemicals*, inert carbon molecules with fluorine substituted for hydrogen, are excellent carriers of oxygen and carbon dioxide.[38] Their discovery has sparked great interest in their potential for stroke therapy. Intravenous administration of perfluorochemical emulsions in experimental animals reduced blood viscosity, improved CBF and oxygen delivery to the ischemic brain, and reduced cerebral infarction in animals subjected to focal ischemia.[116,153] Ventriculocisternal perfusion with oxygenated perfluorochemical emulsions has also effectively reduced infarct volume in animals subjected to focal cerebral ischemia.[148] Preliminary studies in humans suffering vertebral basilar ischemia[194] or cerebral ischemic secondary to vasospasm[85,194] are too sketchy to conclude anything other than that the patents suffered no obvious acute toxicity. Further studies of the perfluorochemicals in experimental animals and in humans with cerebral ischemia are warranted.

Vasodilator Therapy

Despite the increased knowledge of cerebrovascular regulation, there is little understanding of how ischemic conditions affect the brain's arterial-capillary bed and the control of its vascular reactivity. The occlusion of a cerebral artery by a thrombus, embolus, or by vasospasm initiates a complex, often unpredictable sequence of hemodynamic, metabolic, and structural changes in ischemic tissue. The anatomy and vasoreactivity of the ischemic vasculature[130] is but one critical variant that influences outcome. For example, little or no ischemic damage will develop if sufficient collateral vessels open and ischemic vessels dilate maximally to maintain residual blood flow above threshold levels of injury.[7] Alternatively, a relative lack of anastomotic collaterals and/or vascular relaxation, especially when perfusion pressure is marginal, may produce a dense ischemic zone and extensive infarction. With dispersal of the clot, the advent of postischemic hypoperfusion could theoretically exacerbate brain injury. These various premises have stimulated stroke investigators to explore new cerebral vasodilators, but with the exception of calcium antagonists in subarachnoid hemorrhage, the results have been disappointing.[41,42,82,125]

PAPAVERINE AND RELATED DRUGS

Papaverine, an alkaloid with potent, nonspecific vasodilatory properties, increases CBF in patients with cerebrovascular disease.[126,131] Papaverine therapy is short-lived and can be complicated by hypotension. Some patients treated with papaverine develop a "vascular steal," in which blood flow is diverted from ischemic to nonischemic tissue, a potential complication with all vasodilators.[32,94,144] Although Meyer and associates[131] reported clinical benefit in stroke patients treated with papaverine, improvement was not universal and usually of little clinical utility in controlled, double-blind trials.[41] Cyclandelate and nafronyl, "papaverine-like vasodilators" that do not induce significant hypotension at conventional dosages, have similarly shown dubious benefit. A number of other vasodilators, including hexobendine, betahistine, and cinnarizine, have failed to demonstrate consistent practical benefit in adequately controlled, double-blind studies.[41,42] Cyclandelate, however, has emerged more recently as a drug with a multifactorial mode of action that includes improving red blood cell deformability and inhibiting platelet aggregability, perhaps, by blocking calcium entry.[203] Its use might be advantageous during the first few hours of stroke, when ischemic injury is more likely to be reversed by improved circulation, but such remains to be demonstrated.

PROSTAGLANDINS

Prostacyclin (PGI$_2$) is a prostaglandin metabolite with powerful platelet antiaggregant and vasodilatory properties.[109,138] This compound is synthesized and released by the vascular endothelium and smooth-muscle cells to prevent local platelet deposition under normal physiologic conditions (see Fig. 4–4). The onset of ischemia triggers a sharp increase in levels of the PGI$_2$ precursor, arachidonic acid, as the calcium-dependent phospholipases A and C break down membrane lipids. Locally released arachidonic acid is then converted by cyclo-oxygenase to endoperoxide intermediates and prostanoids, or metabolized by lipoxygenase to hydroxy fatty acids and leukotrienes. The latter compounds are capable of altering membrane permeability and inducing vasoconstriction.[135] Among the various metabolites generated, PGI$_2$ stands out as a powerful vasodilator, balanced against the equally potent, platelet-synthesized vasoconstrictor TXA$_2$ (see Fig. 4–3). The opposing influences of endothelial PGI$_2$ and platelet-derived TXA$_2$ may establish a critical balance in pathologic platelet–vessel wall interactions and therefore could be of paramount importance to the integrity of microcirculatory flow.

A strategy in stroke treatment has been to enhance the influence of PGI$_2$ over TXA$_2$ by direct intravenous infusion of PGI$_2$. In very low doses (10^{-7}mol/L), exogenous PGI$_2$ can dilate vascular smooth muscle and reverse the vasoconstriction induced by a variety of vasoactive substances, including serotonin and thrombin, but its effects on ischemic microvasculature are more speculative.[152] An open, nonrandomized study[133] suggested clinical improvement in patients treated within 24 hours after stroke onset. Animal studies[10,205] and two randomized, double-blind clinical studies,[100,124,219] however, have found no useful benefit and even a possible clinical detriment with PGI$_2$ treatment. PGI$_2$ therapy, accordingly, cannot be recommended for clinical use.

CALCIUM CHANNEL ANTAGONISTS

Background. The mechanisms by which calcium channel antagonists can potentially alleviate ischemic brain damage fall into three major categories:

1. Blocking the entry and toxic accumulation of calcium in neurons and other brain cells,

2. Decreasing neurotransmitter release (e.g., EAAs) when presynaptic depolarization becomes pathologically enhanced, and
3. Reversing calcium-mediated vasoconstriction to improve residual blood flow.

The first two of these categories are experimental therapies (see "Calcium Channel Antagonists," p 143).

Three types of voltage-sensitive calcium channels (VSCC) have been identified by their electrophysiologic and pharmacologic properties. These have been labeled "L" for long-lasting calcium conductance, "T" for transient conductance, and "N" for neither L nor T.[132,143] The L- and T-type channels exist in many cells including vascular smooth muscle and neurons, while the N channel may be selectively localized to neurons. It is the L channel that appears sensitive to calcium antagonists, but the mechanisms of blockade differ among the chemically heterogeneous compounds that block the VSCC.

Calcium antagonists can be divided into three chemical classes based on their binding to one of three allosterically interacting receptors closely associated with the VSCC:[185,210]

1. Dihydropyridines, or DHP (e.g., nimodipine, nitrendipine),
2. Phenylalkylamines (e.g., verapamil, flunarizine), and
3. Benzothiazepines (e.g., diltiazem).

When studied in isolated membrane fractions from various tissues, these three stereospecific sites exhibit similar immunochemical and molecular properties.[75] In whole tissue, however, calcium antagonists exhibit sharp differences in activity.[75] Apart from a multiplicity of VSCC subtypes, this tissue selectivity appears influenced by the state of channel activation under differing functional states. Verapamil, for example, is most effective in blocking VSCC that open and close rapidly, whereas DHPs bind inactivated channels 1000 times more avidly than resting channels.[172] Local physiologic and metabolic conditions may thus alter channel-binding properties and result in a striking heterogeneity of VSCC distribution, as detected, for example, by [^{3}H]nitrendipine autoradiography.[77,199] Since the autoradiographic pattern is not homogeneous, VSCC interaction with DHP compounds in the normal brain does not appear to be governed by glia and blood vessels so much as by the influence of various neurotransmitter and neuromodulator systems.[185] In any event, ischemia or hypoxia may modify the VSCC receptor; this could critically influence binding and efficacy of drug action. For example, through modifications of the L channel, ischemia may increase the number of binding sites to DHPs and consequently enhance their pharmacologic action.[122]

Focal cerebral ischemia is often assumed to cause arterial dilation in response to local tissue acidosis and the release of vasoactive metabolites. This appears true for the peripheral territory of a major occluded artery, but in the densely ischemic core that develops into an infarct, a brief vasodilation is characteristically followed by active constriction of pial vessels (i.e., constriction not due to passive collapse of tension in the arterial wall).[129,198,212] The vasoconstriction may be sustained, with evidence of ischemic neuronal damage 2 hours later,[198] or may partly reverse with time, depending on the experimental paradigm.[212] The identity of the vasoconstrictor is unknown; it could involve any of a number of vasoactive substances present in the blood or released by aggregated platelets, by nerve terminals investing the vasculature, by the ischemic nervous tissue, or by the vascular endothelium.[206] Some evidence exists that modest rises in extracellular K^+ concentration (7.7 mmol/L) cause vasodilation, whereas high K^+ concentrations (>40 mmol/L) associated with ischemic damage cause vasoconstriction.[115,197] Hence, the massive release of potassium by ischemic tissue could depolarize the vascular smooth muscle, precipitate calcium entry via voltage-sensitive channels, and cause vasoconstriction. Since the ischemia-induced constriction of pial vessels appears closely associated with impaired blood flow in underlying cortex,[17,129] there is considerable interest in calcium antagonists that can prevent or reverse this vasoconstriction, promote vasodilation, and increase blood flow to the still reversibly-injured brain.

Vascular constriction, regardless of the regulatory mechanism responsible, depends ultimately on an increase in the cytoplasmic calcium concentration in vascular smooth muscle.[206] This can be blocked by a number of calcium antagonists, among which the DHP class is the most potent. Pretreatment of animals with nimodipine (perhaps the most potent cerebral vasodilator of the DHP type,[177,177a,178]) in concentrations that have only a modest effect on blood pressure, will improve residual CBF and attenuate ischemic damage after middle cerebral artery occlusion.[101b,101c,135a] When given after onset of focal ischemia, the usefulness of nimodipine and other calcium channel blockers becomes uncertain, with some experimental studies demonstrating benefit[69,84] and others, none.[76,88]

Pharmacology. As measured in rats, nimodipine is well absorbed after an oral dose and is metabolized rapidly. Its metabolites are excreted in the bile, with its half-life estimated at 90 minutes.[177] Although minor side effects related to vasodilation (e.g., lightheadedness, headache, and flushing) can potentially complicate therapy, these have seldom been observed when nimodipine is given orally at a dosage of 0.35 to 1.5 mg/kg body weight every 4 hours.[2,64,157,177] Unless nimodipine is administered intravenously,[63] hypotension is minimal and of little clinical significance in stroke patients.[57,64]

Clinical Experience and Guidelines. Preliminary data suggest that calcium antagonists of the DHP class may improve neurologic outcome in clinical stroke. After an open study suggested clinical benefit, a Dutch group[64] conducted a double-blind, placebo-controlled, multicentered study and showed nimodipine to reduce mortality and morbidity when given within 24 hours of ischemic onset.

A large US-based, multicentered, randomized study[136] has recently compared nimodipine treatment (60 mg, 120 mg, or 240 mg daily) to placebo in patients suffering a focal ischemic stroke of less than 48 hours duration. No significant difference in outcome was noted for the overall population treated with nimodipine. Further analysis, however, revealed that the 120-mg daily dose reduced the 21-day and 3-month mortality and morbidity (motor paresis) in patients in whom the nimodipine was given within 12 hours of ischemic onset. Studies to confirm this potential benefit with early therapy are currently underway.

Nimodipine has also proved useful in reducing ischemic brain damage attributed to vasospasm in patients with subarachnoid hemorrhage.[2,22] A recent, multicenter trial in Canada[157] demonstrated that nimodipine improved neurologic outcome and decreased ischemic deficits in patients with severe (grade 3 or higher) subarachnoid hemorrhage. Only 46% of the nimodipine group suffered ischemic deficits versus 66% of the placebo group. By 3 months, 29% of the nimodipine-treated patients had good outcomes versus only 10% of the placebo group. Nicardipine is another DHP that may prove useful in ischemic stroke and is currently under study.[13,59,81] In general, the prospects for calcium antagonists as treatment for stroke appear promising, and further experimental and clinical studies are indicated. Particular attention, however, should be paid to starting treatment within hours, if not minutes, of ischemic onset, since timing of vasodilator therapy may be critical for its effectiveness.

EXPERIMENTAL THERAPIES TO MAINTAIN CELLULAR VIABILITY

Calcium Channel Antagonists

Calcium plays a pivotal regulatory role in many of the cell's most fundamental processes (e.g., coupling of external stimuli to mechanical, metabolic, or secretory responses; and maintenance of cytoskeletal organization).[164,207] The biologic effects require that free cytosolic calcium remain very low concentration (10^{-7} mol/L to 10^{-6} mol/L) as compared to the exterior milieu (10^{-3} M). A variety of membrane pumps and exchange systems, such as the smooth endoplasmic reticulum and mitochondria, remove calcium to maintain homeostasis (see Fig. 4–1).[33]

Loss of the calcium-concentration gradient across the cell membrane would be expected to have widespread deleterious effects on cell function, and therefore, to be a major factor in a cell's demise.[176,188] A rapid and early rise of intracellular calcium may also be responsible for a variety of other events exacerbating injury, such as a massive release of excitatory neurotransmitters, epileptic discharges, membrane lipolysis, cytoskeletal disassembly, and loss of ATP production by mitochondria now committed to sequestering calcium. Ischemic-damaged neurons have been shown to accumulate calcium,[51,183] but whether "calcium overload" precedes[48] or passively follows other more critical and "irreversible" cellular damage remains controversial.[36,91,181] Moreover, no clear or consistent relationship has emerged between neuronal necrosis and the density of calcium channels putatively mediating calcium entry.[181]

Under ischemic conditions, the influx of calcium begins abruptly when the external potassium concentration rises to 10 to 15 mmol/L.[86,87,89] The channel(s) of entry into neurons have not been identified, but may occur by the Na/Ca antiporter, by receptor-operated channels, such as the NMDA receptor activated by glutamate, or by the VSCC.

There is some evidence that VSCC blockade with flunarizine can attenuate ischemic brain damage independent of blood flow increases.[49] This could involve multiple neurophysiologic mechanisms, since selected calcium antagonists, including the potent vasodilator nimodipine, have been shown to exert a direct antiepileptic effect on the CNS.[128,178] Agents such as nimodipine may therefore confer cellular protection by several different mechanisms.

EAA Antagonists

Currently, much interest centers on the role of EAA neurotransmitters and their receptors in the pathogenesis of brain injury caused by global and focal cerebral ischemia. New receptor/channel antagonists that cross the blood-brain barrier (BBB) are now available for studies in animals and humans.

Glutamate and aspartate, the best-defined EAA neurotransmitters, are widely distributed in the mammalian CNS. At least three types of membrane receptors that bind these neurotransmitters have been identified: NMDA, quisqualate or AMPA, and kainate. The NMDA receptor is associated with a voltage-dependent ion channel which, when open, allows the entry of sodium and calcium ions into neurons. These ligand-regulated, receptor channel complexes are thought to be importantly involved in the normal workings of long-term potentiation and temporal integration in the hippocampus. Exposed to pathologic conditions, however, these channels may pose a lethal threat to the cell[145,146] by permitting excessive calcium influx.[43]

Neuron cells in culture are relatively insensitive to an hypoxic insult until they have sufficiently matured to establish dendritic connections. Even then, the effects of hypoxia can be attenuated if glutamate or NMDA receptor antagonists, including Mg^{2+}, are applied to the culture media prior to hypoxic exposure. Hypoxia in these mature cultures presumably causes glutamate release, which in turn depolarizes the neurons, unblocks the NMDA-ion complex, and facilitates the influx of Na^+ and Ca^{2+} ions. The influx of Na^+ ions lead to osmotic swelling and cell death.[169,170] If, however, Na^+ ions are removed from the medium, a slower excitotoxic mechanism is revealed, with cell injury dependent on an influx of Ca^{2+} ions.[37] Both competitive (acting at the receptor) and noncompetitive (acting at the ion channel) antagonists of the NMDA receptor can prevent neuron injury in tissue cultures.[37,170]

In vivo, the roles of EAA neurotransmitters and their receptor antagonists in transient, severe ischemia are less clear, and conflicting experimental findings abound. Following transient forebrain ischemia, brain tissue releases glutamate[15] and at least for the hippocampus, some neurons with high concentrations of NMDA receptors, such as the CA1 pyramidal cells,[137] develop irreversible damage. Polar, competitive antagonists, such as D-aminophosphonoheptanoic acid, when injected intracerebrally in the rat, have been reported to protect CA1 hippocampal cells against ischemia.[182] Similarly, the nonpolar, noncompetitive antagonist, MK-801, when given systemically, has been reported to prevent CA1 necrosis in gerbils and rats subjected to forebrain ischemia.[72,193a] However, in other laboratories, competitive[18] and noncompetitive[27] antagonists of the NMDA receptor failed to protect hippocampal neurons against ischemia in several species.[28a] Gerbils treated with MK-801 and exposed to forebrain ischemia developed less hippocampal damage than the saline-treated control group.[27] This neuroprotective effect, however, was entirely the result of hypothermia induced by the combination of MK-801 and brain ischemia. When the gerbils were maintained normothermic, MK-801 exerted no protective effect.[27]

Studies of focal or moderate ischemia in several species have suggested that the volume of cortical infarction caused by middle cerebral artery (MCA) occlusion may be reduced by prior treatment with NMDA receptor antagonists.[51a,150,188a] A study in rats[68] showed a reduction in size of infarct after MCA occlusion by a nonspecific antagonist, kynurenate. Thus, in contrast to severe, transient ischemia, the NMDA-receptor antagonists effectively reduce brain damage from moderate ischemia. Further experiments are needed to resolve these discrepancies and to clarify what role NMDA antagonists will play in the therapy of focal and global brain ischemia.

Recent reports indicate that neuronal damage from transient severe ischemia in rodents is reduced by antagonists of the AMPA receptors.[163a,178a] Such protection was possible even when the drugs were given after the ischemic insult. This class of receptor antagonists is potentially very important, particularly since they are considerably less sedative and may be less likely to induce psychoticlike symptoms than antagonists of the NMDA receptor.

Reduction of Hyperglycemia and Cerebral Acidosis

Augmentation of ischemic brain damage by hyperglycemia has been well documented in many global[73,140,161] and more recently a few focal[45,141] animal models of brain ischemia. Several,[6,127,160] but not all,[1,216] studies of clinical stroke also suggest a correlation between hyperglycemia and a poor neurologic outcome.

The mechanism by which elevated brain carbohydrate levels enhance ischemic brain injury remains unclear. Increasing data, however, implicate the accumulation of hydrogen ions in the brain as at least one contributing factor. Lactate and hydrogen-ion concentrations attained in the ischemic brain are proportionately related to brain glucose and glycogen stores. Tissue lactate levels normally averaging about 1 mmol/L can exceed 40 mmol/L in hyperglycemic animals exposed to global ischemia. By direct measurement, the extracellular pH can fall to 6.1 and the intracellular pH, to 5.5 or lower in similarly treated animals.[112] Such profound degrees of intracellular acidosis can denature enzymes and structural proteins, alter substrate reactivity, and ultimately may kill the cell.

Theoretically, the reduction of cerebral acidosis in the ischemic brain should lessen tissue injury. Therapies to reduce carbohydrate stores in the brain, to treat cerebral acidosis directly, or both include:

1. Reducing blood glucose concentration with hypoglycemic agents, such as insulin,
2. Competitively inhibiting the BBB-glucose transporters using, for example, 2-deoxyglucose or phloretin,
3. Enhancing brain buffers to absorb the acid directly, and
4. Inhibiting brain lactate dehydrogenase to reduce lactic acid formation.

Several of these experimental therapies are being tested in animals, but none thus far have shown clinical practicability. At least in principle, however, tight sugar control in diabetics at risk for stroke and the elimination of glucose-containing infusions in at-risk patients should have prophylactic value.

Antioxidants and Free-Radical Scavengers

Despite the lack of conclusive evidence to support a role for free-radical mechanisms in ischemic brain damage, many studies in animal models of brain ischemia have examined the therapeutic effectiveness of antioxidants and free-radical scavengers.[180,213,221] Protection against ischemia was reported for several agents, including vitamin E, glutathione, allopurinol, desferoxamine, superoxide dismutase, and 21-aminosteroids. Unfortunately, an equal number of experimental studies have reported negative results with most of these agents. Further animal studies are needed to clarify the role of free-radical mechanisms in stroke.

THERAPIES FOR STROKE EDEMA

Therapy, or the lack thereof, for patients with stroke-related brain edema has changed little since this subject was reviewed in 1977 by the Study Group on Brain Edema in Stroke.[192] They were unable to recommend for or against the use of osmotic agents, steroids, or diuretics. This conclusion was remarkably temperate in view of what appears to be overwhelmingly negative clinical data. Aside from a brief reduction of brain water content by osmotic agents, no studies indicate that therapy with low[4] or high[142] doses of steroids or diuretic agents provides significant amelioration of brain edema from stroke. Moreover, recent experimental data suggest that glucocorticoids may, in fact, be deleterious to the ischemic brain.[173] We question whether further efforts to identify pharmacologic agents to reduce stroke edema, short of protecting brain cells against irreversible injury, is warranted. Occasionally, such measures may slightly reduce stroke mortality, but almost always they lead to severely disabled survivors.

SELECTION OF ESTABLISHED PHARMACOTHERAPIES

Therapies that reduce stroke risk factors such as atherosclerosis, hypertension, diabetes mellitus, rheumatic heart disease, and smoking are partly responsible for the 46% decline in the incidence of stroke registered in a representative US population between 1950 and 1980.[26] Unfortunately, the most recent analysis of this same population[26] indicates that the stroke incidence has stabilized at a level that maintains stroke as the leading cause of neurologic morbidity and the third leading cause of medical-related deaths in the United States. Improving the treatment of stroke risk factors is important, but short of a cure for atherosclerosis, such therapies are unlikely to reduce the incidence of stroke much further.

Stroke pharmacotherapies considered to be *established, possibly effective*, or *experimental* are summarized in Table 4 – 7. The *established* and *possibly effective* therapies are intended to prevent an initial stroke or its recur-

Table 4-7 STROKE PHARMACOTHERAPIES*

Condition	Established	Possibly Effective	Experimental
TIA	Aspirin[31] Ticlopidine[91]+	Warfarin[28]	
ACUTE PROGRESSIVE STROKE			
Thromboembolic		Heparin[179]	Thrombolysis (tPA, APSAC, etc.) Calcium channel antagonists Voltage-dependent (e.g., nimodipine) Ligand-dependent (e.g., MK-801) Free-radical agents (Superoxide dismutase, 21-Aminosteroids)
Complicating SAH	Nimodipine[157]	Volume expansion[107]	
Complicating vasculitis	Glucocorticoids		
COMPLETED STROKE		Aspirin[21] Ticlopidine[65]	
CARDIOGENIC EMBOLI			
Myocardial infarction	Heparin/warfarin[54]		
RHD and AF	Warfarin or heparin/warfarin[117]		
Nonvalvular AF	Warfarin or aspirin[191]		
Prosthetic valves	Warfarin plus dipyridamole[188]		
CEREBRAL VEIN THROMBOSIS		Heparin[113]	

+Pending FDA approval
Abbreviations: TPA = tissue plasminogen activator; APSAC = anisoylated plasminogen-streptokinase complex; SAH = subarachnoid hemorrhage; RHD = rheumatic heart disease; AF = atrial fibrillation.

rence. Therapies to improve cerebral circulation or reduce brain damage in the face of active cerebral ischemia all remain *experimental*. The following conclusions and therapeutic recommendations are drawn only from stroke pharmacotherapies that are considered established and are intended only to identify appropriate treatment populations and modalities. It is assumed that appropriate diagnostic procedures have been taken to identify and segregate patients with TIAs caused by atherothrombosis versus those caused by cardiogenic emboli.

1. Prophylactic antiplatelet therapy does not reduce the risk of stroke in asymptomatic individuals, as shown in 27,000 physicians in the United Kingdom and the United States.[156,189] Since MI is a risk factor for stroke, however, patients older than the age of 40 who have never suffered a cerebral vascular event, but who have documented risk factors (e.g., atherosclerosis, hypertension), should receive alternate-day therapy with 325 mg of aspirin to reduce the risk of myocardial ischemia.

2. Patients with a history of TIA or completed stroke should be treated with an antiplatelet agent to lessen the chances of either an initial stroke or its recurrence.[5] While neuroprotective results were obtained only at an aspirin dose of 1300 mg daily, 325 mg of aspirin has fewer side effects and may be equally effective. Ticlopidine at a dose of 250 mg twice daily may be considered as an alternative to aspirin prophylaxis.[92,65]

3. Patients with MI plus an anterior or septal wall infarct or an intramural thrombus demonstrated with two-dimensional echocardiography (2D-echo) should be heparinized (PTT = 1.5 to 2 times control) and converted to warfarin therapy (PT = 1.3 to 1.7 times control) until such time that the 2D-echo indicates resolution of the thrombus.[54]

4. In patients with rheumatic heart disease, as defined by either mitral or aortic valve involvement, the presence of systemic or cerebral embolism or atrial fibrillation (AF) are clear indications for anticoagulation.[117] To prevent recurrent thromboemboli to brain, the patient should be heparinized and converted to warfarin therapy. Anticoagulants should be delayed for approximately 1 week in patients who are severely hypertensive, who have large areas of infarction on CT scans, or who show evidence of hemorrhagic conversion.

5. Patients with nonvalvular AF are candidates for anticoagulation if they present with evidence of systemic embolism, a left atrial thrombus on 2D-echo, or dilated or hypertrophic cardiomyopathy. Patients who undergo DC conversion of AF are also candidates for anticoagulation prior to the procedure.[191] Asymptomatic patients older than the age of 60 with isolated AF may be considered for prophylactic anticoagulation or aspirin on an individual basis, since these individuals face a fivefold to sixfold increase in the risk of stroke.[53] Patients older than the age of 75 showed no risk reduction with aspirin,[53] and data on warfarin therapy in this subpopulation are not yet available.

SUMMARY

Effective therapy for stroke and hypoxic-ischemic disorders has been an elusive goal of neurologic therapy. Recent progress, however, justifies an optimistic approach to these disorders. Clinical trials conducted during the past decade have enhanced our understanding of the role of anticoagulation and antiplatelet therapy in preventing cerebral infarction. Both aspirin and warfarin sodium are effective for prevention of stroke in patients with TIA.

Thrombolytic therapy is currently undergoing clinical trials for stroke.

Much more has been learned about the details of the cascade of biochemical events that cause neuron injury and death in ischemic tissue. Combinations of intracellular calcium overload, energy failure, generation of toxic free radicals, and acidosis appear to be major events that lead to neuronal death. Therapeutic strategies to block entry of calcium into cells through VSCC (e.g., nimodipine) reduce brain injury in animal tests, and several clinical trials also have had positive results. Other approaches, including attempts to block calcium entry through EAA-operated calcium channels and to reduce energy failure and free radicals, are promising but remain experimental.

REFERENCES

1. Adams, H, Olinger, C, Marler, J, Biller, J, Brott, T, Barsan, W, and Banwart, K: Comparison of admission serum glucose concentration with neurologic outcome in acute cerebral infarction. Stroke 19:455–458, 1988.
2. Allen, GS, Ahn, HS, Preziosi, TJ, Battye, MB, Boone, S, Chou, S, Kelly, D, Weir, B, Crabbe, R, Lavek, P, Rosenbloom, S, Dorsey, F, Ingram, C, Mellits, D, Bertsh, L, Boisvert, D, Hundley, M, Johnson, R, Strom, J, and Transou, C: Cerebral arterial spasm—A controlled trial of nimodipine in patients with subarachnoid hemorrhage. N Engl J Med 308:619–624, 1983.
3. American-Canadian Cooperative Study Group: Persantine-aspirin trial in cerebral ischemia, Part II: Endpoint Results. Stroke 16:406–415, 1985.
4. Anderson, D and Cranford, R: Corticosteroids in ischemic stroke. Stroke 10:68–71, 1979.
5. Antiplatelet Trialists' Collaboration: Secondary prevention of vascular disease by prolonged antiplatelet treatment. Br Med J 296:320–331, 1988.
6. Asplund, K, Hagg, E, Helmers, C, Lithner, F et al: The natural history of stroke in diabetic patients. Acta Med Scand 207:417–424, 1980.
7. Astrup, J, Siesjö, B, and Symon, L: Editorial: Thresholds in cerebral ischemia —the ischemic penumbra. Stroke 12:723–725, 1981.
8. Astrup, J, Symon, L, Branston, NM, and Lassen, NA: Cortical evoked potential and extracellular potassium and hydrogen at critical levels of brain ischemia. Stroke 8:51, 1977.
9. Aveldano, M and Bazan, N: Rapid production of diacylglycerols enriched in arachidonate and stearate during early brain ischemia. J Neurochem 25:919–920, 1975.
10. Awad, I, Little, JR, Lucas, F, Skrinska, V, Slugg, R, and Lesser, R: Treatment of acute focal cerebral ischemia with prostacyclin. Stroke 14:203–209, 1983.
11. Barnett, HJM and Hyland, JJ: Noninfective intracranial venous thrombosis. Brain 76:36–49, 1953.
12. Baumgartner, HR and Muggli, R: Adhesion and aggregation: Morphological demonstration and quantification in vivo and in vitro. In Gordon, JL (ed): Platelets in Biology and Pathology. North-Holland Publishing Co, New York, 1976, pp 23–57.
13. Beck, DW, Adams, HP, Flamm, ES, Godersky, JC, and Loftus, CM: Combination of aminocaproic acid and nicardipine in treatment of aneurysmal subarachnoid hemorrhage. Stroke 19:63–67, 1988.
14. Bell, BA, Symon, L, and Branston, NM: CBF and time thresholds for the formation of ischemic cerebral edema and the effects of reperfusion in baboons. J Neurosurg 62:31–46, 1985.
15. Benveniste, H, Drejer, J, Schousboe, A, and Diemer, NH: Elevation of the extracellular concentrations of glutamate and aspartate in rat hippocampus during transient cerebral ischemia monitored by intracerebral microdialysis. J Neurochem 43:1369–1374, 1984.
16. Biller, J, Massey, E, Marler, J, Adam, H, Davie, J, Bruno, P, Herriksen, R, Linhardt, R, Goldstein, L, Alberts, M, Kisker, C, Toffol, G, Greenberg, C, Banwart, K, Bertels, C, Beck, D, Walker, M, and Magnani, H: A dose escalation

study of ORG 10172 (low molecular weight heparinoid in stroke). Neurology 39:262–265, 1989.

17. Blair, RDG and Waltz, AG: Regional cerebral blood flow during acute ischemia. Neurology 20:802–808, 1970.

18. Block, G and Pulsinelli, W: N-methyl-D-aspartate receptor antagonists: Failure to prevent ischemia-induced selective neuronal damage. In Raichle, M and Powers, W (eds): Cerebrovascular Diseases, Fifteenth Princeton Conference. Raven Press, New York, 1987, pp 37–42.

19. Bosley, TM, Woodhams, PL, Gordon, RD, and Balazs, R: Effects of anoxia on the stimulated release of amino acid neurotransmitters in the cerebellum in vitro. J Neurochem 40:189–201, 1983.

20. Bousser, MG, Chiras, J, Bories, J, and Castaigne, P: Cerebral venous thrombosis: A review of 38 cases. Stroke 16:199–213, 1985.

21. Bousser, MG, Eschwege, E, Haguenau, M, Lefauconnier, N, Thibult, D, Touboul, D, and Touboul, P: "AICLIA" controlled trial of aspirin and dipyridamole in the secondary prevention of atherothrombotic cerebral ischemia. Stroke 14:5–14, 1983.

22. Brandt, L, Ljunggren, B, Saveland, H, and Andersson, KE: Use of a calcium channel antagonist in aneurysmal subarachnoid hemorrhage. In Vanhoutte, PM, Paoletti, R, and Govoni, S (eds): Calcium Antagonists. Pharmacology and Clinical Research. New York Academy of Sciences, New York, 1988, pp 667–675.

23. Breckinridge, AN: Clinical pharmacology of anticoagulants. In Mead, TW (ed): Anticoagulants and Myocardial Infarction: A Reappraisal. John Wiley & Sons, New York, 1984, pp 63–90.

24. Brierley, JB and Graham, DI: Hypoxia and vascular disorders of the central system. In Adams, JH, Corsellis, JAN, and Duchen, LW (eds): Greenfield's Neuropathology. John Wiley & Sons, New York, 1984, pp 125–207.

25. Brott, T, Haley, EC, Levy, DE, Barsan, WG, Reed, R, Olinger, C, and Marker, J: Very early therapy for cerebral infarction with tissue plasminogen activator (TPA). Stroke 19:133, 1988.

26. Broderick, J, Phillips, S, Whisnant, J, O'Fallon, W, and Bergstralh, E: Incidence rates of stroke in the eighties: The end of the decline in stroke? Stroke 20:577–582, 1989.

27. Buchan, A and Pulsinelli, W: Hypothermia but not the N-methy-D-aspartate antagonist, MK-801, attenuates neuronal damage in gerbils subjected to transient global ischemia. J Neurosci 10:311–316, 1990.

28. Buchan, AM and Barnett, HJM: The management of stroke. In Oxbury, JM and Swash, M (eds): Clinical Neurology. Churchill Livingstone, New York, 1991, pp 924–952.

28a. Buchan, A, Li, H, Pulsinelli, W: The N-methyl-D-aspartate antagonist, MK-801, fails to protect against neuronal damage caused by transient, severe forebrain ischemia in the adult rat. J Neurosci 11:1049–1056, 1991.

29. Buchanan, DS and Brazinsky, JH: Dural sinus and cerebral venous thrombosis. Incidence in young women receiving oral contraceptives. Arch Neurol 22:440–444, 1970.

30. Buckler, PW and Douglas, AS: The pathological and clinical basis for anticoagulants in ischemic heart disease. In Mead, TW (ed): Anticoagulants and Myocardial Infarction: A Reappraisal. John Wiley & Sons, New York, 1984, pp 1–28.

31. Canadian Cooperative Study Group: A randomized trial of aspirin and sulfinpyrazone in threatened stroke. N Engl J Med 299:53–59, 1978.

32. Capon, A, de Rood, M, Verbist, A, and Fruhling, J: Action of vasodilators on regional cerebral blood flow in subacute or chronic cerebral ischemia. Stroke 8:25–29, 1977.

33. Carafoli, E: Intracellular calcium homeostasis. Annu Rev Biochem 56:395–433, 1987.

34. Cerebral Embolism Study Group: Immediate anticoagulation of embolic stroke: A randomized trial. Stroke 14:668–676, 1983.

35. Cerebral Embolism Study Group: Immediate anticoagulation of embolic stroke: Brain hemorrhage and management options. Stroke 15:779–789, 1984.

36. Cheung, JY, Bonventre, JV, Malis, CD, and Leaf, A: Calcium and ischemic injury. N Engl J Med 314:1670–1676, 1986.

37. Choi, D: Ionic dependence of glutamate neurotoxicity. J Neurol Sci 7:369–379, 1987.

38. Clark, LC and Gollan, F: Survival of mammals breathing organic liquids equilibrated with oxygen at atmospheric pressure. Science 152:1755–1756, 1966.

39. Clouse, LH and Comp, PC: The regulation of hemostasis: The protein C system. N Engl J Med 314:1298–1304, 1986.

40. Collen, D: Biological properties of plasminogen activators. In Sobel, B, Collen, D, and Grossbard, EB (eds): Tissue Plasminogen Activator in Thrombolytic Therapy. Marcel Dekker, Inc, New York, 1987, pp 3–24.

41. Cook, P and James, I: Cerebral Vasodilators, Part I. N Engl J Med 305:1508–1513, 1981.

42. Cook, P and James, I: Cerebral Vasodilators, Part II. N Engl J Med 305:1560–1564, 1981.

43. Cotman, C and Iversen, L: Excitatory amino acids in the brain: Focus on NMDA receptors. Trends in Neuroscience 10:263–265, 1987.

44. Coulshed, N, Epstein, EJ, McKendrick, CS, Galloway, R, and Walker, E: Systemic embolism in mitral valve disease. Br Heart J 32:26, 1970.

44a. Crowell, R, Marcoux, F, and DeGirolami, U: Variability and reversibility of focal cerebral ischemia in unanesthetized monkeys. Neurology 31:1295–1302, 1981.

45. deCourten-Myers, G, Myers, R, and Schoofield, L: Hyperglycemia enlarges infarct size in cerebrovascular occlusion in cats. Stroke 19:623–630, 1988.

46. Del Zoppo, G: Thrombolytic therapy in cerebrovascular disease. Stroke 19:1174–1179, 1988.

46a. Del Zoppo, G: An open multicenter trial of recombinant tissue plasminogen activator in acute stroke: A progress report. Stroke 21:174–175, 1990.

47. Del Zoppo, G, Ferbert, A, Otis, S, Bruchmann, H, Brückmann, H, Hacke, W, Zynoff, J, Harker, L, and Zeumer, H: Local intra-arterial fibrinolytic therapy in acute carotid territory stroke: A pilot study. Stroke 19:307–313, 1988.

48. Deshpande, JK, Siesjö, BK, and Wieloch, T: Calcium accumulation and neuronal damage in the rat hippocampus following cerebral ischemia. Journal of Cerebral Blood Flow and Metabolism 7:89–95, 1987.

49. Deshpande, JK and Wieloch, T: Flunarizine, a calcium entry blocker, ameliorates ischemic brain damage in the rat. Anesthesiology 64:215–224, 1986.

50. Di Rocco, C, Iannelli, A, Leone, G, Moschini, M, and Valori, VM: Heparin-urokinase treatment in aseptic dural sinus thrombosis. Arch Neurol 38:431–435, 1981.

51. Dienel, GA: Regional accumulation of calcium in postischemic rat brain. J Neurochem 43:913–925, 1984.

51a. Dirragl, U, Tanabe, J, and Pulsinelli, W: Pre- and posttreatment with MK-801 but not pretreatment alone reduces neocortical damage after focal cerebral ischemia in the rat. Brain Res 527:62–68, 1990.

52. Duke, RJ, Bloch, RF, Turpie, AGG, Trebilcock, R, and Bayer, N: Intravenous heparin for the prevention of stroke progression in acute partial stable stroke: A randomized controlled trial. Ann Intern Med 105:825–828, 1986.

53. Dunn, M, Alexander, J, de Silva, R, and Hildner, F: Antithrombotic therapy in atrial fibrillation. Chest 95(Suppl 2):118S–127S, 1989.

54. Editorial. Left ventricular thrombosis and stroke following myocardial infarction. Lancet 335:759–760, 1990.

55. Estanol, B, Rodriquez, A, Conte, G, Aleman, JM, Loyo, M, and Pizzato, J: Intracranial venous thrombosis in young women. Stroke 10:680–684, 1979.

56. Estol, D and Pessin, M: Anticoagulation: Is there still a role in atherothrombotic stroke? Stroke 21:820–824, 1990.

57. Fagan, SC, Gengo, FM, Bates, V, Levine, SR, and Kinkel, WR: Effect of nimodipine on blood pressure in acute ischemic stroke in humans. Stroke 19:401–402, 1988.

58. Fields, WS, Lehak, NA, Frankowski,

RF, and Hardy, RJ: Controlled trial of aspirin in cerebral ischemia. Stroke 8:301–316, 1977; 9:309–318, 1978.

59. Flamm, ES, Adams, HP, Beck, DW, Pinto, RS, Marler, J, Walker, M, Godersky, J, Loftus, C, Biller, J, Boarini, D, O'Del, C, Banwart, K, Kongable, G: Dose-escalation study of intravenous nicardipine in patients with aneurysmal subarachnoid hemorrhage. J Neurosurg 68:393–400, 1988.

60. Gaehtgens, P and Marx, P: Hemorheological aspects of the pathophysiology of cerebral ischemia. Journal of Cerebral Blood Flow and Metabolism 7:259–265, 1987.

61. Garde, A, Samuelsson, K, Fahlgren, H, Hedbert, E, Hjerne, L-G, and Ostman, J: Treatment after transient ischemic attack: A comparison between anticoagulant drug and inhibition of platelet aggregation. Stroke 14:677–681, 1983.

62. Gardiner, M, Nilsson, B, Rehncrona, S, and Siesjö, B: Free fatty acids in the rat brain in moderate and severe hypoxia. J Neurochem 36:1500–1505, 1981.

63. Gelmers, HJ: Effects of nimodipine (Baye e 9736) on postischemic cerebrovascular reactivity, as revealed by measuring regional cerebral blood flow (rCBF). Acta Neurochir (Wien) 63:283–290, 1982.

64. Gelmers, HJ, Gorter, K, de Weerdt, CJ, and Wiezer, HJ: A controlled trial of nimodipine in acute ischemic stroke. N Engl J Med 318:203–207, 1988.

65. Gent, M, Easton, JD, Hachinski, VC, Panak, E, Sicurella, J, Blakely, J, Ellis, D, Harbison, J, Roberts, R, and Turpie, A: The Canadian American Ticlopidine study (CATS) in thromboembolic stroke. Lancet 2:1215–1220, 1989.

66. Gent, M, Blakely, JA, Hachinski, V, Roberts, R, Barnett, H, Bauyer, N, Carruthers, S, Collins, S, Gawel, M, Giroux-Klimek, M, Hopkins, M, Jain, P, Larry, M, Meloche, J, Saerens, E, Sicurella, J, and Turpil, A: A secondary prevention, randomized trial of suloctidil in patients with a recent history of thromboembolic stroke. Stroke 16:416–424, 1985.

67. Genton, E, Barnett, HJM, Fields, WS,

Gent, M, and Hoak, J: Cerebral ischemia: Role of thrombosis and antithrombotic therapy. Study Group on Antithrombotic Therapy. Stroke 8:150–175, 1977.

68. Germano, I, Pitts, L, Meldrum, B, Bartkowski, H, and Simon, R: Kynurenate inhibition of cell excitation decreases stroke size and deficits. Ann Neurol 22:730–734, 1987.

69. Germano, IM, Bartkowski, HM, Cassel, ME, and Pitts, LH: The therapeutic value of nimodipine in experimental focal cerebral ischemia. Neurological outcome and histopathologic findings. J Neurosurg 67:81–87, 1987.

70. Gettelfinger, DM and Kokmen, E: Superior sagittal sinus thrombosis. Arch Neurol 34:2–6, 1977.

71. Gibson, G, Pulsinelli, W, Blass, J, and Duffy, T: Brain dysfunction in mild to moderate hypoxia. Am J Med 70:1247–1254, 1981.

72. Gill, R, Foster, A, and Woodruff, G: Systemic administration of MK-801 protects against ischemia-induced hippocampal neurodegeneration in the gerbil. J Neurosci 7:3343–3349, 1987.

73. Ginsberg, M, Welsh, F, and Budd, W: Deleterious effect of glucose pretreatment on recovery from diffuse cerebral ischemia in the cat. Stroke 11:347–354, 1980.

74. Ginsberg, MD, Budd, WW, and Welsh, FA: Diffuse cerebral ischemia in the cat: I. Local blood flow during severe ischemia and recirculation. Ann Neurol 3:482–492, 1978.

75. Godfraind, T, Norel, N, and Wibo, M: Tissue specificity of dihydropyridine-type calcium antagonists in human isolated tissues. Trends in Pharmacological Science 9:37–39, 1988.

76. Gotoh, O, Mohamed, AA, McCulloch, J, Graham, DI, Harper, M, and Teasdale, G: Nimodipine and the hemodynamic and histopathological consequences of middle cerebral artery occlusion in the rat. Journal of Cerebral Blood Flow and Metabolism 6:321–331, 1986

77. Gould, RJ, Murphy, KMM, and Snyder, SH: Autoradiographic localization of calcium channel antagonist re-

ceptors in rat brain with 3H-nitrendipine. Brain Res 330:217–223, 1985.

78. Greenberg, DA: Calcium channels and calcium channel antagonists. Ann Neurol 21:317–330, 1987.

79. Grotta, J, Ackerman, R, Correia, J, Fallick, G, and Chang, J: Whole blood viscosity parameters and cerebral blood flow. Stroke 13:296–301, 1982.

80. Grotta, J, Ostrow, P, Fraifeld, E, Hartman, D, and Gary, H: Fibrinogen, blood viscosity, and cerebral ischemia. Stroke 16:192–8, 1985.

81. Grotta, J, Spydell, J, Pettigrew, C, Ostrow, P, and Hunter, D: The effect of nicardipine on neuronal function following ischemia. Stroke 17:213–219, 1986.

82. Grotta, JC: Can raising cerebral blood flow improve outcome after acute cerebral infarction? Stroke 18:264–267, 1987.

83. Grotta, JC: Current status of hemodilution in acute cerebral ischemia. Stroke 18:689–90, 1987.

84. Hakim, AM: Cerebral acidosis in focal ischemia: II. Nimodipine and verapamil normalize cerebral pH following middle cerebral artery occlusion in the rat. Journal of Cerebral Blood Flow and Metabolism 6:676–683, 1986.

84a. Hall, E, Pazara, K, and Braughler, J: 21-aminosteroid lipid perioxidation inhibitor μ74006F protects against cerebral ischemia in the gerbil. Stroke 19:997–1002, 1989.

85. Handa, H, Nagasawa, S, and Yonekawa, Y: New treatment of cerebral vasospasm with fluorosol-DA 20%. In Bolin, RB, Geyer, R, and Nemo, G (eds): Advances in Blood Substitute Research. Alan R Liss, New York, 1983, pp 299–303.

86. Harris, R and Symon, L: Extracellular pH, potassium, and calcium activities in progressive ischemia of rat cortex. Journal Cerebral Blood Flow and Metabolism 4:178–186, 1984.

87. Harris, R, Symon, L, Wieloch, T, Siesjö, B, and Bramton, N: Calcium fluxes in ischemia and hypoglycemia. Relationship to energy failure. In Bes, A, Braquet, P, Paoletti, R, and Siesja, B (eds): Cerebral Ischemia. Ex-

cerpta Medica, New York, 1984, pp 147–155.

88. Harris, RJ, Branston, NM, Symon, L, Bayhan, M, and Watson, A: The effects of a calcium antagonist, nimodipine, upon physiological response of the cerebral vasculature and its possible influence upon focal cerebral ischaemia. Stroke 13:759–766, 1982.

89. Harris, RJ, Symon, L, Branston, NM, and Bayhan, M: Changes in extracellular calcium activity in cerebral ischaemia. Journal of Cerebral Blood Flow and Metabolism 1:203–209, 1981.

90. Harrison, MJG, Pollock, S, Kendell, BE, and Marshall, J: Effect of haematocrit on carotid stenosis and cerebral infarction. Lancet 2:114–115, 1981.

91. Hass, WK: Beyond cerebral blood flow, metabolism and ischemic thresholds: Examination of the role of calcium in the initiation of cerebral infarction. In Meyer, US, Lechner, H, Reivich, M, Oh, E, and Arabinar, A (eds): Cerebral Vascular Disease, vol. 3. Excerpta Medica, Amsterdam, 1981, pp 3–17.

92. Hass, WK, Easton, DJ, Adams, HP, Jr, Pryse-Phillips, W, Molony, B, Anderson, S, and Kamm, B: A randomized trial comparing ticlopidine hydrochloride with aspirin for the prevention of stroke in high-risk patients. N Engl J Med 321:501–507, 1989.

93. Hawkins, R: Cerebral energy metabolism. In McCandless, DW (ed): Cerebral Energy Metabolism and Metabolic Encephalopathy. Plenum Press, New York, 1985, pp 3–17.

94. Heiss, W-D and Podreka, I: Assessment of pharmacological effects on cerebral blood flow. Eur Neurol 17(Suppl 1): 135–143, 1978.

95. Hemodilution in Stroke Study Group: Effect of hypervolemic hemodilution treatment of acute stroke. Stroke 19:150, 1988.

96. Hirsch, J: Anti-coagulant and platelet anti-aggregant agents. In Barnett, H, Stein, BM, Mohr, JP, and Yatsu, FM (eds): Churchill Livingstone, New York, 1986, pp 925–966.

97. Horrocks, L, Dorman, R, and Porcellati, G: Fatty acids and phospholipids in brain during ischemia. In Bes, A, Bra-

quet, P, Paoletti, R, and Siesjö, BK (eds): Cerebral Ischemia. Excerpta Medica, New York, 1984, pp 211–222.

98. Hossmann, KA, van den Kerckhoff, W, and Mastuoka, Y: Treatment of cerebral ischemia by hemodilution. Bibl Haematologica 47:77–85, 1981.

99. Hsu, CY, Norris, JW, Hogan, EL, Bladin, P, Dinsdale, H, Yatsu, F, Ernest, M, Scheinberg, P, Caplan, L, Karp, H, Swanson, P, Feldman, R, Cohen, M, Mayman, C, Cobert, B, and Savitsky, J: Pentoxifylline in acute non-hemorrhagic stroke: A randomized, placebo controlled double blind trial. Stroke 19:716–722, 1988.

100. Huczynski, J, Kostka-Trabka, E, Sotowska, W, Bieron, K, Grodzinska, L, Dembinska-Kiec, A, Pykosz-Mazur, E, Peczak, E, and Gryglewski, R: Double-blind controlled trial of the therapeutic effects of prostacyclin in patients with completed ischaemic stroke. Stroke 16:810–814, 1985.

101. Italian Acute Stroke Study Group: Haemodilution in acute stroke: Results of the Italian haemodilution trial. Lancet 1:318–320, 1988.

101a. Jacewicz, M and Plum, F: Aseptic Cerebral Venous Thrombosis. In Einhaupl, K, Kempski, O, and Baethmann, A (eds): Cerebral Venous Thrombosis: Experimental and Clinical Aspects. Plenum Press, New York, 1990, pp 157–170.

102. Janaki, S: Pentoxifylline in strokes: A clinical study. J Int Med Res 8:56–62, 1980.

103. Johansson, BB: Pentoxifylline: Cerebral blood flow and glucose utilization in conscious spontaneously hypertensive rats. Stroke 17:744–747, 1986.

104. Johnson, PC: Autoregulation of blood flow. Proceedings of an international symposium. Circ Res 15(Suppl 1):1–291, 1964.

104a. Jones, H and Millikan, C: Temporal profile of acute carotid system cerebral infarction. Stroke 7:64–72, 1976

104b. Jones, H, Millikan, C, and Sandok, B: Temporal profile of acute vertebrobasilar system cerebral infarction. Stroke 11:173–177, 1980

104c. Patrick, B, Ramirez-Lassepaz, M,

and Snyder, B: Temporal profile of vertebrobasilar territory infarction. Stroke 11:643–648, 1980

105. Kagstrom, E, Smith, M-L, and Siesjö, BK: Local cerebral blood flow in the recovery period following complete cerebral ischemia in the rat. Journal of Cerebral Blood Flow and Metabolism 3:170–182, 1983.

106. Kannel, WB, Gordon, T, Wolf, PA, and McNamara, P: Hemoglobin and the risk of cerebral infarction. Stroke 3:409–420, 1972.

107. Kassell, NF, Peerless, SJ, Durward, QJ, Beck, DW, Drake, CG, and Adams, HP: Treatment of ischemic deficits from vasospasm with intravascular volume expansion and induced arterial hypertension. Neurosurgery 11:337–343, 1982.

108. Keating, EC, Gross, SA, Schlamowitz, RA, Mazur, JH, Pitt, W, and Miller, D: Mural thrombi in myocardial infarctions: Prospective evaluation by two-dimensional echocardiography. Am J Med 74:989–995, 1983.

109. Kiwak, KJ, Coughlin, SR, and Moskowitz, MA: Arachidonic acid metabolism in brain blood vessels: Implications for the pathogenesis and treatment of cerebrovascular diseases. In Barnett, HJM, Mohr, JP, Stein, BM, and Yatsu, FM (eds): Stroke Pathophysiology, Diagnosis, and Management. Churchill Livingstone, New York, 1986, pp 141–163.

110. Kontos, HA: Cerebral microcirculation in stroke. In Barnett, HJM, Mohr, JP, Stein, BM, and Yatsu, FM (eds): Stroke Pathophysiology, Diagnosis, and Management. Churchill Livingstone, New York, 1986, pp 91–95.

111. Koppenhagen, K, Wenig, HG, and Muller, K: The effect of pentoxyfylline (Trental) on cerebral blood flow: A double-blind study. Curr Med Res Opin 4:681–687, 1977.

112. Kraig, R and Nicholson, C: Profound acidosis in presumed glia during ischemia. In Powers, W and Raichle, M (eds): Cerebrovascular Diseases. Raven Press, New York, 1987, pp 97–102.

113. Krayenbuhl, HA: Cerebral venous and

sinus thrombosis. Clin Neurosurg 14:1–24, 1966.

114. Kuschinsky, W: Coupling of Blood Flow and Metabolism in the Brain — the Classical View. In Seylaz, A and Sercombe, R (eds): Neurotransmission and Cerebrovasacular Functions II. Elsevier, New York, 1989, pp 331–342.

115. Kuschinsky, W, Wahl, M, Bosse, O, and Thurau, K: Perivascular potassium and pH as determinants of local pial arterial diameter in cats. A microapplication study. Circ Res 31:240–247, 1972.

116. Laycock, JR, Coakham, HB, Silver, IA, and Walters, FJ: Effect of carotid artery ligation and infusion of Fluosol FC-43 emulsion on brain surface oxygen tension. Stroke 17:1242–1246, 1986.

117. Levine, H, Pauker, S, and Salzman, E: Antithrombotic therapy in valvular heart disease. Chest 95(Suppl 2):98S–106S, 1989.

118. Levine, M, Raskob, G, and Hirsh, J: Hemorrhagic complications of long-term anticoagulant therapy. Chest 95:26S–35S, 1989.

118a. Liu, T, Beckman, J, Freeman, B, Hogan, E, and Hsu, C: Polyethylene glycol-conjugated superoxidase dismutase and catalase reduce ischemic brain injury. Am J Physiol 256:H589–593, 1989.

119. Lou, HC, Edvinsson, L, and MacKenzie, ET: The concept of coupling blood flow to brain function: Revision required? Ann Neurol 22:289–297, 1987.

120. Lowry, OH, Passonneau, JV, Hasselberger, FX, and Schulz, DW: Effect of ischemia on known substrates and cofactors of the glycolytic pathway in brain. J Biol Chem 239:18–30, 1964.

121. MacIntyre, DE: The platelet release reaction: Association with adhesion and aggregation and comparison with secretory responses in other cells. In Gordon, JL (ed): Platelets in Biology and Pathology. North-Holland Publishing Co, New York, 1976, pp 23–57.

122. Magnoni, MS, Govoni, S, Battaini, F, and Trabucchi, M: L-type calcium channels are modified in rat hippocampus by short-term experimental ischemia. Journal of Cerebral Blood Flow and Metabolism 8:96–99, 1988.

123. Marcum, JM, Dedman, JR, Brinkley, BR, and Means, AR: Control of microtubule assembly-disassembly by calcium-dependent regulator protein. Proc Natl Acad Sci USA, 75:3771–3775, 1978.

124. Martin, JF, Hamdy, N, Nicholl, J, Lewtas, N, Bergvall, U, Owen, P, Syder, D, and Holroyd, M: Double-blind controlled trial of prostacyclin in cerebral infarction. Stroke 16:386–390, 1985.

125. McHenry, LC, Jr: Cerebral vasodilator therapy in stroke. Stroke 3:686–691, 1972.

126. McHenry, LC, Jr, Jaffe, ME, Kawamura, J, and Goldberg, HI: Effect on papaverine on regional blood flow in focal vascular disease of the brain. N Engl J Med 282:1167–1170, 1970.

126a. Meister, W, Einhaupl, K, Villbringer, A, Schmiechek, P, Haber, R, Pfister, H, Pellkofer, M, Steinhoff, H, Deckert, M, and Anneser, F: Treatment of Patients with Cerebral Sinus and Vein Thrombosis with Heparin. In Einhaupl, K, Kempski, O, and Baethmann, A (eds): Cerebral Venous Thrombosis: Experimental and Clinical Aspects. Plenum Press, New York, 1990, pp 225–230.

127. Melamed, E: Reactive hyperglycaemia in patients with acute stroke. J Neurol Sci 29:267–275, 1976.

128. Meyer, FB, Anderson, RE, Sundt, TM, Jr, and Sharbrough, FW: Selective central nervous system calcium channel blockers — A new class of anticonvulsant agents. Mayo Clin Proc 61:239–247, 1986.

129. Meyer, FB, Sundt, TM, Jr, Anderson, RE, and Tally, P: Ischemic vasoconstriction and parenchymal brain pH. In Vanhoutte, PM, Paoletti, R, and Govoni, S (eds): Calcium Antagonists. Pharmacology and Clinical Research. New York Academy of Sciences, New York 1988, pp 502–515.

130. Meyer, FB, Sundt, TM, Jr, Yanagihara, T, and Anderson, RE: Focal cerebral ischemia: Pathophysiological mechanisms and rationale for future avenues of treatment. Mayo Clin Proc 62:35–55, 1987.

131. Meyer, JS, Gotoh, F, Gilroy, J, and Nara, N: Improvement in brain oxygenation and clinical improvement in pa-

tients with strokes treated with papaverine hydrochloride. JAMA 194:957–961, 1965.

132. Miller, RJ: Multiple calcium channels and neuronal function. Science 235:46–52, 1987.

133. Miller, VT, Coull, BM, Yatsu, FM, Shah, AB, and Beamer, NB: Prostacyclin infusion in acute cerebral infarction. Neurology 34:1431–1435, 1984.

134. Miller, VT and Hart, RG: Heparin anticoagulation in acute brain ischemia. Stroke 19:403–406, 1988.

135. Minamisawa, H, Terashi, A, Katayama, Y, Kanda, Y, Shimizu, J, Shiratori, T, Inamura, K, Kaseki, H, and Yoshino, Y: Brain eicosanoid levels in spontaneously hypertensive rats after ischemia with reperfusion: Leukotriene C4 as a possible cause of cerebral edema. Stroke 19:372–377, 1988.

135a. Mohamed, A, Gatoh, O, Graham, D, Osborne, K, McCulloch, J, Mendelow, A, Teasdale, G, and Harper, A: Effect of pretreatment with the calcium antagonist nimodipine on local blood flow and histopathology after middle cerebral artery occlusion. Ann Neurol 18:705–711, 1985.

136. Mohr, JP: Nimodipine and Other Calcium Antagonists in Acute Ischemic Stroke. In Nimodipine Pharmacological and Clinical Results in Cerebral Ischemia. Springer-Verlag, Berlin, 1991, pp 151–161.

137. Monaghan, DT and Cotman, CW: Distribution of N-methyl-D-aspartate sensitive L-[3H]-glutamine binding sites in rat brain. J Neurosci 5:2909–2919, 1985.

138. Moncada, S: Biology and therapeutic potential of prostacyclin. Stroke 14:157–168, 1983.

139. Monk, JP and Heel, RC: Anisoylated plasminogen streptokinase activator complex (APSAC): A review of its mechanism of action, clinical pharmacology and therapeutic use in acute myocardial infarction. Drugs 34:25–49, 1987.

140. Myers, RE and Yamaguchi, S: Nervous system effects of cardiac arrest in monkeys. Arch Neurol 34:65–74, 1977.

141. Nedergaard, M: Transient focal ischemia in hyperglycemic rats is associated with increased cerebral infarction. Brain Res 408:79–85, 1987.

142. Norris, JW and Hachinski, VC: High dose steroid treatment in cerebral infarction. Br Med J 292:21–23, 1986.

143. Nowcyky, MC, Fox, AP, and Tsien, RW: Three types of neuronal calcium channel with different calcium agonist sensitivity. Nature 316:440–443, 1985.

144. Olesen, J and Paulson, OB: The effect of intra-arterial papaverine on the regional cerebral blood flow in patients with stroke or intracranial tumor. Stroke 2:148–159, 1971.

145. Olney, JW: Neurotoxicity of excitatory amino acids. In McGeer, EG, Olney, JW, and McGeer, PL (eds): Kainic Acid as a Tool in Neurobiology. Raven Press, New York, 1978, pp 37–70.

146. Olney, JW: Excitotoxins: An overview. In Fuxe, K, Roberts, P, and Schwarcz, R (eds): Excitotoxins. Plenum Press, New York, 1983, pp 82–96.

147. Olsson, JE, Brechter, C, Bäcklund, D, Krook, H, Müller, R, Nitelius, E, Olsson, O, and Tornberg, A: Anticoagulant vs. antiplatelet therapy as prophylactic against cerebral infarction in transient ischemic attacks. Stroke 11:4–9, 1980.

148. Osterholm, JL, Alderman, JB, Triolo, AJ, D'Amore, BR, Williams, HD, and Frazer, G: Severe cerebral ischemia treatment by ventriculosubarachnoid perfusion with an oxygenated fluorocarbon emulsion. Neurosurgery 13:381–387, 1983.

149. Ott, EO, Lechner, H, and Aranibar, A: High blood viscosity syndrome in cerebral infarction. Stroke 5:330–333, 1974.

150. Ozyurt, E, Graham, DI, Woodruff, GN, and McCulloch, J: Protective effect of the glutamate antagonist, MK-801, in focal cerebral ischemia in the cat. Journal of Cerebral Blood Flow and Metabolism 8:138–143, 1988.

151. Patrignani, P, Filabozzi, P, and Patrono, C: Selective cumulative inhibition of platelet thromboxane production by low-dose aspirin in healthy subjects. J Clin Invest 69:1366–1372, 1982.

152. Paul, KS, Whalley, ET, Forster, C, Lye, R, and Dutton, J: Prostacyclin and cere-

bral vessel relaxation. J Neurosurg 57:334–40, 1982.

153. Peerless, SJ, Ishikawar, R, Hunter, IG, and Peerless, MJ: Protective effect of fluosol-DA in acute cerebral ischemia. Stroke 12:558–563, 1981.

153a. Pessin, M, Del Zoppo, G, and Estol, C: Thrombolytic agents in the treatment of stroke. Clin Neuropharm 13:271–289, 1990.

154. Petersen, P, Boysen, G, Godtfredsen, J, Andersen, E, and Andersen, B: Placebo-controlled, randomised trial of warfarin and aspirin for prevention of thromboembolic complications in chronic atrial fibrillation. Lancet 1:175–179, 1989.

155. Petito, CK, Feldmann, E, Pulsinelli, WA, and Plum, F: Delayed hippocampal damage in human following cardiorespiratory arrest. Neurology 37:1281–1286, 1987.

156. Peto, R, Gray, R, Collins, R, Whealey, K, Hennekens, C, Jamrozikt, K, Warlow, C, Hafner, B, Thompson, E, Norton, S, Gilliband, J, and Doll, R: Randomized trial of prophylactic daily aspirin in male doctors. Br Med J 296:313–316, 1988.

157. Petruk, KC, West, M, Mohr, G, Bryce, K, and Weir, A. Nimodipine treatment in poor grade aneurysm patients. J Neurosurg 68:505–517, 1988.

158. Plum, F and Pulsinelli, W: Cerebral metabolism and hypoxic-ischemic brain injury. In Asbury, A, McKhann, G, and McDonald, A (eds): Diseases of the Nervous System. WB Saunders, Philadelphia, 1986, pp 1086–1101.

159. Poller, L: Therapeutic ranges in anticoagulation administration. Br Med J 290:1683–1686, 1985.

160. Pulsinelli, W, Levy, D, Sigsbee, B, Scherer, P, and Plum, F: Increased damage after ischemic stroke in patients with hyperglycemia with or without established diabetes mellitus. Am J Med 74:540–544, 1983.

161. Pulsinelli, W, Waldman, S, and Rawlinson, D: Moderate hyperglycemia augments ischemic brain damage: A neuropathological study in the rat. Neurology 32:1239–1246, 1982.

162. Pulsinelli, WA: Selective neuronal vul-

nerability: Morphological and molecular characteristics. Prog Brain Res 63:29–37, 1985.

163. Pulsinelli, WA, Brierley, JB, and Plum, F: Temporal profile of neuronal damage in a model of transient forebrain ischemia. Ann Neurol 11:491–498, 1982.

163a. Pulsinelli, W and Buchan, A: In vivo Brain Ischemia and Amino Acid Neurotransmitters: A Comparison of Focal and Global Ischemia. In Schousboe, A, Diener, N, and Kofoel, H (eds): Drug Research Related to Neuroactive Amino Acids. Alfred Benzon Symposium 32. Munksgaard, Copenhagen, 1991, in press.

164. Rassmussen, H: The calcium messenger system. N Engl J Med 314:1094–1101, 1986.

165. Reis, DJ and Iadecola, C: Regulation by the brain of its blood flow and metabolism: Role of intrinsic neuronal networks and circulating. In Owman, C and Hardebo, JE (eds): Neural Regulation of Brain Circulation. Elsevier Science Publishers, Amsterdam, 1986, pp 129–145.

166. Robins, M and Baum, HM: Incidence. The National Survey of Stroke. Stroke 12(Suppl 1):45–55, 1981.

167. Rosenberg, RD, Oosta, GM, Jordan, RE, and Gardner, WT: Mechanism of anti-thrombin action and the structural basis of heparin's anticoagulant function. In Lindblad, RL, Brown, WV, and Mann, KG (eds): Chemistry and Biology of Heparin. Elsevier, Amsterdam, 1981, pp 249–269.

168. Rothman, SM: Synaptic activity mediates death of hypoxic neurons. Science 220:536–537, 1983.

169. Rothman, SM: The neurotoxicity of excitatory amino acids is produced by passive chloride influx. J Neurosci 5:1483–1489, 1985.

170. Rothman, SM and Olney, JW: Glutamate and the pathophysiology of hypoxic-ischemic brain damage. Ann Neurol 19:105–111, 1986.

171. Ruether, R and Dorndorf, W: Aspirin in patients with cerebral ischemia and normal angiograms. The results of a double blind trial. In Breddin, K, Dorndoff, W, Lew, D, and Marks, R (eds): Ace-

tyl salicyclic acid in cerebral ischemia coronary heart disease. Schattauer Verlag, Stuttgart, 1978, pp 97–106.

172. Sanguinetti, MC and Kass, RS: Voltage-dependent block of calcium channel current in the calf cardiac Purkinje fiber by dihydropyridine calcium channel antagonists. Circ Res 55:336–348, 1984.

173. Sapolsky, R and Pulsinelli, W: Glucocorticoids potentiate ischemic injury to neurons: Therapeutic implications. Science 229:1397–1400, 1985.

174. Scandanavian Stroke Study Group: Multicenter trial of hemodilution in acute ischemic stroke. I. Results in the total patient population. Stroke 18:691–699, 1987.

175. Scandanavian Stroke Study Group: Multicenter trial of hemodilution in acute ischemic stroke. Results of subgroup analysis. Stroke 19:464–471, 1988.

176. Schanne, FA, Kane, AB, Young, EE, and Farber, JL: Calcium dependence of toxic cell death: A final common pathway. Science 206:700–702, 1979.

177. Scriabine, A, Battye, R, Hoffmeister, F, Kazda, S, Robertson, T, Garthoff, B, Schlüter, G, Rämsch, K-D, and Scherling, D: Nimodipine. New Drugs Annual: Cardiovascular Drugs 3:197–218, 1985.

177a. Scriabine, A, Tearsdale, G, Tettenborn, D, and Young, W (eds): Nimodipine Pharmacological and Clinical Results in Cerebral Ischemia. Springer-Verlag, Berlin, 1991, pp 1–273.

178. Scriabine, A and van den Kerckhoff, W: Pharmacology of nimodipine: A review. In Vanhoutte, PM, Poaletti, R, and Govoni, S (eds): Calcium Antagonists: Pharmacology and Clinical Research. New York Academy of Sciences, New York, 1988, pp 698–706.

178a. Shearderon, M, Nielson, E, Hansen, A, Jacobson P, and Honore, T: 2-3, Dihydroxy-6-nitro-7-sulfamoyl-benzo (F) quinoxaline: A neuroprotectant for cerebral ischemia. Science 247:571–574, 1990.

179. Sherman, D, Dyken, M, Fisher, M, Harrison, M, and Hart, R: Antithrombotic therapy for cerebrovascular dis-

orders. Chest 95(Suppl 2):140S–155S, 1989.

180. Siesjö, B: Cell damage in the brain: A speculative synthesis. Journal of Cerebral Blood Flow and Metabolism 1:155–185, 1981.

181. Siesjö, B. Historical overview. Calcium, ischemia, and death of brain cells. In Vanhoutte, PM, Poaletti, R, and Govoni, S (eds): Calcium Antagonists. Pharmacology and Clinical Research. New York Academy of Sciences, New York, 1988, pp 638–661.

181a. Siesjö, B, Agardh, C-D, and Bengtsson, F: Free radicals and brain damage. Cerebrovascular and Brain Metabolism Reviews. 1:165–211, 1989.

182. Simon, R, Swan, J, Griffith, T, and Meldrum, B: Blockade of N-methyl-D-aspartate receptors may protect against ischemic damage in the brain. Science 226:850–852, 1984.

183. Simon, RP, Griffiths, T, Evan, MC, Swan, JH, and Meldrum, BS: Calcium overload in selectively vulnerable neurons of the hippocampus during and after ischemia: An electron microscopy study in the rat. Journal of Cerebral Blood Flow and Metabolism 4:350–361, 1984.

184. Sixty-Plus Reinfarction Study Research Group: A double blind-trial to assess long-term oral anticoagulant therapy in elderly patients with myocardial infarction. Lancet 1:64–68, 1982.

185. Snyder, SH and Reynolds, IJ: Calcium-antagonist drugs: Receptor interactions that clarify therapeutic effects. N Engl J Med 313:995–1002, 1985.

186. Sokoloff, L: Circulation and energy metabolism of the brain. In Siegel, GJ (ed): Basic Neurochemistry. Little, Brown & Co, Boston, 1981, p 471.

187. Sorensen, PS, Pedersen, H, Marquardsen, J, Petersson, H, Heltberg, A, Simonsess, N, Munck, O, and Andersen, L: Acetylsalicylic acid in the prevention of stroke in patients with reversible cerebral ischemic attack. A Danish cooperative study. Stroke 14:15–22, 1983.

188. Stein, P and Kantrowitz, A: Antithrombotic therapy in mechanical and biological prostethic heart valves and

saphenous vein bypass grafts. Chest 95(Suppl 2):107S–116S, 1989.

188a. Steinberg, G, Salch, J, and Kumis, D: Delayed treatment with dextromethorphan and dextrophan reduces cerebral damage after transient focal ischemia. Neurosci Lett 89:193–197, 1988.

189. Steering and Committee of the Physicians Health Study Research Group: Brief Report: Findings in the aspirin component of the ongoing physicians' health study. N Engl J Med 318:262–264, 1988.

190. Strand, T, Asplund, K, Eriksson, S, Hagg, E et al: A randomized controlled trial of hemodilution therapy in acute ischemic stroke. Stroke 15:980–989, 1984.

191. Stroke Prevention in Atrial Fibrillation Study: Preliminary Report. N Engl J Med 322:863–869, 1990.

192. Study Group on Brain Edema in Stroke: Brain edema in stroke. Stroke 8:512–540, 1977.

193. Sundt, TM, Sharbrough, FW, Anderson, RE, and Michenfelder, JD: Cerebral blood flow measurement and electroencephalograms during carotid endarterectomy. J Neurosurg 41:310–320, 1974.

193a. Swann, J and Meldrum, B: Protection by NMDA antagonists against selective neuronal loss following transient ischemia. Journal of Cerebral Blood Flow and Metabolism 10:343–351, 1990.

194. Swann, KW, Ropper, AH, and Zervans, T: Initial results of a chemical trial of fluorosol-DA 20% in acute cerebral ischemia. In Bolin, RB, Geyer, R, and Nemo, G (eds): Advances in Blood Substitute Research. Alan R. Liss, New York, 1983, pp 399–404.

195. Swedish Cooperative Study Group: High-dose acetylsalicyclic acid after cerebral infarction. Stroke 18:325–334, 1987.

196. Symon, L, Crockard, HA, Dorsch, NW, Branston, NM, and Juhacz, J: Local cerebral blood flow and vascular reactivity in a chronic stable stroke in baboons. Stroke 6:482–492, 1975.

197. Teasdale, G, Legrain, Y, MacKenzie, E, and Graham, DI: Potassium release and vascular events in focal cerebral ischae-

mia. Journal of Cerebral Blood Flow and Metabolism 3(Suppl 1):S395–S396, 1983.

198. Teasdale, G, Tamura, A, Graham, D, Rabow, L, and MacKenzie, E: Vasoconstriction in focal cerebral ischemia. In Cervos-Navarra, J and Fritschka, E (eds): Cerebral Microcirculation and Metabolism. Raven Press, New York 1981, pp 77–81.

199. Thayer, SA, Murphy, SN, and Miller, RJ: Widespread distribution of dihydropyridine-sensitive calcium channels in the central nervous system. Mol Pharmacol 30:505–509, 1987.

200. The European Stroke Prevention Study Group: The European prevention study (ESPS): Principal endpoints. Lancet 2:1351–1354, 1987.

201. The tPA-Acute Stroke Study Group: An open multicenter study of the safety and efficacy of various doses of r-tPA in patients with acute stroke: Preliminary results. Stroke 19:134, 1988.

202. Thomas, DJ: Hemodilution in acute stroke. Stroke 16:763–764, 1985.

203. Timmerman, H: Calcium modulation and clinical effect profile of cyclandelate. Drugs 33(Suppl 2):1–3, 1987.

204. UK-TIA Study Group: Transient ischemic attack: (UK-TIA) aspirin trial: Interim results. Br Med J 296:316–320, 1988.

205. van den Kerckhoff, W, Hossman, KA, and Hossman, V: No effect of prostacyclin on blood flow and blood coagulation following global cerebral ischemia. Stroke 14:724–730, 1983.

206. Van Nueten, JM, Janssens, WJ, and Vanhoutte, PM: Calcium antagonism and vascular smooth muscle. In Vanhoutte, PM, Paoletti, R, and Govoni, S (eds): Calcium Antagonists. Pharmacology and Clinical Research. New York Academy of Sciences, New York, 1988, pp 234–247.

207. Vanhoutte, PM, Paoletti, R, and Govoni, S: Calcium Antagonists: Pharmacology and Clinical Research. New York Academy of Sciences, New York, 1988, pp 1–796.

208. Vanhoutte, PM, Rubanyi, GM, Miller, VM, and Houston, DS: Modulation of vascular smooth muscle contraction by

the endothelium. Annu Rev Physiol 48:307–320, 1986.

209. Villringer, A, Garner, C, Meister, W, Haberl, R, and Einhaupl, K: High-dose heparin treatment in cerebral sinus-venous thrombosis. Stroke 19:135, 1988.

210. Wagner, JA, Guggino, SE, Reynolds, IJ, Snowman, AM, Biswas, A, Olivera, BM, and Snyder, SH: Calcium antagonist receptors: Clinical and physiological relevance. In Vanhoutte, PM, Paoletti, R, and Govoni, S (eds): Calcium Antagonists: Pharmacology and Clinical Research. New York Academy of Sciences, New York, 1988, pp 117–133.

211. Walker, AE, Robins, M, and Weinfeld, FD: Clinical findings: The National Survey of Stroke. Stroke 12(Suppl 1): 13–44, 1981.

212. Waltz, AG and Sundt, TM: The microvasculature and microcirculation of the cerebral cortex after arterial occlusion. Brain 90:681–696, 1967.

213. Watson, BD, Busto, R, Goldberg, WJ, Santiso, M, Yoshida, S, and Ginsberg, M: Lipid peroxidation in vivo induced by reversible global ischemia in the rat. J Neurochem 42:268–274, 1984.

214. Weinreich, DJ, Burke, JF, and Pauletto, FJ: Left ventricular mural thrombit complicating acute myocardial infarction. Ann Intern Med 100:789–794, 1984.

215. Wolf, PA, Dawber, TR, and Thomas HE, Jr: Epidemiologic assessment of chronic atrial fibrillation and risk of stroke: The Framingham study. Neurology 28:973–977, 1978.

216. Woo, E, Ma, J, Robinson, J, and Yu, L: Hyperglycemia as a stress response in acute stroke. Stroke 19:1359–1364, 1988.

217. Wood, JH, Polyzoidis, KS, Epstein, CM, Gibby, GL, and Tindall, GT: Quantitative EEG alterations after isovolemic hemodilutional augmentation of cerebral perfusion in stroke patients. Neurology 34:764–768, 1984.

218. Wood, JH, Polyzoidis, KS, Kee, DB, Jr, Prats, AR, Gibby, G, and Tindall, G: Augmentation of cerebral blood flow induced by hemodilution in stroke patients after superficial temporal-middle cerebral arterial bypass operation. Neurosurgery 15:535–539, 1984.

219. Yatsu, FM, Pettigrew, LC, and Grotta, JC: Medical therapy of ischemic stroke. In Barnett, HJM, Stein, BM, Mohr, JP, and Yatsu, F (eds): Stroke: Pathophysiology, Diagnosis and Management. Churchill Livingstone, New York, 1986, pp 1069–1084.

220. Yanagisawa, M, Kurihara, H, Kimura, S, Tomobe, Y, Kobayashi, M, Mitsiu, Y, Yazaki, Y, Goto, K, and Masaki, T: A novel potent vasoconstrictor peptide produced by vascular endothelial cells. Nature 332:411–415, 1988.

221. Yoshida, S, Abe, K, Busto, R, Watson, B, Kogure, K, and Ginsberg, M: Influence of transient ischemia on lipid-soluble antioxidants, free fatty acids and energy metabolites in rat brain. Brain Res 245:307–316, 1982.

Chapter 5

MIGRAINE

Stephen J. Peroutka, M.D., Ph.D.

THEORIES OF MIGRAINE
  PATHOGENESIS
PHARMACOLOGIC APPROACHES TO
  MIGRAINE
FUTURE APPROACHES

Headache is probably the most common human ailment. It is also the most common complaint of patients evaluated by neurologists.[24] A large percentage of these patients will be diagnosed as having migraine, a specific subtype of headache afflicting approximately 10% to 20% of the population. The morbidity associated with the 40 million migraine sufferers in the United States is staggering. It is estimated that approximately 64 million workdays are lost each year in this country due to migraine. Therefore, it is imperative that physicians can easily distinguish migraine from other types of headache so that appropriate treatment can be initiated.

All debilitating headaches should be evaluated for a possibly more malignant neurologic etiology prior to the consideration of migraine (Table 5–1). For example, meningitis, an uncommon disease in the adult, is particularly easy to mistake for migraine in that the cardinal symptoms of pounding headache, photophobia, nausea, and vomiting are present. A ruptured aneurysm, arteriovenous malformation, or intraparenchymal hemorrhage may also present with symptoms of headache only and a normal head computed tomography

(CT) scan. A lumbar puncture often is required to make the definitive diagnosis of a subarachnoid hemorrhage. In an elderly person presenting with a severe and frequently pounding headache, perhaps complicated by visual changes, temporal arteritis should be the major diagnostic consideration. A tender temporal artery, elevated erythrocyte sedimentation rate, or monocular blindness should be particularly alerting to this diagnosis. By contrast, it is unlikely that an intracranial tumor will be misdiagnosed as migraine in the emergency room although a tumor can present as a pounding unilateral headache associated with nausea. Other head pains such as cluster headache, trigeminal neuralgia, or sinus headache are rarely confused with migraine. The diagnosis of migraine should be considered only after each of the aforementioned diagnoses has been considered and eliminated.

Migraine is a specific neurologic syndrome that has a wide variety of manifestations.[26,37] At the most basic level, migraine can be defined as a throbbing (usually unilateral) headache with associated nausea. A premonitory phase may last as long as 24 hours before the headache and may consist of mood and appetite changes. The headache itself is often accompanied by photophobia, hyperacusis, polyuria, and/or diarrhea. A migraine attack usually lasts from hours to days and is followed by prolonged pain-free intervals. The headache frequency is extremely variable

Table 5–1 DIFFERENTIAL DIAGNOSIS OF DEBILITATING NONMIGRAINOUS HEADACHES

MENINGITIS
Nuchal rigidity, headache, photophobia, and prostration; may not be febrile. Lumbar puncture is diagnostic.

INTRACRANIAL HEMORRHAGE
Nuchal rigidity, headache; may not have clouded consciousness or seizures. Hemorrhage may not be seen on CT scan. Lumbar puncture shows "bloody tap," which does not clear by the last tube. A fresh hemorrhage is not xanthochromic.

ARTERIOVENOUS MALFORMATION
May have symptoms identical to migraine headaches. Contrast CT scan or magnetic resonance imaging may be diagnostic.

TUMOR
May present with prostrating pounding headaches that are associated with nausea and vomiting. Should be suspected in new "migraine," which is invariably unilateral.

TEMPORAL ARTERITIS
May present with a unilateral pounding headache. Onset generally in older patients (>50 years) and frequently associated with visual changes. The erythrocyte sedimentation rate is the best screening test and is usually markedly elevated (>50). Definitive diagnosis can be made by arterial biopsy.

Table 5–2 CLASSIFICATION OF MIGRAINE

Types of Migraine	Symptoms
Common	Unilateral (80%), throbbing headache with associated nausea
Classic	Same as common migraine but preceded by a visual aura
Complicated Hemiplegic	Sudden onset of hemiparesis followed by a contralateral throbbing headache
Ophthalmoplegic	Unilateral eye pain and ipsilateral ophthalmoplegia
Basilar artery	Visual aura with alterations in consciousness prior to headache

but usually ranges from 1 to 2 per year to 1 to 4 per month.

A commonly used classification system for migraine is summarized in Table 5–2. A "classic" migraine begins with neurologic symptoms that constitute the *aura* or *prodrome* of the headache. Visual distortions are the most common complaint of patients and usually consist of blurred vision, scintillating scotoma (a blind spot with shimmering edges), and/or fortification spectra (zigzag lines). These symptoms evolve during the course of 15 to 20 minutes. A severe, throbbing pain then begins on the side of the head contralateral to the visual distortions. In 80% of patients, the pain is unilateral and, in most patients, the headache tends to recur on the same side of the head. Importantly, there is associated nausea and the patient may occasionally vomit. A "common" migraine is identical to the "classic" headache except that it lacks the aura or prodrome phase. If the patient has focal neurologic deficits other than visual distortions, the migraine is designated "complicated." A rarer form of migraine, basilar artery migraine, produces alterations in consciousness (see Table 5–2).

A major problem confronting the physician is that migraine therapy is extremely confusing. First of all, migraine patients represent only a subpopulation of patients with headache complaints. Because of the wide variation in migraine symptomatology, it is often difficult to distinguish migraine from other types of headache. In particular, muscle-contraction or tension headaches may be coincident with migraine (i.e., mixed headache syndrome). Second, there is no known common mechanism of action for the agents used in migraine therapy. Drugs such as anti-inflammatory agents, ergots, antidepressants, beta-adrenergic blockers, serotonergic agents, and calcium channel blockers are reportedly effective in migraine therapy yet do not appear to share any common pharmacologic action. Third, the pathophysiology of migraine remains unknown. There are no serologic or radiologic tests for migraine. By necessity, the diagnosis of migraine is based on the clinical history. Moreover, the evaluation of the efficacy of pharmacologic therapies must depend on subjective patient reports.

Nonetheless, the successful treatment of migraine can often result in a dramatic decrease in the morbidity associated with the headache. This chapter will initially focus on a review of current theories of migraine pathogenesis. Discussion of a wide variety of pharmacologic approaches to the acute and prophylactic treatment of migraine will follow. These therapies will be presented in a sequence that is recommended for use in the pharmacologic treatment of patients with migraine.

THEORIES OF MIGRAINE PATHOGENESIS

Vascular Theory of Wolff

Abnormalities of cerebral blood flow (CBF) appear to play a pivotal role in the pathogenesis of migraine. Based on the theory of Wolff, migraine was considered to be a vasospastic disorder. It was hypothesized that cerebral vasoconstriction occurs during the migraine prodrome and vasodilation occurs during the headache phase. In apparent support of this theory, a number of CBF studies have documented a decrease in CBF during the aura and an increase in CBF during the headache phase of migraine.[25] These data demonstrate that vasomotor dysregulation occurs during the two phases of classic migraine.

The ability of these changes to induce the symptoms of migraine, however, has been questioned. Specifically, the decrease in CBF that is observed does not appear to be significant enough to cause focal neurologic symptoms. Also, the increase in CBF per se is not painful, and vasodilation alone cannot account for the local edema and focal tenderness often observed in migraineurs. Thus, it is likely that simple vasoconstriction and vasodilation are the basic pathophysiologic abnormalities in migraine.

It is clear, though, that CBF is altered during certain migraine attacks.

Spreading Depression of Leao

Recently, the work of Olesen and colleagues[38] has led to the suggestion that migraine results from spreading depression of cortical electrical activity (i.e., "spreading depression of Leao"). Spreading depression is an electrical phenomenon observed in nonhuman species that occurs in the cerebral cortex in response to noxious stimuli. A focal reduction in electrical activity and increase in blood flow occurs and then spreads across the hemisphere at the rate of 2 to 3 mm/min.[31] The electroencephalogram (EEG) of the animal returns to normal within approximately 10 minutes, but evoked cortical responses may be depressed for as long as an hour after the noxious stimulation. Cerebral blood flow during and after spreading depression in rats has been studied by autoradiographic methods.[29] These studies demonstrated that cortical blood flow is reduced by 20% to 25% following induced spreading depression.

Olesen and co-workers[39,40] studied gional blood flow changes in patients during a classic migraine attack. A gradual spread of reduced blood flow was observed starting in the occipital region and advancing anteriorly. Importantly, these blood flow changes did not correspond to the distribution of the major intracranial arteries, but the observed flow changes were similar to the electrical phenomenon of spreading depression of Leao. The researchers[40] speculated that the aura of classic migraine may occur secondary to the spreading oligemia observed in classic migraine patients. This theory states that migraine results from an evolving process in the cerebral cortex that occurs secondary to decreased cortical function, decreased cortical metabolism and/or vasoconstriction of cortical arterioles.[38]

Regional oligemia has not been observed in common migraine patients. Lauritzen and Olesen[30] studied 12 patients within 20 hours of the onset of a common migraine. There were no changes in focal or global CBF in any of the patients. In addition, Olesen's group[41] studied 12 patients in whom attacks could be provoked by red wine. In studies of patients in which migraine could be induced, regional CBF studies were all within normal limits. Regional blood flow thus seems to be normal during a common migraine attack, in contrast to the changes that have been reported in a classic migraine attack. While the theory of spreading depression is interesting, it must be noted that this electrical phenomenon has never been recorded in humans during a migraine attack.

Serotonergic Abnormalities

Serotonin (5-hydroxytryptamine; 5-HT) is a biogenic amine neurotransmitter that has been implicated in the pathogenesis of migraine. Serotonin neurons innervate many regions of the brain, including the cerebral cortex (see Chapter 8) and cerebral blood vessels. Biochemical studies have documented abnormalities of serotonergic systems in migraine (Table 5–3).[12,16,28,49] For example, plasma and platelet levels of 5-HT rise during the migraine aura, fall rapidly at the onset of the headache, and remain low during the migraine attack. At the same time, increased amounts of 5-HT and its metabolites are excreted in the urine during most headache attacks. The observation that migraine may be precipitated by drugs that cause release of this biogenic amine from tissue stores, such as reserpine and fenfluramine, also support a role for 5-HT in the disorder.[16,49]

Recent research has focused on the role of 5-HT receptor subtypes in the mechanism of action of antimigraine drugs. A variety of molecular, biochemical, and physiologic observations suggest that multiple 5-HT receptors exist in the central nervous system (CNS).[46,54] 5-HT receptors can be generally divided into three main "families:" $5\text{-}HT_1$, $5\text{-}HT_2$, and $5\text{-}HT_3$ receptors. Within each of the 3 "families," receptor subtypes have been described. The diversity of 5-HT receptor subtypes offers a unique opportunity to clinical neuropharmacologists. Theoretically, each receptor subtype provides a target site in the CNS that can be pharmacologically manipulated. The goal of the basic scientific research is to identify the potential functional significance of each 5-HT receptor subtype. The evolving hypothesis is that the clinical efficacy of abortive antimigraine agents derives from their ability to stimulate a specific 5-HT receptor subtype (i.e., the $5\text{-}HT_1$ receptor family), whereas prophylactic antimigraine agents share an ability to block $5\text{-}HT_2$ and/or $5\text{-}HT_{1C}$ receptors (Table 5–3).

$5\text{-}HT_1$ RECEPTORS

The $5\text{-}HT_{1D}$ receptor is a $5\text{-}HT_1$ receptor subtype that was initially characterized in 1987 through binding studies performed with radiolabeled serotonin[20] and has been shown to be widespread in the human brain.[48,55,56] In fact, $5\text{-}HT_{1D}$ receptors are the most

Table 5–3 HYPOTHETICAL ROLE OF 5-HT RECEPTOR "FAMILIES" IN MIGRAINE THERAPY

"Family"	Subtypes Included	Type of Activity	Type of Migraine Relief
$5\text{-}HT_1$	$5\text{-}HT_{1D}$	Agonist	Acute
$5\text{-}HT_2$	$5\text{-}HT_2$	Antagonist	Prophylactic
	$5\text{-}HT_{1C}$*		

*Although originally classified as a $5\text{-}HT_1$ receptor, the $5\text{-}HT_{1C}$ receptor was reclassified on the basis of molecular biologic studies.

common type of 5-HT receptor subtype observed in the human brain.[48] The $5-HT_{1D}$ receptor also functions as the "autoreceptor" that controls the release of 5-HT and other neurotransmitters.[22] $5-HT_{1D}$ receptors are distinguished from $5-HT_{1A}$ and $5-HT_{1C}$ receptors using specific 5-HT analogue drugs. $5-HT_{1B}$ receptors resemble $5-HT_D$ receptors but are not present in the human brain.

At the same time, vascular studies have identified a "5-HT_1-like" receptor in the cranial vasculature that may be identical to the $5-HT_{1D}$ receptor.[7,15,23,42] Multiple vascular studies have implicated this "5-HT_1-like" receptor in the constriction of cerebral blood vessels. In particular, a novel serotonergic agent, sumatriptan (formerly called GR 43175), appears to be an extremely selective agonist of these vascular 5-HT receptors.[15] Moreover, recent studies have indicated that sumatriptan is a potent and selective $5-HT_{1D}$ receptor agent.[34,47] Therefore, the "5-HT_1-like" receptor in certain cerebral vessels may, in fact, be the $5-HT_{1D}$ receptor. This observation is important since sumatriptan has recently been reported to be extremely effective in the acute treatment of migraine.[13]

Two theories have been proposed to explain the efficacy of $5-HT_1$ receptor agonists in migraine. On one hand, the receptor(s) stimulated by both ergots and sumatriptan has been implicated in the constriction of arteriovenous anastomoses.[53] Under the migraine model proposed by Heyck,[21] as yet unknown events lead to the opening of carotid arteriovenous anastomoses in the head. Blood is diverted from the capillary beds, and ischemia and hypoxia result. Based on this hypothesis of migraine, an effective antimigraine agent would close the shunts and restore blood blow. Indeed, Feniuk and colleagues[15] have shown that sumatriptan is a selective vasoconstrictor of the carotid circulation in the dog. As noted above, these "5-HT_1-like" receptors display marked pharmacologic similarities to $5-HT_{1D}$ receptors defined in radioligand-binding studies.

The $5-HT_{1D}$ agonists like dihydroergotamine (DHE) and sumatriptan may act by blocking the release, at the nerve terminal, of transmitters such as 5-HT, norepinephrine, and/or acetylcholine. Indeed, Saito and associates[52] have demonstrated that ergotamine and DHE are able to block the development of neurogenic plasma extravasation in the dura mater that follows depolarization of perivascular axons following capsaicin injection or unilateral electrical stimulation of the trigeminal nerve. The ability of potent $5-HT_{1D}$ agonists to antagonize endogenous transmitter release may, theoretically, account for both this effect and for their efficacy in the acute treatment of migraine.[35,52]

5-HT_2 RECEPTORS

The $5-HT_2$ receptor "family" has been extensively characterized in vitro, and a number of potent $5-HT_2$ antagonists have been marketed as prophylactic antimigraine agents. Methysergide, cyproheptadine, pizotifen, and amitriptyline are potent agents at the $5-HT_2$ receptor in the human brain, whereas verapamil and nifedipine display slightly lower affinities for these sites. These data demonstrate that a number of antimigraine drugs display high or moderate affinity for the $5-HT_2$ receptor subtype in the human brain.

Hypotheses have been proposed that may explain the efficacy of $5-HT_2$ antagonists in the prophylactic treatment of migraine. First, the $5-HT_2$ receptor has been shown to mediate contraction of smooth muscle in many vascular beds.[45] Second, Moskowitz and colleagues[10,11] have demonstrated that 5-HT can stimulate production of prostacyclin and other products of arachidonic acid metabolism in smooth muscle cells in vitro. This action of 5-HT appears to be mediated by $5-HT_2$ receptors since methysergide, cyproheptadine, and pizotifen potently prevent this effect. The significance of this finding is that modulation of prostacyclin and arachidonic acid metabolism may have important effects on vascular tone[10] and/or local inflammation.[43] In essence, 5-HT (via $5-HT_2$ receptors) could stimulate arachidonic acid metabolism at the onset of a migraine attack, and this would be expected to lead to a "sterile inflammatory reaction" in the brain vasculature. Theoretically, $5-HT_2$ antagonists are able to inhibit 5-HT from inducing the inflammatory state. Once the inflammatory reaction is initiated (i.e., once the migraine begins), however, $5-HT_2$ antagonists would be of little benefit.

Recently, it has been suggested that $5-HT_{1C}$ receptor antagonists, as opposed to the $5-HT_2$ receptor antagonists, may play an important role in the pathophysiology of migraine.[17] This suggestion derives from the fact that $5-HT_{1C}$ receptors share similar pharmacologic characteristics to $5-HT_2$ receptors, since both sites are subtypes of the $5-HT_2$ "family" of receptors. Unfortunately, currently available prophylactic antimigraine agents do not differentiate between $5-HT_{1C}$ and $5-HT_2$ receptors. Therefore, selective $5-HT_{1C}$ antagonists must be identified and developed before this interesting hypothesis can be tested in clinical trials.

Role of the Trigeminovascular System

The trigeminal nerve provides the principal afferent pathway for the transmission of head pain in humans. Ray and Wolff[51] subjected human volunteers to stimulation of the pial and dural arteries and sinuses to determine the pain-sensitive intracranial structures. Large pial arteries composing the circle of Willis were extremely sensitive to stimulation of their proximal segments but became progressively less sensitive over the cortical convexities. The pain was described as throbbing, aching, burning, or crushing.

The trigeminal nerve projects to both pial and arachnoidal structures in nonhuman species. This system has been termed the *trigeminovascular system*.[35] In their peripheral unmyelinated fibers, these neurons contain the neurotransmitter peptide substance P. Neuronal depolarization induces release of substance P into the wall of cerebral blood vessels. Substance P is known to dilate pial arteries, increase vascular permeability, and activate cells that participate in the inflammatory response. Thus, a "sterile" inflammation of the vasculature may result.[35] Stimulation of dural blood vessels also has been shown to activate nociceptive trigeminal nuclei.[32] Moskowitz and colleagues[36] suggested that the headache phase of migraine may result from the abnormal interaction of neurotransmitters released from trigeminal neurons with cranial blood vessels. This hypothesis may be useful in understanding some of the clinical aspects of migraine in humans. First, the mediation of migraine by the trigeminovascular system could account for the fact that the majority of migraines are unilateral. Second, this system would explain why the pain in migraine is usually referred to areas innervated by the trigeminal nerve. Third, the most common aura of migraine results from "posterior circulation" dysfunction, an area in which the vasculature is densely innervated by the first division of the trigeminal nerve. Most importantly, this theory of migraine allows for the development of animal models in which drug efficacy could be determined.

PHARMACOLOGIC APPROACHES TO MIGRAINE

Acute Treatments

SYMPTOMATIC TREATMENT

The vast majority of migraine attacks can be treated solely with symptomatic measures (Table 5–4). At the first onset of symptoms, mild analgesics such as aspirin or acetaminophen should be taken. Aspirin, for example, has been used in migraine for more than 50 years and remains the drug used most frequently in abortive therapy. Other non-

Table 5-4 ACUTE MIGRAINE THERAPIES

Drug	Trade Name	Dosage
Aspirin	—	650 mg q4h
Acetaminophen	—	650 mg q4h
Acetaminophen (325 mg), Isometheptene (65 mg), Dichloralphenazone (100 mg)	Midrin, Isocom	2 capsules at onset followed by 1 capsule q1h (maximum 5 capsules)
Aspirin (650 mg), Butalbital (50 mg)	Axotal*	1 tablet q4h (maximum 6 tablets)
Aspirin (325 mg), Caffeine (40 mg), Butalbital (50 mg)	Fiorinal*	1 or 2 tablets q4h (maximum 6 tablets)
Acetaminophen (325 mg), Butalbital (50 mg)	Phrenilin*	1 or 2 tablets q4h (6 capsules maximum)
Ergotamine (1 mg), Caffeine (100 mg)	Wigraine; Cafergot	2 tablets at onset then 1 table q½h (maximum 6/d or 10/wk)
Ergotamine (2 mg), Caffeine (100 mg), Belladonna (0.25 mg), Pentobarbital (30 mg)	Cafergot P-B	1 suppository at onset then 1 h later (maximum 2/d or 5/wk)
Ergotamine (2 mg), Caffeine (100 mg), Tartaric Acid (21.5 mg)	Wigraine P-B	1 suppository at onset then 1 h later (maximum 2/d or 5/wk)
Ergotamine (2 mg)	Ergostat; Ergomar	1 sublingual tablet at onset and q½h (maximum 3/d or 5/wk)
Ergotamine (9 mg/mL)	Medihaler Ergotamine Aerosol	Single inhalation at onset followed by q5min (maximum 6/d; or 15/wk)
Dihydroergotamine (1 mg/mL)	D.H.E. 45	1 mL IM or IV at onset and q1h (maximum 3 mL/d or 6 mL/wk)

*Not specifically indicated by the Food and Drug Administration for migraine.

steroidal anti-inflammatory agents are also effective pain relievers and differ from aspirin primarily in cost to the patient. Mild analgesics should be taken at the first sign of the onset of an acute attack and then every 4 hours until the headache is completely relieved. They are most effective if taken very early in the course of the headache, but rarely are able to relieve completely the pain associated with moderate-to-severe migraine attacks.

A number of stronger but non-narcotic analgesics have been developed. In general, each preparation contains a combination of aspirin or acetaminophen with sedatives such as butalbital or mild vasoconstrictors like isometheptene. Two of these commercial products (Midrin and Migralam) have been officially indicated for use in migraine. By contrast, combination agents such as Axotal, Fiorinal, and Phrenilin, although officially indicated for muscle-contraction headaches, can be used to treat relatively mild migraines.

In addition, the patient should be advised to enter a dark and quiet room. An attempt should be made to sleep, since patients will often awaken without a headache.[58] Antiemetics are another important yet infrequently used symptomatic treatment. Since nausea is a discomforting, nearly constant component of migraine, concurrent treatment with antiemetic medications such as prochlorperazine (Compazine), promethazine (Phenergan), or metoclopramide (Reglan) is indicated. In Europe, metoclopramide is considered the antiemetic of choice due to its putative ability to stimulate gastric motility.

ERGOTS

A large proportion of migraine patients will respond to mild analgesics, antiemetics, and sleep. For refractory patients, ergot preparations are recommended. The drugs have potent vasoconstrictor effects and interact with a number of neurotransmitter receptors. The use of ergots for acute migraine attacks should be restricted to patients having infrequent but severe migraine. Ergot preparations can be taken orally, sublingually, rectally, intramuscularly, intravenously, or via inhalers.

As with other medications used to abort an attack, the patient should be advised to take ergot preparations as soon as possible after the onset of a headache. Gastrointestinal absorption of ergots is erratic; this fact may explain the large variation in patient response to these drugs.[16,43] Co-administration of caffeine has been reported to increase intestinal absorption of ergots, which provides a rationale for the use of combination pills containing caffeine.[1] Various preparations of ergots are available (see Table 5–4), most of which contain additional ingredients such as caffeine and/or barbiturate derivatives.

With ergotamine preparations, a 1- or 2-mg dose should be taken at the onset of the headache and can be followed by as many as four additional 1-mg tablets, each taken 30 minutes apart. No more than 10 mg/wk of ergotamine should be taken by a single patient. Of concern is the fact that ergotamine has a relatively long biologic half-life. The administration of doses greater than 1 mg/d may cause peripheral vasospasm and can, rarely, lead to serious side effects such as gangrene (Table 5–5).[43] Therefore, the manifestations of ergotism should be evaluated in patients on long-term therapy. Ergotamine preparations are also contraindicated in pregnancy, peripheral vascular disease, angina, and hypertension. It is also recommended that ergots not be used in complicated migraine. Nausea and vomiting are probably the most common side effects of ergots. This presents a significant problem given that these symptoms are usually part of the migraine syndrome itself.

Because nausea and vomiting are such a problem in migraine, sublingual, rectal, and inhalation forms of ergotamine have been recommended (see Table 5–4). The effectiveness of drug administered by these different routes has not been rigorously evaluated. Clinical experience indicates, however, that orally administered ergotamine is erratically absorbed and sublingual preparations are frequently swallowed. Rectal absorption is more reliable, although many patients and clinicians prefer bronchial inhalation for acute therapy. Several preparations are available that combine ergotamine with other drugs such as caffeine, belladonna, and phenobarbital (see Table 5–4). The relative efficacy of these preparations has not been well studied.

Table 5–5 MAJOR SIDE EFFECTS OF DRUGS USED TO TREAT MIGRAINE

Agent	Adults and Children	Pregnant Women
Ergots	Nausea, vomiting, weakness, diarrhea, numbness, tingling, arterial spasm; chronic administration and withdrawal lead to rebound headache and depression; propranolol and ergots may worsen arterial spasm.	Contraindicated in pregnancy; transported into breast milk.
Metoclopramide	Restlessness, drowsiness in 10%; Extrapyramidal reactions more frequent in children, respond to anticholinergics.	Use cautiously in pregnancy; transported into breast milk.
Beta-adrenergic blockers	May worsen congestive failure, heart block, asthma, diabetes, and Raynaud's syndrome.	May affect fetal development, use only if necessary; transported into breast milk.
Calcium channel blockers	Dizziness, hypotension, headache, peripheral edema, bradycardia, skin eruptions.	Generally not used in pregnancy; transported into breast milk.
Tricyclic antidepressants	Anticholinergic effects, drowsiness, agitation, postural hypotension, nausea, vomiting.	Use cautiously in pregnancy.
Cyproheptadine	Drowsiness, CNS depression, paradoxic excitement.	Use cautiously in pregnancy; transported into breast milk.
Methysergide	Retroperitoneal pleuropulmonary and cardiac fibrosis after prolonged use; insomnia, lightheadedness, vascular spasm.	Contraindicated.

SUMATRIPTAN

Recently, sumatriptan (formerly called GR 43175) has been reported to be extremely effective in the acute treatment of migraine. Doenicke and associates[13] reported that 2 mg of intravenous sumatriptan completely abolished migraine symptoms in 71% of 24 migraine attacks and significantly reduced headache symptoms in the remaining patients. Only minor side effects (transient pressure in the head, feeling of warmth, or tingling) were observed. As of early 1990, sumatriptan is in phase III trials in the United States, and it continues to show great promise as an acute migraine therapy with minimal side effects. Although its mechanism of action was initially unclear, it has been suggested that sumatriptan may selectively stimulate a subpopulation of 5-HT receptors.[23,24] Indeed, the hypothesis to be tested is that the ability of sumatriptan to stimulate 5-HT_{1D} receptors might account for its antimigraine efficacy.

OTHER AGENTS

A variety of other medications has been recommended for acute migraine attacks. For example, corticosteroids have been reported to be effective in some refractory migraine cases, but the actual use of steroids in acute migraine is quite rare. By contrast, many patients are routinely treated with potent narcotics, despite the fact that such addicting drugs have no effect on the underlying migraine process. Therefore, the use of narcotics such as meperidine (Demerol) should be limited to severe acute migraine cases in which all other measures have failed. Long-term use of narcotics to treat migraine is never indicated.

EMERGENCY MANAGEMENT
OF MIGRAINE

A protocol for the emergency abortive management of severe migraine is outlined in Table 5–6. Although narcotic analgesics are commonly administered in emergency room management of migraine, it is best to avoid them for chronic recurrent episodes. Instead, a combination of intravenous ergot and antiemetic agent is preferred. For otherwise healthy adults, a useful regimen is 10 mg of intravenous metoclopramide followed by intravenous DHE mesylate (D.H.E. 45). Raskin and colleagues[5,50] have recommended 0.5 to 1 mg intravenous DHE initially, which may be repeated in 1 hour. This group reported that 49 of 55 patients were headache-free within 48 hours after receiving 0.5 mg DHE and 10 mg metoclopramide every 8 hours. Up to 3 mg of DHE may be given in the first 3 hours. Eight hours later, DHE in doses up to 2 mg may be repeated every 8 hours for 3 days. Metoclopramide in doses of 10 to 20 mg may be repeated every 4 hours as needed intravenously or orally. Metoclopramide has serotonin- and dopamine-blocking activity, which may contribute to its apparent synergism with ergot to abort migraine. Induction of sleep is often desirable as pain is subsiding and this can be safely accomplished using triazolam in a dose of 0.125 to 0.25 mg. Variations on this protocol can be tailored to the needs of patients with less severe episodes. For example, a combination of rectal or inhaled ergotamine (Medihaler Ergotamine Aerosol) and oral metoclopramide may be effective. The ordinary precautions for ergots need to be followed; avoid giving them to patients with coronary artery disease; peripheral vascular disease; hepatic or renal disease; or during pregnancy. If attacks have recurred, consideration should be given to starting prophylactic treatment as described in the next section.

A special problem is frequently presented by patients who are taking chronic narcotic analgesics for their headaches. Narcotics do not act upon the primary headache mechanism, and narcotic addiction can lead to confusing headache from withdrawal. One approach to this problem is to institute specific abortive and prophylactic migraine treatment, start the patient on a dose of oral methadone equivalent to their current dose of narcotics, and taper it during 10 days (Table 5–7).

Prophylactic Treatments

A small proportion of migraine patients have frequent headache attacks. A consensus among neurologists is to treat prophylactically patients having three or more migraines per month. The following section lists, in order of current usage, the medications that have consistently been shown effective in the prophylactic treatment of migraine (Table 5–8). Importantly, none of these agents is effective in greater than 60% to 70% of patients. Prophylactic medications should be given for a period of 6

Table 5–6 EMERGENCY TREATMENT OF SEVERE MIGRAINE

Avoid narcotics if possible.
Begin:	Metoclopramide, 10 mg IV over 1–2 min, followed by dihydroergotamine mesylate (D.H.E. 45) 0.5–1.0 mg IV

Evaluate for relief and side effects.
Continue:	Repeat D.H.E. 45 in 1 h and give up to 3.0 mg in the first 3 h: May repeat 0.5–2 mg q8h for 3 d. Repeat metoclopramide, 10–20 mg q4h.
For sleep:	Triazolam, 0.125–0.25 mg PO.
Prophylaxis:	Evaluate need and prescribe as soon as stable.

Table 5–7 EQUIVALENCY OF ORAL NARCOTICS WITH METHADONE

Drug	Dose Equivalent to 10 mg of methadone PO
Codeine	100 mg
Meperidine	150 mg
Propoxyphene	65 mg
Oxycodone	15 mg
Hydromorphone	3.75 mg

Table 5–8 PROPHYLACTIC MIGRAINE THERAPIES

Drug	Trade Name	Dosage
BETA-ADRENERGIC AGENTS		
Propranolol	Inderal	80–320 mg/d
Atenolol	Tenormin*	50–100 mg/d
Nadolol	Corgard*	40–80 mg/d
Metoprolol	Lopressor*	100–450 mg/d
Timolol	Blocadren*	20–60 mg/d
ANTIDEPRESSANTS		
Amitriptyline	Elavil*	50–200 mg/d
Phenelzine	Nardil*	15 mg tid
Isocarboxazid	Marplan*	10 mg qid
SEROTONERGIC DRUGS		
Methysergide	Sansert	4–8 mg/d
Cyproheptadine	Periactin*	4–16 mg/d
CALCIUM CHANNEL BLOCKERS		
Diltiazem	Cardizem*	180–240 mg/d
Nifedipine	Procardia*	10–40 mg tid
Verapamil	Isoptin*	80–120 mg tid
OTHER AGENTS		
Aspirin		75 mg/d (children)
Chlorpromazine	Thorazine*	50–150 mg/d
Naproxen	Naprosyn*	550 mg bid

*Not specifically indicated by the Food and Drug Administration for migraine.

months and then discontinued, due to the high incidence of complete remission in migraine. If a rebound of headache occurs after discontinuation of prophylactic therapy, then the medication regimen should be re-instituted for another 6-month trial.

BETA-ADRENERGIC ANTAGONISTS

A serendipitous finding in patients with exertional angina showed that propranolol (Inderal) was able to prevent frequent migraine attacks.[59,59] Approximately 50% to 70% of patients will derive some benefit from prophylactic propranolol therapy. Approximately one third of the patients report greater than 50% reduction in the number of attacks. A dose of 40 mg twice a day or one long-acting 80-mg tablet is usually begun, with as much as 320 mg/d being given for at least 4 to 6 weeks before deciding that the patient is nonresponsive to therapy.

A variety of other beta-adrenergic agents have been used in the treatment of migraine.[57] Atenolol (Tenormin), metoprolol (Lopressor), nadolol (Corgard), and timolol (Blocadren) appear to be at least as effective as propranolol in migraine prophylaxis. More variable results have been obtained with pindolol (Visken). By contrast, a number of other beta-adrenergic antagonists (e.g., acebutolol, oxprenolol, alprenolol) do not appear to be effective in migraine therapy.[57]

The pathophysiologic basis for the effectiveness of certain beta-adrenergic antagonists is not known; no single pharmacologic property of this class of drugs can explain their apparent clinical efficacy.[43] Antimigraine effects of these drugs do not correlate with their potency a beta-adrenergic receptors, since not all beta-adrenergic antagonists are effective migraine agents. The ability of certain beta-adrenergic agents to modulate serotonergic systems has also been suggested to be the basis of their antimigraine efficacy.[43,49] Alternatively, it has been suggested that only pure beta-adrenergic antagonists are effective agents in migraine therapy.[14,57] Drugs that display "intrinsic sympathomimetic activity" (i.e., partial agonist activity) at the beta-adrenergic receptor may be less effective migraine prophylactic agents.

Side effects with beta-adrenergic agents are seldom severe (see Table 5–5), but these drugs are contraindicated in asthma, sinus bradycardia, congestive heart failure, and diabetes mellitus. They should be used cautiously in pregnancy only if absolutely necessary. Relatively selective beta$_1$-blocking drugs such as atenolol may be relatively safer in patients with asthma and diabetes than nonselective beta blockers, but they should still be used very cautiously. They are not approved for use for migraine. Common side effects include lethargy, gastrointestinal upset, and orthostatic hypotension. Agents with lower lipid solubility than propranolol, such as atenolol and nadolol, may cause fewer CNS side effects because of their poorer penetration into the brain. These side effects rarely necessitate discontinuation of the drug, however.

AMITRIPTYLINE

The tricyclic antidepressant, amitriptyline, is an effective prophylactic agent in migraine, independent of its antidepressant actions.[8,9,18] Amitriptyline is a potent blocker of 5-HT uptake and is also an antagonist of multiple neurotransmitter receptors, but its mechanism of action in migraine prophylaxis remains unknown. Despite its widespread clinical use in this disorder, the drug is not specifically indicated for the treatment of migraine. It may offer advantages for patients with diabetes or asthma in whom beta-adrenergic blockers are contraindicated.

Amitriptyline is commonly used in "mixed" headache cases (i.e., patients having symptoms of both migraine and muscle-contraction headaches). Patients are started on a 25- to 50-mg dose at bedtime, and the dose may be increased to 150 to 200 mg/d. A significant proportion of patients complain of extreme sedation caused by the drug. If this problem occurs, the dose should be halved. A 6-week trial is recommended before the drug is considered ineffective. Side effects are usually related to the anticholinergic properties of the drug (i.e., dry mouth, dizziness, blurred vision, urinary retention). The sedation and weight gain occasionally encountered may limit patient compliance. Finally, since amitriptyline may predispose to cardiac arrhythmias, it is contraindicated in heart disease.

SEROTONIN (5-HT) RECEPTOR ANTAGONISTS

Serotonergic antagonists such as methysergide represent the first class of drugs to be shown effective in migraine prophylaxis.[26,27] Methysergide is an ergot derivative that has complex effects on serotonergic and other neurotransmitter systems. Methysergide has been shown effective in 60% to 80% of patients with migraine and should be given for at least a 3-week trial.[27] Routine side effects include nausea, vomiting, and diarrhea. Unfortunately, as experience developed with this agent, a small number of patients developed retroperitoneal fibrosis (see Table 5–5). Therefore, it is recommended that this drug be administered only for a period of 6 months. The patient should then discontinue the medication for at least 4 to 8 weeks.

Other 5-HT antagonists have also been reported effective in migraine prophylaxis, but cyproheptadine (Periactin) is the only other serotonergic agent available currently in the United States. Used primarily as an antihistamine with anticholinergic properties, it is employed successfully by many clinicians for migraine prophylaxis, especially in children and in adults with asthma who cannot take beta blockers safely. Adults generally require 10 to 16 mg/d; the dose for children is approximately 0.25 mg/kg per day, or about 2 to 4 mg, two or three times a day. Frequent side effects include sleepiness, dry mouth, and increased appetite.

CALCIUM CHANNEL BLOCKERS

Calcium channel blockers represent a potentially novel class of antimigraine agents.[19,44] These drugs block the entrance of extracellular calcium into vascular smooth-muscle cells and thereby prevent vasoconstriction. In fact, no known endogenous vasoactive agent can contract intracranial blood vessels in the presence of an adequate concentration of a calcium channel antagonist drug.[44] Although generally considered as a group of agents, the calcium channel blockers are structurally diverse. At least three classes have been described: dihydropyridines (e.g., nifedipine, nimodipine), phenalkylamines (e.g., verapamil), and benzothiazepines (e.g., diltiazem). Each class appears to block a distinct subtype of calcium channel and/or different part of the calcium channel.[19] Regardless of their exact locus of action, these agents share the ability to prevent contractions of vascular smooth muscle, and the drugs appear to increase neuronal viability under hypoxic conditions (see Chapter 4).[3,19]

Beginning in 1981, a variety of clinical studies reported that calcium channel blockers were effective in migraine prophylaxis. The most extensive clinical studies to date have analyzed the effects of flunarizine, a relatively weak calcium channel antagonist.[4] As described in a recent review, the drug was found to be safe and effective in the treatment of both classic and common migraine. Although approved in Europe, it is not available in the United States. In addition, a number of recent case reports and studies have documented the effectiveness of diltiazem, verapamil, nifedipine, and nimodipine in the prophylactic treatment of migraine. These drugs appear to decrease both the frequency and severity of classic and common migraine.

Although a number of clinical studies suggest that calcium channel block-ers are effective migraine prophylaxis agents, it should be stressed that none of these agents has been specifically approved for use in migraine in the United States. Moreover, recent studies[2,33] have questioned the effectiveness of calcium channel blockers in migraine and, in addition, have reported a high incidence of side effects in migraine patients treated with these agents. Side effects can be expected to develop in 20% to 60% of the patients but are usually mild and consist of constipation and mild orthostatic hypotension.[2] Diltiazem appears to have marginally fewer side effects than verapamil and both are superior in this regard to nifedipine. The drugs are contraindicated in pregnancy.

OTHER AGENTS

A variety of other medications have been reported effective in migraine prophylaxis. In children, low-dose aspirin (75 mg/d) is often effective. Chlorpromazine, a phenothiazine with antiemetic properties, has been recommended as a first-line drug in migraine prophylaxis.[6] The nonsteroidal anti-inflammatory agent naproxen (Naprosyn) also has been reported to be an effective migraine prophylactic agent.[60] Monoamine oxidase (MAO) inhibitors such as phenelzine (Nardil) and isocarboxazid (Marplan) have been reported to be effective in migraine prophylaxis.[43] There is also evidence that MAO inhibitors are valuable in migraine prophylaxis, possibly due to their ability to increase levels of endogenous 5-HT. Frequent side effects include orthostatic hypotension, insomnia, and nausea. Narcotics are definitely contraindicated in migraine prophylaxis due to their addictive potential.

FUTURE APPROACHES

Future progress in migraine therapy is likely to be focused on more effective abortive therapies. The "ideal" migraine drug of the future would be taken at the onset of the headache and provide complete relief of symptoms, thereby eliminating the need for prophylactic medications. The drugs would have minimal side effects and would allow the patient to continue to function normally. Ultimately, neurologic drug therapy would eliminate the significant morbidity currently experienced with migraine.

As summarized in Table 5–3, antimigraine drugs share an ability to interact with specific 5-HT receptor subtypes. These observations offer a novel approach to the analysis to antimigraine agents. Drugs could be selected for use in clinical migraine studies based on their selectivity for a specific 5-HT receptor subtype. For example, an agent that displays both high affinity and selectivity for 5-HT$_{1D}$ receptors could be clinically evaluated. Its effectiveness, or lack thereof, could indicate the importance of this specific 5-HT receptor site in the pathogenesis of migraine. Future attempts to determine a common mechanism of action for effective antimigraine agents should elucidate the pathogenesis of this neurologic syndrome.

SUMMARY

Migraine remains the most common yet least understood neurologic syndrome. Unlike most neurologic illnesses, the diagnosis of migraine essentially rests on the clinical history. There are no serologic or radiologic tests to document the disease. Although pain is a highly subjective phenomenon, it is the only available guide to the severity of the illness. In addition, an extremely large number of patients complain of headache that is unrelated to migraine. It is therefore not surprising that the treatment of migraine can be frustrating for the clinician.

At the basic science level, the lack of animal models and objective therapeutic response criteria has hindered migraine research. Significant progress has been made in the past decade, how-

ever, and current studies should greatly elucidate the pathogenesis of migraine. First of all, the documentation of vasomotor dysregulation in human with migraine suggests that changes in blood flow may be a primary or secondary manifestation of a migraine attack. Second, the analysis of endogenous pain-producing substances and the response of nociceptive neurons indicate that the trigeminovascular system plays a crucial role in migraine pathogenesis. Finally, the determination of the exact mechanism of action of seemingly diverse agents such as propranolol, amitriptyline, and methysergide may provide important insights into migraine etiology.

ACKNOWLEDGMENTS

I would like to thank Faith Smith and Mary T. Keller for their excellent assistance in preparation of the manuscript. This work was supported in part by the John A. Hartford Foundation, Inc., the Alfred P. Sloan Foundation, and the National Migraine Foundation.

REFERENCES

1. Ala-Hurula, V: Correlation between pharmacokinetics and clinical effects of ergotamine in patients suffering from migraine. Eur J Clin Pharmacol 21: 397, 1982.
2. Albers, GW, Simon, LT, Hamik, A, and Peroutka, SJ: Nifedipine versus propranol for the initial prophylaxis of migraine. Headache 29:215–218, 1989.
3. Amery, WK: Brain hypoxia: The turning-point in the genesis of the migraine attack? Cephalalgia 2:83–109, 1982.
4. Amery, WK: Flunarizine, a calcium channel blocker: A new prophylactic drug in migraine. Headache 23:70–74, 1983.
5. Callaham, M and Raskin, N: A controlled study of dihydroergotamine in the treatment of acute migraine headache. Headache 26:168–171, 1986.

6. Caviness, VS, Jr and O'Brien, P: Headache. N Engl J Med 302:446–450, 1980.

7. Connor, HE, Feniuk, W, and Humphrey, PPA: Characterization of 5-HT receptors mediating contraction of canine and primate basilar artery by use of GR43175, a selective 5-HT$_1$-like receptor agonist. Br J Pharmacol 96:379–387, 1989.

8. Couch, JR and Hassanein, RS: Amitriptyline in migraine prophylaxis. Arch Neurol 36:695–699, 1979.

9. Couch, JR, Ziegler, DK, and Hassanein, RS: Amitriptyline in migraine prophylaxis. Neurology 26:121–127, 1976.

10. Coughlin, SR, Moskowitz, MA, Antoniades, HN, and Levine, L: Serotonin receptor-mediated stimulation of bovine smooth muscle cell prostacyclin synthesis and its modulation by platelet-derived growth factor. Proc Natl Acad Sci USA 78:7134–7138, 1981.

11. Coughlin, SR, Moskowitz, MA, and Levine, L: Identification of a serotonin type 2 receptor linked to prostacyclin synthesis in vascular smooth muscle cells. Biochem Pharmacol 33:692–695, 1984.

12. Dalessio, DJ: On migraine headache: Serotonin and serotonin antagonism. JAMA 181:318–321, 1962.

13. Doenicke, A, Brand, J, and Perrin, VL: Possible benefit of GR43175, a novel 5-HT$_1$-like receptor agonist, for the acute treatment of severe migraine. Lancet 1:1309–1311, 1988.

14. Fanchamps, A: Why do not all beta-blockers prevent migraine? Headache 25:61–62, 1985.

15. Feniuk, W, Humphrey, PPA, and Perren, MJ: The selective carotid arterial vasoconstrictor action of GR43175 in anaesthetized dogs. Br J Pharmacol 96:83–90, 1989.

16. Fozard, JR: 5-Hydroxytryptamine in the pathophysiology of migraine. In Bevan, JA, Godfraind, T, Maxwell, RA, Stoclet, JC, and Worcel, M (eds): Vascular neuroeffector mechanisms. Elsevier Science Publishers, Amsterdam, 1985, pp 321–328.

17. Fozard, JR and Gray, JA: 5-HT$_{1C}$ receptor activation: A key step in the initia-

tion of migraine? TIPS 10:307–309, 1989.

18. Gomersall, JD and Stuart, A: Amitriptyline in migraine prophylaxis. J Neurol Neurosurg Psychiatry 36:684–690, 1973.

19. Greenberg, DA: Calcium channel antagonists and the treatment of migraine. Clin Neuropharmacol 9:311–328, 1986.

20. Heuring, RE and Peroutka, SJ: Characterization of a novel ^{3}H-5-hydroxytryptamine binding site subtype in bovine brain membranes. J Neurosci 7:894–903, 1987.

21. Heyck, H: Pathogenesis of migraine. Res Clin Stud Headache 2:1–28, 1969.

22. Hoyer, D and Middlemiss, DN: Species differences in the pharmacology of terminal 5-HT autoreceptors in mammalian brain. Trends in Pharmacological Sciences 10:130–132, 1989.

23. Humphrey, PPA, Feniuk, W, Perren, MJ, Connor, HE, Oxford, AW, Coates, IH, and Butina, D: GR43175, a selective agonist for the 5-HT$_1$-like receptor in dog isolated saphenous vein. Br J Pharmacol 94:1123–1132, 1988.

24. Kurtzke, JF, Bennett, DR, Berg, BO, Beringer, GB, Goldstein, DO, and Vates, TS: On national needs for neurologists in the United States. Neurology 36:383–388, 1986.

25. Lance, JW: Headache. Ann Neurol 10:1–10, 1981.

26. Lance, JW and Anthony, M: Some clinical aspects of migraine. Arch Neurol 15:356–361, 1966.

27. Lance, JW, Anthony, M, and Somerville, B: Comparative trial of serotonin antagonists in the management of migraine. Br Med J 2:327–330, 1970.

28. Lance, JW, Lambert, GA, Goadsby, PJ, and Zagami, AS: 5-Hydroxytryptamine and its putative aetiological involvement in migraine. Cephalalgia (Suppl 9):7–13, 1989.

29. Lauritzen, M, Jorgensen, MB, Diemer, NH, Gjedde, A, and Hansen, AJ: Persistent oligemia of rat cerebral cortex in the wake of spreading depression. Ann Neurol 12:469–474, 1982.

30. Lauritzen, M and Olesen, J: Regional cerebral blood flow during migraine at-

tacks by xenon-133 inhalation and emission tomography. Brain 107:447–461, 1984.

31. Leao, AAP: Pial circulation and spreading depression of activity in the cerebral cortex. J Neurophysiol 7:391–396, 1944.

32. Maciewicz, R, Strassman, A, Mason, P, and Moskowitz, M: Activation of nociceptive neurons in the spinal; trigeminal nucleus by stimulation of dural blood vessels. Society of Neuroscience Abstracts 12:30–1986.

33. McArthur, JC, Marek, K, Pestronk, A, McArthur, J, and Peroutka, SJ: Nifedipine in the prophylaxis of classic migraine: A crossover, double-masked, placebo-controlled study of headache frequency and side effects. Neurology 39:284–286, 1989.

34. McCarthy, BG and Peroutka, SJ: Comparative neuropharmacology of dihydroergotamine and sumatriptan (GR 43175). Headache 29:420–422, 1989.

35. Moskowitz, MA: The neurobiology of vascular head pain. Ann Neurol 16:157–168, 1984.

36. Moskowitz, MA, Romero, J, Reinhard, JF, Melamed, E, and Pettibone, DJ: Neurotransmitters and the fifth cranial nerve: Is there a relation to the headache phase of migraine? Lancet 2:883–885, 1979.

37. Olesen, J: Some clinical features of the acute migraine attack. An analysis of 750 patients. Headache 18:268–271, 1978.

38. Olesen, J: Migraine and regional cerebral blood flow. Trends in Neuroscience 8:318–321, 1985.

39. Olesen, J, Larsen, B, and Lauritzen, M: Focal hyperemia followed by spreading oligemia and impaired activation of rCBF in classic migraine. Ann Neurol 9:344–352, 1981.

40. Olesen, J, Lauritzen, M, Tfelt-Hansen, P, Henriksen, L, and Larsen, B: Spreading cerebral oligemia in classical and normal cerebral blood flow in common migraine. Headache 22:242–248, 1982.

41. Olesen, J, Tfelt-Hansen, P, Henriksen, L, and Larsen, B: The common migraine attack may not be initiated by cerebral ischaemia. Lancet 2:438–440, 1981.

42. Parsons, AA, Whalley, ET, Feniuk, W, Connor, HE, and Humphrey, PPA: 5-HT$_1$-like receptors mediate 5-hydroxytryptamine-induced contraction of human isolated basilar artery. Br J Pharmacol 96:434–449, 1989.

43. Peatfield, RC, Fozard, JR, and Rose, FC: Drug treatment of migraine. In Rose, FC (ed): Handbook of Clinical Neurology. Raven Press, New York, 1986, pp 173–216.

44. Peroutka, ST: The pharmacology of calcium channel antagonists: A novel class of anti-migraine agents? Headache 23:278–283, 1983.

45. Peroutka, SJ: Vascular serotonin receptors: Correlation with 5-HT$_1$ and 5-HT$_2$ binding sites. Biochem Pharmacol 33:2349–2353, 1984.

46. Peroutka, SJ: 5-Hydroxytryptamine receptor subtypes. Annu Rev Neurosci 11:45–60, 1988.

47. Peroutka, SJ and McCarthy, BG: Sumatriptan (GR 43175) interacts selectively with 5-HT$_{1B}$ and 5-HT$_{1D}$ binding sites. Eur J Pharmacol 163:133–136, 1989.

48. Peroutka, SJ, Switzer, JA, and Hamik, A: Identification of 5-hydroxytryptamine$_{1D}$ binding sites in human brain membranes. Synapse 3:61–66, 1989.

49. Raskin, NH: Pharmacology of migraine. Annu Rev Pharmacol Toxicol 21:463–478, 1981.

50. Raskin, NH: Repetitive intravenous dihydroergotamine as therapy for intractable migraine. Neurology 36:995–997, 1986.

51. Ray, BS and Wolff, HG: Experimental studies on headache. Arch Surg 41:813–856, 1940.

52. Saito, K, Markowitz, S, and Moskowitz, MA: Ergot alkaloids block neurogenic extravasation in dura mater: Proposed action in vascular headaches. Ann Neurol 24:732–737, 1988.

53. Saxena, PR and Ferrari, MD: 5-HT$_1$-like receptor agonists and the pathophysiology of migraine. Trends in Pharmacological Sciences 10:200–204, 1989.

54. Schmidt, AW and Peroutke, SJ: 5-Hydroxytryptamine receptor "families". FASEB Journal 3:2242–2249, 1989.

55. Waeber, C, Dietl, MM, Hoyer, D, Probst, A, and Palacios, JM: Visualization of a novel serotonin recognition site

(5-HT$_{1D}$) in the human brain by autoradiography. Neurosci Lett 88:11–16, 1988.

56. Waeber, C, Schoeffter, P, Palacios, JM, and Hoyer, D: Molecular pharmacology of 5-HT$_{1D}$ recognition sites: Radioligand binding studies in human, pig and calf brain membranes. Naunyn Schmiedebergs Arch Pharmacol 337:595–601, 1988.

57. Weerasuriya, K, Patel, L, and Turner, P: B-adrenoceptor blockade and migraine. Cephalalgia 2:33–45, 1982.

58. Wilkinson, M: Treatment of the acute migraine attack—Current status. Cephalalgia 3:61–67, 1983.

59. Wykes, P: The treatment of angina pectoris with coexistent migraine. Practitioner 200:702–704, 1968.

60. Ziegler, DK and Ellis, DJ: Naproxen in prophylaxis of migraine. Arch Neurol 42:582–584, 1985.

Chapter 6

IMMUNE-MEDIATED DISORDERS

Mark S. Freedman, M.D.,
Jack P. Antel, M.D., and
David P. Richman, M.D.

ORGANIZATION OF THE IMMUNE SYSTEM
CNS–IMMUNE SYSTEM INTERACTIONS
AUTOIMMUNE NEUROLOGIC DISEASES
IMMUNOTHERAPIES

The healthy immune system is a complex series of lymphocyte-monocyte cell subsets that interact in a precisely regulated manner to recognize and remove exogenous agents from the body. Specific mechanisms enable the cellular components of the immune system to recognize exogenous agents (antigens), to distinguish self from nonself products, to interact with each other, to home to the site where the antigen is located, to destroy the antigen, and finally to terminate the response. Clinical disorders of the immune system can result either from deficiencies that make the host susceptible to infection or from injury inflicted on self-tissue by the immune mediators themselves (i.e., autoimmune disease). Increased understanding of these processes provides insight into the pathogenesis of immunologic diseases and identifies opportunities for designing appropriate and nontoxic therapies. This chapter addresses these issues by considering (1) the organization of the immune system in general, (2) unique properties of the cellular components of the central nervous system (CNS) that may influence their interaction with the immune system, (3) human neurologic disorders and corresponding animal disease models in which immune mechanisms are established or postulated to be involved in their pathogenesis, and (4) pharmacologic approaches to manipulating immune function. A glossary of the acronyms used appears as Table 6–1.

ORGANIZATION OF THE IMMUNE SYSTEM

Lymphocytes can be considered in two major categories: the B cells, which mature in various lymphoid organs (e.g., spleen, lymph nodes), and the T cells, which mature in the thymus.[36] B cells secrete immunoglobulin (Ig) or antibodies and are the mediators of *humoral immunity* (Table 6–2). T cells mediate their effects via direct cell-target interactions, usually an antigen-specific process, or via release of soluble mediators (cytokines) that lack antigen specificity. T-cell-mediated immunity is commonly termed *cell-mediated immunity.*

178

Table 6–1 GLOSSARY OF ACRONYMS

Acronym	Meaning
AChR	Acetylcholine receptor
ACTH	Adrenocorticotropic hormone
ADCC	Antibody-dependent cell cytotoxicity
ADEM	Acute disseminated encephalomyelitis
AMP	Adenosine monophosphate
C	Constant region
CD2, CD3, etc.	Receptors located on lymphocytes
CD4+, CD8+	Major classes of T cells
CIDPN	Chronic inflammatory demyelinating polyneuropathy
COP-1	Copolymer-1 (synthetic compound resembling MBP)
CREAE	Chronic relapsing EAE
DTH	Delayed type hypersensitivity
EAE	Experimental allergic encephalomyelitis
EAMG	Experimental autoimmune myasthenia gravis
EAN	Experimental allergic neuritis
Fab	Immunoglobulin fragment at antigen-binding end
Fc	Immunoglobulin fragment opposite antigen-binding end
GBS	Guillain-Barré syndrome
GMP	Guanosine monophosphate
H chain	Heavy chain of immunoglobulin molecule
HLA	Human leukocyte antigen
IC	Immune complex
IFN	Interferon
Ig	Immunoglobulin
IL-2	Interleukin-2
K cells	Killer cells
L chain	Light chain of immunoglobulin molecule
LAK	Lymphokine-activated killer
LES	Lambert-Eaton syndrome
LFA	Lymphocyte function associated
mAbs	Monoclonal antibodies
MBP	Myelin basic protein
MG	Myasthenia gravis
MHC	Major histocompatibility complex
mRNA	Messenger RNA
MS	Multiple sclerosis
NK cells	Natural killer cells
TcR	T-cell receptor
TLI	Total lymphoid irradiation
V	Variable region

Table 6–2 MAJOR COMPONENTS OF THE B-CELL MEDIATED (HUMORAL) IMMUNE SYSTEM

Stimulation of antigen receptors on B cells activates antibody (Ig) production
Antibody (Ig) molecules are composed of a protein tetramer:
  2 polypeptide light (L) chains each containing
    a constant (C) region and
    a variable (V) region
  2 polypeptide heavy (H) chains
    several C domains
    single V domain
Antibody class (IgG, IgM, IgA) determined by C domain of H chains
Antibody variable regions determine its idiotype

B-Cell-Mediated Immunity (Humoral Immunity)

Interaction of antigen with the antigen receptor on the surface of resting B cells, usually in conjunction with T-cell-secreted soluble factors, results in proliferation and differentiation of these B cells into Ig-(antibody) secreting cells. The interaction of antibody molecule with antigen, classically described as a lock-and-key arrangement, is highly specific, with the specificity determined by the unique structure of the variable region of Ig molecule. The variable region of the antigen receptor, and hence its antigen specificity, is identical to that of the antibody molecule secreted by the cell.

Each Ig molecule is a tetramer comprised of two polypeptide heavy (H) chains and two light (L) chains covalently joined by disulfide bonds (Fig. 6–1). The L chains, which can be either of the kappa or lambda type, consist of a constant (C) region, that is, a domain identical for all L chains of a given type; and a variable (V) region, whose structure varies from one Ig molecule to the next. The H chains are each comprised of several C domains and a single V region. The H-chain C region determines the class of the Ig (IgG, IgA, IgM) and accounts for its biologic properties, such as complement fixation. Within the V regions of both the H and L chains are segments in which the amino acid sequence variability is concentrated (hypervariable regions); the less variable regions are designated as framework regions. Amino acid sequences from the hypervariable regions of each pair of linked H and L chains contribute to a

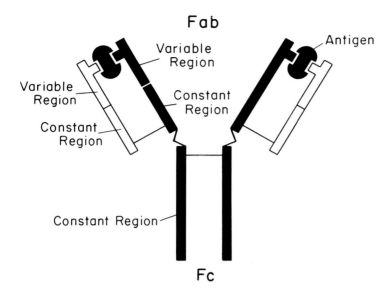

Figure 6-1. An antibody (Ig) molecule, composed of two heavy chains (shown in black) and two light chains (shown in white) linked by disulfide bonds. The variable and constant regions of the chains are labeled on the left side of the diagram only. Variable regions of both chains determine the specificity of antigen binding. The unique structural sequences of the V-regions comprise the antibody's idiotype.

single antigen-combining site (complementarity-determining region); therefore, each IgG molecule has two potential antigen combining sites.

The almost limitless structural possibilities of the variable region of Ig molecules results, to a great extent, from the highly polymorphic nature of multiple genes encoding each of the two or three regions (V and J for L chains; V, D, and J for H chains), that make up the entire V region. The gene loci for each region lie in separate segments of the chromosomal DNA. The process of translocation of one gene from each separated locus in the germline DNA, to lie in proximity with each other, and then with the appropriate C-region gene, occurs during B-cell development. The final result is an mRNA encoding an entire H or L chain.

The unique structural amino acid sequences of the Ig V regions are themselves antigenic; each of these sites on an Ig molecule is referred to as an *idiotope*, and collectively they make up an Ig molecule's *idiotype*. An idiotope may or may not be included in the antigen combining site. The variable region of the cell surface antigen receptor on a B cell, which is identical to the variable region of the cell's antibody product, expresses the identical idiotypes as the

antibody. Antibodies recognizing idiotypes either on antibody molecules or antigen receptors (i.e., anti-id antibody) are postulated to play important roles in regulating immune reactivity ("network theory of the immune response"). Anti-id antibodies interacting with the cell receptor can result in either increased or decreased antibody production. The subset of anti-id directed against epitopes (antigenic determinants) within the antigen-binding site, so-called internal image anti-ids, can mimic the effects of the antigen, which may include agonist activity at neurotransmitter, hormone, or viral receptors. Therapeutic strategies based on the use of anti-id antibody to down-regulate autoimmune B cells are discussed in a later section (Immunotherapies).

Autoantibodies act through a number of pathogenic mechanisms, from simple blockade of antigen function to lysis of the cells' expressing the specific target antigen. The cytotoxic effects frequently are the result of induction of the membrane attack complex through activation of the complement cascade. Complement activation also results in release of soluble mediators of inflammation from the tissues and recruitment of other inflammation-mediating cells. Antibody combining with either circulating or tissue-bound antigen can result in immune complex (IC) formation. In endothelium or choroid plexus, IC deposition per se can result in disruption of function. It also can lead to complement pathway activation and inflammation. Immune complex formation and deposition contribute heavily to the clinical features of lymphocytic choriomeningitis virus disease and probably to some of the cerebral manifestations of systemic lupus erythematosus.

T-Cell-Mediated Immunity (Cell-Mediated Immunity)

T-cell interaction with antigen, as with B cells, also occurs via a specific site on the cell surface, namely the T-cell receptor (TcR) (Fig. 6–2). The TcR complex is a macromolecular structure comprised of a T_i heterodimer, which bears structural similarities to that of the B-cell receptor molecule (i.e., Ig) and which is in noncovalent association with a collection of proteins of invariant structure, referred to as the CD3 complex (Table 6–3). The T_i heterodimer for most cells is made up of an α and β chain, each of which has a V and C region. In analogy with the Ig molecules (and associated B-cell antigen receptors), the V regions of TcRs are encoded by multiple genes, which undergo rearrangements during T-cell differentiation to generate a single variable-region-encoding gene. The homologies noted between sequences of Ig and TcR genes suggest their derivation from a common ancestral gene. In a small proportion of T cells, the T_i heterodimer is comprised of a γ and a δ chain, indicating separate lineage of these cells. The precise functional properties of these cells remain to be defined, with natural killer activity being one implicated function.

Unlike the case for B cells, antigen alone is insufficient to activate T cells, but rather requires interaction with antigen complexed with major histocompatibility complex (MHC) molecules (Fig. 6–2). T-cell receptors identify peptide fragments of protein antigens. The fragments are produced in the course of intracellular-antigen processing by antigen-presenting cells.[17] Such cells include B cells, macrophages, and specialized cells within different body tissues. In the nervous system, astrocytes, microglia, and cerebral endothelial cells all can serve as antigen-presenting cells. The processed peptide fragments are then bound to the MHC molecule on the surface of the presenting cell, and it is the complex that is recognized by the appropriate TcR. For the classic T-cell-mediated autoimmune

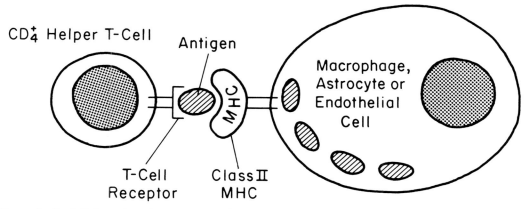

Figure 6–2. Cellular interaction necessary for T cell–mediated cellular immunity. For a helper (CD4+) cell to be activated, the antigen must be presented to the T-cell receptor by another cell that also expresses the same MHC-antigen class, in this case the Class II MHC antigen.

Table 6-3 MAJOR COMPONENTS OF THE T-CELL MEDIATED (CELLULAR) IMMUNE SYSTEM

T-cell activation results from ligation of the T-cell antigen receptor by a peptide associated with a major histocompatibility complex (MHC) molecule present on the surface of antigen-presenting cells, which have initially processed antigen into the required peptide form.

CD4+ T CELLS i.e., HELPER (INDUCER) T CELLS

- Recognize class II MHC antigen
- Promote effector responses of cytotoxic T cells and B cells
- Release cytokines required for T-cell proliferation, B-cell maturation, and macrophage activation

CD8+ T CELLS, i.e., CYTOTOXIC AND SUPPRESSOR T CELLS

- Recognize class I MHC molecules
- Cytotoxic cells lyse cell targets expressing specific antigen plus MHC class I molecules
- Suppressor cells down-regulate reactivity of B and T cells

ANTIGEN-PRESENTING CELLS (APCs)

- Express MHC class II molecules
- Present antigen to CD4+ T cells
- Secrete cytokines that contribute to T-cell activation (e.g., IL-1)
- Macrophages—Other properties include phagocytosis and release of cytotoxic soluble factors (e.g., complement, tumor necrosis factor, proteases)
- B cells, dendritic cells, CNS glia (microglia, astrocytes)

NATURAL KILLER (NK) CELLS

- Lymphoid origin but without T-cell receptor gene products
- Lyse targets (mainly tumor cells) without MHC restriction

LYMPHOKINE-ACTIVATED KILLER (LAK) CELLS

- Generated in vitro by culture with IL-2
- Probably share lineage and effector function with NK cells

KILLER (K) CELLS

- Bear Fc receptors
- Can be T or non-T cells
- Mediate antibody-dependent cell cytotoxicity

---

disease, experimental allergic encephalomyelitis (EAE), recent studies have demonstrated that the TcRs of the majority (at least for inbred mice and rats) of the T cells reacting with immuno-genic peptide fragments of the antigen, myelin basic protein (MBP), are encoded by a small number of available V-region genes.[31,40,54] In these studies, antibodies ("anti-idiotype") directed against the highly represented TcRs markedly reduced the autoimmune response to MBP.[31,53,54] These results raise the possibility that the host factors involved in autoimmunity include particular TcR V-region gene repertoires.

The MHC antigens are also critical for permitting cell-cell interaction involving T cells. The two major classes of T cells, namely CD4+ and CD8+ cells, initially were identified on the basis of function, helper and suppressor cytotoxic, respectively (see section entitled "Immune Regulation"). Each has been shown to interact with specific MHC-antigen classes, that is, CD4+ cells recognize class II MHC antigens, whereas CD8+ cells recognize class I. The CD4 and CD8 molecules on T cells are closely associated with the TcR and through their interactions with MHC molecules contribute to the T-cell activation process. The CD4 molecule is also the receptor for the acquired immune deficiency syndrome (AIDS)

Other T-cell surface molecules also influence T-cell activation and T-cell interactions with other cells. The CD2 complex found on all T cells is now known to be the receptor site on the T cells for sheep red blood cells and serves as an alternate T-cell activation site. A group of T-cell surface antigens termed *lymphocyte-function-associated antigens*, which belong to the Ig supergene family, further contribute to the efficiency of T-cell adherence to other cells. A promising immunopharmacologic strategy is the use of monoclonal antibodies (mAbs) specifically recognizing the above T-cell surface antigens to modify T-cell reactivity during the course of immune-mediated disease.

T-cell activation and proliferation, which follow the cell's interaction with antigen, depend on two signal pathways.[19,24] The first pathway of cellular events follows antigen interaction with the TcR. The series of resultant cellular events includes phosphatidylinositol turnover, calcium influx, a brief increase in cyclic adenosine monophosphate, and induction of interleukin-2 (IL-2) receptors on the cells. The second pathway, activated by accessory cells or interleukin (IL-1), results in protein kinase activation, increase in cyclic guanosine monophosphate and IL-2 production. This second pathway can be initiated by direct stimulation of the CD2, CD5, and CD28 complexes, which are found on all T cells, at sites distinct from the TcR-associated CD3 complex. Lymphocytes use the purine salvage pathway rather than "de novo" synthesis to generate nucleoside monophosphates. Deficiencies of adenosine deaminase and purine nucleoside phosphorylase, enzymes involved in the purine salvage pathway, are associated with devastating immunodeficiency states.

T cells can effect their responses in several ways. A specific mechanism of T-cell-mediated target-cell killing is termed *antigen-specific cytotoxicity.* This effector response involves direct cell-cell interaction between a cell target and a T cell that has been sensitized to an antigen expressed on the surface of the cell. Cytolytic T-cell activity has classically been ascribed to cells bearing the CD8 phenotype, which see their target in the presence of class I MHC antigens. Data from both animal and human tissue culture studies indicate that glial cells, including oligodendrocytes, express a sufficient density of class I MHC antigens, at least under certain conditions, to be vulnerable targets of cytotoxic T cells.[42] Phenotypic CD4+ cells, which recognize their targets in the presence of class II MHC antigens, are now also shown to mediate cytotoxicity.

The CD4+ T cells are the central cell type involved in initiating the classic T-cell-dependent delayed-type hypersensitivity (DTH) reaction, so called because of the several-day delay seen between administration of antigen (e.g., skin test antigen) and development of the immune response (i.e., inflammation) at the tissue site (see Fig. 6–2). In mice, this function can be further local-

ized to a subset of CD4+ cells, T_{H1}. The DTH response requires that antigen-sensitized T cells migrate from the systemic circulation to the site of antigen deposition, where subsequent recruitment of additional lymphocyte and monocyte populations occurs. This issue of trafficking of lymphocytes is a central one when considering pharmacologic strategies to selectively inhibit a tissue-specific immune-mediated disease.[13]

Studies in which antigen-specific CD4+ cell lines are used for the passive transfer of inflammatory disease such as EAE or adjuvant arthritis indicate that T cells, particularly when activated, release soluble factors such as endoglycosidases, which disrupt the vascular endothelium, contributing to the cells' ability to enter the tissues.[29] Soluble T-cell factors, especially interferon (IFN) gamma, released by activated T cells, can induce class II MHC antigen expression on endothelial cells composing the blood-brain barrier, as well as on astrocytes and microglia within the CNS parenchyma; such induction may be crucial for T-cell homing to their tissue targets. MHC class II antigen expression on the above-mentioned CNS cells has especially been observed in disease states featuring active inflammation.[44] The T-helper cells, once reaching the target site, release a host of soluble factors (cytokines) that can further increase vascular permeability, recruit and activate other non-antigen-sensitized lymphocytes and macrophages, and damage cell targets directly.

The macrophage, in addition to its function in antigen presentation, plays a central role in mediating tissue injury during the course of inflammation (see Table 6–3).[22] Macrophages release lysosomal hydrolases that mediate proteolytic functions. They also release the products of the arachidonic acid pathway, namely prostaglandins and leukotrienes, which contribute to tissue injury and modify immune reactivity. Other macrophage-released products include oxygen radicals, complement components, IL-1, and tumor necrosis factor. Thus, the overall tissue injury reflects the combined effects of antigen-specific and nonspecific responses.

The DTH reaction may have specific relevance to central and peripheral nervous system demyelinating disease in view of data indicating that a DTH reaction occurring in response to tuberculin injection into rabbit eye and brain can induce demyelination, a phenomenon termed *bystander demyelination.*[22] Therapies that inhibit the activity of the cellular and soluble mediators of inflammation might well be expected to reduce the extent of tissue damage that occurs during the course of inflammatory immune diseases.

Cell-mediated cytotoxicity can also be mediated by other cells of the lymphocyte-monocyte lineage (see Table 6–3). These include the natural killer (NK), lymphokine-activated killer (LAK), and killer (K) cells. The NK cells can induce target-cell killing without the need for prior sensitization against a specific antigen. These cells both produce and respond to IFN-gamma. The NK cells were initially defined by their ability to kill tumor cells in vitro; their role in mediating tissue injury in autoimmune disease or in controlling viral diseases of the CNS is less clear. More recently, NK cells were shown to function as antigen presenting cells and to play a role in immune regulation. The LAK cells are a cell type generated in vitro in response to IL-2 stimulation. They can mediate nonantigen non-MHC-restricted lysis of selected cell targets, including tumor cells. Combined administration of LAK cells and IL-2 is being evaluated as biologic therapy for cancers, including gliomas.

The K cells are the cellular mediators of antibody-dependent cell cytotoxicity (ADCC). This form of target-cell lysis requires that a specific antibody coat an antigen on the cell target, making the cell susceptible to lysis. ADCC-mediated lysis would present a form of immune injury combining humoral and cell-mediated mechanisms. Researchers postulate that ADCC occurs in multiple sclerosis (MS); it has been

demonstrated that mouse glial cells exposed to MS sera and lymphocytes are subject to lysis. A distinct possibility in many chronic inflammatory disorders is that multiple immune effector mechanisms contribute to the overall extent of tissue damage.

Immune Regulation

T-CELL-MEDIATED REGULATION

Induction of effective T- and usually B-cell responses requires the presence of a specific subset of T cells, termed *T-inducer* or *T-helper cells*, contained within the CD4+ cell population. The helper/inducer function of these cells in vitro can be replaced, at least in part, by soluble mediators secreted by the cells. The central role of CD4 cells in initiating and augmenting immune reactivity has made these cells a key target for immunotherapy protocols.

Specific subsets of T cells, termed suppressor cells, have been demonstrated to inhibit immune reactivity of both B and T cells.[51] In humans, these cells are found within the CD8+ cell population, which also contains the antigen-specific cytotoxicity-mediating cells. Defining phenotypically distinct subsets mediating selective suppressor versus cytotoxic functions remains an ongoing problem. The CD28 and CD11b molecules have been shown to define mutually exclusive subsets subserving cytotoxic or suppressor functions respectively in some (but not all) in vitro assay systems. In multiple sclerosis, one can find aberrant suppressor function in the face of preserved cytotoxic function.

Induction of CD8+ suppressor function may depend on input from a subpopulation of CD4+ cells, termed *suppressor/inducer cells*. This subset of CD4+ cells was initially defined by the expression of the CD45RA molecule antigen complex; subsequent data have suggested that CD45RA expression is characteristic of naive T cells and may thus reflect a maturation phase of the cell rather than a fixed functional property.[36] Additional "markers" for the suppressor/inducer subset, such as Leu8 and CD29, are being evaluated. Quantitative deficiencies in suppressor inducer cells, as determined using anti-CD45RA mAbs, are reported to occur in MS, perhaps contributing to the observed defect in suppressor effector function. These findings could reflect that naive T cells have been transformed into "memory" cells with the attendant loss of expression of the CD45RA antigen. Suppressor cells also are influenced by contra-suppressor cells and by products of the immune system themselves, including antibody and immune complexes, and a variety of soluble molecules, including prostaglandins and IFN.

The roles of immunoregulatory mechanisms in preventing self-directed immune responses or in contributing to states of immune nonresponsiveness continue to be defined. The demonstration that one can recover autoreactive T cells from normal individuals indicates that active regulatory mechanisms, rather than total elimination of self-directed cell clones during development, account for the observed absence of autoimmune tissue injury in the normal condition. Levels of immune response to a wide range of antigens by a given host have been shown to be a reflection of active suppressor mechanisms.

Immunologic unresponsiveness to a specific antigen against which the host is initially capable of responding (i.e., tolerance) can develop after exposure to the antigen. In the EAE disease model, resistance to development of disease can be induced in animals by passive transfer of lymphoid cells derived from animals recovered from EAE, by active immunization with myelin proteins in incomplete adjuvant, or by oral feeding of MBP. The concept of T-cell vaccination to prevent autoimmune disease has arisen from demonstrations that injection of animals with disease-mediating, autoreactive T cells, exposed to hydrostatic pressure or glutaraldehyde-in-

duced cross-linking, results in resistance to subsequent disease induction, and that this resistance can be passively transferred.[8] Sun and colleagues[46] have suggested that an anticlonotype CD8 cytotoxic cell directed against autoreactive disease-mediating T cells accounts for the resistance.

Mechanisms other than active suppression may also be involved in tolerance and resistance to autoimmune disease. Tolerance can be induced in cloned helper T-cell lines, indicating that intrinsic cellular mechanisms can underlie development of nonresponsiveness in the absence of any suppressor influences. For example, Levich and associates[28] demonstrated that exposure of T-helper cells to monomeric antigen (human γglobulin) resulted in the cells' no longer being able to provide help. The effect seemingly was independent of any effects on cell proliferative capacity. Recovery from acute EAE does occur in animals depleted of suppressor cells.

B-CELL-MEDIATED REGULATION

The regulation of B-cell responses by their own products (antibodies) has been classically described as the *network theory*.[36] This theory postulates that antibody produced by a clonal B-cell population is recognized as antigen by another B-cell population, which produces an anti-id antibody (see Fig. 6–1). Anti-id antibody directed against the antigen-combining site of the original B cells' Ig molecule, or antigen receptor, might be expected to inhibit the immune response by blocking antigen access to the B cell. As mentioned, however, the anti-id might also mimic antigen. In this regard, anti-id antibodies have been used as vaccines for prevention of specific viral diseases. Noncombining, site-directed anti-id antibodies can also modify immune reactivity. Anti-id antibody has been detected in sera of patients with myasthenia gravis (MG) and in the cerebrospinal fluid of patients with MS and subacute sclerosing panencephalitis.[34] The anti-id antibody itself can induce anti-anti-id, which may resemble the original antibody. Evidence also exists that B-cell idiotypes interact with T-cell idiotypes (i.e., unique antigenic regions of the TcR of a given T cell), a process that potentially could result in augmentation or inhibition of an immune response. Knowledge regarding mechanisms of induction and regulation of the immune response has opened further means to institute immunotherapy in autoimmune disorders.

Cell-Cell Interaction in the Immune System

The previous descriptions of the components of the immune system and their interdependence clearly indicates the need for mechanisms whereby the involved cell subsets can (1) recognize each other and their targets and (2) communicate with each other.

ROLE OF MHC ANTIGENS

The MHC complex (in man, termed the human leukocyte antigen [*HLA*] *region*) is divided into two classes (I and II) based on structure and function of the gene products and their tissue distribution.[3] Class I HLA antigens, encoded by three different polymorphic gene loci, are found on all nucleated cells except, as discussed below, on neural cells, and are composed of a chain associated noncovalently with β2-microglobulin. Class I MHC antigens are the restriction element for $CD8^+$ cells. Class II HLA antigens are encoded by three "families" of polymorphic gene loci, DR, DQ and DP; are more limited in their tissue distribution than are class I antigens, being found mainly on specialized antigen-presenting cells such as macrophages and B cells; are made up of α and β chains; and function as the restriction element for $CD4^+$ cells. The class II MHC antigens are critical for efficient antigen presentation by accessory cells to $CD4^+$ T cells. The MHC Class II repertoire of animals and man, as well as the TcR repertoire, significantly influence levels of immune responsiveness to specific antigens and susceptibility to development of autoimmune disease. Within the CNS, both class I and II MHC antigen expression by endothelial and glial cells is at low or undetectable levels, as measured by usual immunohistochemical techniques; however, high levels of expression can be induced by IFN-gamma and perhaps other soluble lymphokines. Increased expression of MHC antigens on glial cells and possibly on endothelial cells is observed in both MS and EAE, as well as on peripheral nerve and muscle in the region of inflammation. Treatment of animals with anti – class II antibody reduces the severity of EAE and experimental autoimmune MG.

SOLUBLE MEDIATORS ACTING AS INTERCELLULAR SIGNALS

Interaction between cellular components of the immune system is to a large extent mediated by soluble factors produced by the involved cell subsets. The number of identified soluble mediators is continually expanding. Among these are soluble factors released by monocytes, which can activate T cells (IL-1, IL-6, tumor necrosis factor [TNF]) or modify suppressor T-cell function (prostaglandins); and soluble factors released by T lymphocytes, which can amplify T-cell proliferation (IL-2), promote B-cell growth and differentiation (B-cell growth factors, IL-3 – IL7), suppress B-cell and T-cell responses (soluble immune suppressor factors), induce MHC expression (IFN-gamma) and affect nonlymphoid tissues (e.g., astrocyte and oligodendrocyte-activating and differentiating factors). Availability of these factors in cloned form and of mAbs against these factors or their receptors again widens one's capacity to modulate immune reactivity.

CNS-IMMUNE SYSTEM INTERACTIONS

The brain has traditionally been considered an immunologically privileged site and yet, paradoxically, it is the site of the most studied autoimmune experimental disease, EAE.[35] Experience with implanting allografts within the CNS indicates that by augmenting immune reactivity systemically, such as by addition of a skin allograft on host skin, one can dramatically augment allograft rejection within the brain. Understanding what properties of the lymphocytes, cell surface, and cytokine repertoire determine their capacity to "home" to the CNS is likely to be central to defining the basis of CNS-specific autoimmune disease. It is also necessary to define the interactions of the "homing" lymphocytes with the components of the blood-brain barrier. The capacity of activated lymphocytes to induce MHC antigens on cells composing the blood-brain barrier and to release soluble factors that disrupt the blood-brain barrier likely are central processes in the migration of T cells into the CNS. Susceptibility to EAE is influenced by genetically determined properties of the blood-brain barrier, particularly its response to biogenic amines.[30] Therapeutic manipulation of the trafficking process could be highly tissue specific, and thus it could avoid some of the systemic complications to be expected with agents directed at the overall immune system.

The nervous system itself can exert profound influences on the immune system, likely via release of neurohormones and neurotransmitters.[18] The autonomic nervous system is known to innervate lymphoid organs. A wide range of neural-derived substances, including beta-adrenergic agonists, serotonin, histamine, and neuropeptides (e.g., enkephalins, vasoactive intestinal peptide [VIP], somatostatin), are known to affect monocyte, lymphocyte, and NK cell functions. Lymphocytes have receptors for, and secrete, a number of hormones, neurotransmitters, and growth factors. For example, lymphocytes contain mRNA for adrenocorticotropic hormone (ACTH) and actually produce and secrete it. These lymphocyte products not only are controlled by the usual endocrine mechanisms, but also are induced by exposure to viral infection, likely due to the effects of IFN-γ. The role of neurochemicals in underlying the effects of behavior states on immune status and on immune diseases forms the field of psychoneuroimmunology. The possibility exists that disordered immune function can be manipulated using neurohormone-neurotransmitter agonists and antagonists, working either directly on the immune system or indirectly on the nervous system control of immune function.

AUTOIMMUNE NEUROLOGIC DISEASES

Myasthenia gravis is the prototype human antibody-mediated autoimmune neurologic disease[11,12] (Table 6–4). The antigen in MG and in its animal model, EAMG, is the nicotinic acetylcholine receptor (AChR), the neurotransmitter receptor at the neuromuscular junction. Antibodies directed against the AChR mediate target injury via a number of mechanisms. They produce complement-mediated lysis of the postsynaptic membrane. In addition, cross-linking of AChRs increases their turnover. Finally, the function of the remaining AChRs can be blocked by antibodies binding to crucial portions of the AChR molecule. A second autoimmune disease of this synapse, Lambert-Eaton syndrome (LES) (see Table 6–4) also is antibody mediated. The antigen in LES appears to be the voltage-gated calcium channel in the membrane of the presynaptic motor nerve terminal. It appears that membrane lysis and direct blockade of channel function play an insignificant role in LES; the major pathogenic mechanism is down-regu-

Table 6–4 AUTOIMMUNE NEUROLOGIC DISEASES—PERIPHERAL

Disease	Immunogenetic Susceptibility	Pathology	Specific Antigen Sensitivity	Passive Transfer	Animal Model
Peripheral Nerve					
• Myelin					
Guillain-Barré syndrome	?−	Inflammation, demyelination	?	Serum-induced demyelination	Experimental allergic neuritis
• Chronic inflammatory polyneuritis	?+	" "	?		C57 aged mice
• IgM paraprotein-associated neuropathy	?	IgM deposition, noninflammatory widened myelin lamellae	?	?	
• Motor neuropathy with multifocal conduction block ± IgM paraprotein	?	Noninflammatory neuropathy vs neuronopathy	GM., GD1b	?	
• ?Axonal neuropathy with paraproteinemia	?	Axonopathy, noninflammatory			
Neuromuscular junction					
• Myasthenia gravis	+	Motor endplate destruction	Acetylcholine receptor	+	Experimental autoimmune myasthenia gravis
• Lambert-Eaton syndrome		Reduced number of nerve terminal active zones	Pre-synaptic CA^{2+} channel (frequently associated with small-cell lung tumor [? common antigen])	+	—

lation of channels by antibody cross-linking.

EAMG was initially induced by injection of rabbits with nicotinic AChR purified from the electric organ of electric fish.[12] The disease can be transferred either with antibodies or AChR-sensitized T-cell lines (helper phenotype), and has been induced in many species, including primates. The most highly studied form, that induced in inbred rats or mice, is biphasic. A short-lived acute phase begins about 1 week after injection and is characterized by necrosis and inflammatory cell infiltration of the postsynaptic portion of the neuromuscular junction. The antibody titer is relatively low during this phase. This acute phase clears within a few days to be followed by a chronic phase beginning about 2 weeks later and generally progressing to death. Histologically, there is no longer inflammation or necrosis in the endplate region, but rather a simplification of the highly folded postsynaptic membrane and a reduction in the amount of AChR. The antibody titer is high during this phase, and continues to rise. Evidence suggests that the lack of inflammation in the chronic phase relates to the reduced density of antigen in the postsynaptic membrane following the first exposure to antibody and the accompanying severe inflammation. The histologic findings in human MG are identical to those in the chronic phase, although recent studies have demonstrated the occasional presence of inflammation and necrosis at endplates.[11,12]

In other apparently antibody-mediated conditions, such as the paraneoplastic syndromes, subacute cerebellar degeneration, and subacute sensory neuritis, and in the syndromes of IgM paraproteinemia associated with demyelinating motor/sensory neuropathy or multifocal conduction block and motor neuropathy, tissue-specific antibodies also can be demonstrated (Table 6–5).[2] In contrast with MG and LES, however, these diseases are not yet readily transferable to animals, perhaps because the autoantibodies are species specific. In addition, the demonstration that antibodies, particularly those directed against lipid moieties, can induce target tissue injury in disorders currently postulated to involve T-cell-mediated mechanisms (e.g., Guillain-Barré syndrome or GBS, EAE, and possible MS) indicates that humoral factors may become involved in contributing to tissue injury, regardless of the primary initiating event. Antibodies arising presumably secondary to tissue injury, and which may not themselves induce tissue injury, are found in multiple disease states.

Multiple sclerosis has been considered the prototype T-cell-mediated disorder of the CNS (see Table 6–5). In MS, the initiating event remains in question. It may be autosensitization to an antigen present on the oligodendrocytes or its myelin membrane, or exposure to a specific viral infection. T-cell sensitization to myelin antigens, as follows immunization with neural tissue-containing vaccines or as a consequence of certain viral infections, particularly measles, can result in an inflammatory demyelinating disorder, namely acute disseminated encephalomyelitis (ADEM). However, ADEM is a uniphasic illness. The evidence supporting MS as an autoimmune disorder includes the pathologic findings of inflammatory infiltrates (T cells, B cells, and macrophage cells) at the lesion sites, overrepresentation of the disease in individuals with specific genetically determined properties of their immune system, specifically those related to their MHC and T-cell receptor repertoires, and the apparent state of immune activation (increased intrathecal IgG synthesis, proportion of T cells expressing activation antigens) coupled with demonstrable defects in immune regulatory mechanisms. As with EAMG, the existence of a model immune-mediated CNS demyelinating disease, EAE, has provided major insights into the basic cellular mechanisms likely to be operative. This disease model also has been used to test the efficacy of potentially therapeutic

Table 6-5 AUTOIMMUNE NEUROLOGIC DISEASES—CNS

Disease	Immunogenetic Susceptibility	Pathology	Specific Antigen Sensitivity	Passive Transfer	Animal Model
CNS—Neuronal					
• Systemic lupus erythematosus	+	Primary vascular, noninflammatory	Multiple autoantibodies including antineuronal	—	Spontaneous lupus in mice
• Paraneuroplastic syndromes					
• Subacute cerebellar degeneration	?	Inflammation, neuronal loss	Common neuronal-tumor antigen (Hμ)	—	—
• Dorsal root ganglionitis	?	" "	" "	—	—
• Opsoclonus-myoclonus	?	" "	"?	—	—
• Limbic encephalitis	?	" "	?	—	—
• Amyotrophic lateral sclerosis	Doubtful	Noninflammatory	None known	—	Experimental autoimmune motor neuron disease?
CNS—Myelin					
• Acute disseminated encephalomyelitis	?	Inflammation, demyelination	Myelin basic protein	—	Experimental allergic encephalomyelitis
• Multiple sclerosis	+	" "	?	—	" "?

agents, with the results leading directly to their application to their presumed human counterparts. Throughout the following section on specific therapeutic agents, the effect of such agents on these disease models will be discussed.

Experimental allergic encephalomyelitis is an inflammatory disease of the CNS that can be induced in a variety of animal species by *systemic* immunization using as antigen either whole CNS, MBP, or proteolipid protein suspended in adjuvant.[31] Susceptibility to EAE for a given species is strain- and age-specific. Multiple genes contribute to overall susceptibility, including ones affecting immune responsiveness (MHC class II and TcR repertoire), genes affecting blood-brain barrier properties, and perhaps those regulating intrinsic neural-cell properties such as inductibility of MHC antigens on glial cells. Although "classic" EAE is a uniphasic disease, conditions can be selected that result in a chronic relapsing disease (CREAE) featuring marked amounts of CNS demyelination. In the acute phase of the disease, one can demonstrate T-cell sensitivity to the inducing antigen, particularly specific regions of the MBP molecule. In CREAE, clinical relapses may or may not be associated with appearance of MBP-reactive blood T cells. EAE has been passively transferred by use of T-cell lines bearing the T-helper phenotype, which are sensitized to the specific encephalitic portion of the MBP molecule.[54] Within the lesions, however, the majority of T cells are host derived, indicating the importance of cell recruitment to lesion formation.

Indeed, T-cell lines must be injected systemically, not intracerebrally, to obtain the disease. At lesion sites, one can find T cells of both T-helper and T-suppressor/cytotoxic phenotypes. Astrocytes, and perhaps endothelial cells, in and near lesions express MHC antigens even prior to the appearance of clinical disease; increased permeability of the blood-brain barrier can also be demonstrated early on. Interactions of immune-mediating cells with astrocytes and endothelial cells, both of which contribute to the blood-brain barrier, may be critical for permitting systemic T cells to interact with, modify, and cross the blood-brain barrier and to reach their target sites within the CNS.

Macrophage accumulation is a hallmark of the EAE lesions. Their soluble products likely contribute significantly to the myelin destruction ("bystander demyelination"). Systemic macrophage depletion, even after onset of clinical signs, retards further development of EAE.

Although EAE cannot be transferred using antibody alone, one can demonstrate that sera derived from animals developing EAE after immunization with white matter will mediate myelin-toxic effects; such effects seemingly involve antimyelin antibodies, particularly directed against glycolipids. The extent of tissue injury (demyelination) in EAE reflects the combined effects of multiple immune mediators. B-cell-depleted animals reportedly are resistant to EAE, likely as a result of the loss of B-cell antigen-presenting function.

Guillain-Barré syndrome is considered an autoimmune disorder of the peripheral nervous system. Pathologic findings of inflammatory infiltrates in affected nerves and the development of an animal model, experimental allergic neuritis, which can be induced by immunization with peripheral nerve antigen and passively transferred by T cells, implicates cell-mediated immune mechanisms in the pathogenesis of GBS. Most of the principles described regarding the immunopathogenesis of EAE can also be applied to experimental allergic neuritis. In GBS, no convincing HLA association is demonstrated, nor has a specific antigen to which T cells are sensitized yet been found. The involvement of antibody in the nerve injury process is indicated by findings of neurotoxic effects of GBS serum, the presence of the previously mentioned glycolipid antibodies, and the possible beneficial effect of plasmapheresis. Current opinion suggests that GBS is a T-cell-initiated disorder in which B cells and macrophages contribute to the destruction of peripheral nerve myelin.

IMMUNOTHERAPIES

The overall aim of immune-directed therapy is control of the immune-mediated disorder with little or no toxicity to the host. A general principle to be followed is that the more selective an agent is with regard to its effect on the putative disease-mediating immune process, the more likely it is to fulfill the above criterion. Immune-directed therapy has evolved in parallel with advances in understanding of the mechanisms underlying immune reactivity, and with development or identification of agents targeting ever more selective sites within the immune response pathway (Table 6–6). One might consider the previously used, current, and anticipated immune-suppressive therapies as falling into several categories: (1) nonantigen specific therapies that affect overall activity of lymphocytes — these include the classic cytotoxic agents and radiation therapy; (2) agents affecting precise intracellular or extracellular immune pathways that become activated during the process of an immune response — that is, biologic response modifiers; (3) specific antigen- or antibody-directed therapies; (4) autoreactive T-cell therapy; (5) agents interfering with final soluble effector mediators of tissue damage — that is, antibody secreted by B cells or soluble mediators released by T cells and macrophages such as anti-inflammatory agents; and (6) corticosteroids, which exert multiple effects on the immune system. As a converse to immunosuppressive agents, one need consider agents that may augment selected components of the immune response.

Nonantigen-Specific Directed Therapy

CYTOTOXIC DRUGS

The prototypes of these agents, which have received widest use in treatment of human neurologic disease, are cyclophosphamide (Cytoxan) and azathio-

Table 6–6 IMMUNOTHERAPIES FOR NEUROLOGIC DISEASE

NONANTIGEN-SPECIFIC DIRECTED THERAPY

- Cytotoxic drugs (See Table 6–7)

   Cyclophosphamide (alkylating agent)
   Azathioprine (purine antimetabolite)

- Lymphoid irradiation

BIOLOGIC RESPONSE MODIFIERS

- Intracellular agents (e.g., isoprinosine — disrupts purine salvage pathway)
- Cyclosporine — inhibits the production of cytokines by T cells

SPECIFIC ANTIGEN- OR ANTIBODY-DIRECTED THERAPY

- Antigen-directed therapy

   Eliminate antigen
   Induce suppressor mechanisms
   Reduce antigen-reactive T or B cells

- Antibody-directed therapy (plasmapheresis)

AUTOREACTIVE CELL IMMUNOTHERAPY

- Monoclonal antibodies used to remove specific T cells
- Interfere with lymphocyte-monocyte migration
- Vaccination with altered autoreactive T-cell lines

ANTI-INFLAMMATORY AGENTS

- Inhibitors of arachidonic acid cascade
- Protease inhibitors

CORTICOSTEROIDS

AUGMENTATION OF IMMUNE RESPONSE (e.g., administration of IFN-γ)

prine (Imuran) (Table 6–7).[34] Cyclophosphamide is the prototype of the alkylating agents.[25,27] The drug affects both resting and cycling lymphocytes. Alkylation of the nitrogen of the purine guanine of DNA can lead to miscoding of DNA replication. The presence of two or more alkyl radicals per molecule of drug permits covalent cross-linking reactions of other molecules. Cross-linking of DNA prevents cell replication. The functional effects of cyclophosphamide on the immune system are dose related and, in animal model systems, related to the time interval between antigenic

Table 6–7 ACTION OF CYTOTOXIC DRUGS

CYCLOPHOSPHAMIDE (CYTOXAN)

- Short-term, intensive treatment: 600 mg/ m^2 × 5 d;[50] intermittent "boosters" or chronic oral therapy (2–4/mg/kg per day)
- Activated by liver metabolism
- Affects resting and cycling lymphocytes
- Alkylation of guanine in DNA causes miscoding and destruction of purine guanines
- Produces cross-linking of DNA strands
- Low dose effects — may abrogate suppressor function and augment immune response
- High dose effect — inhibits humoral and cell-mediated responses

AZATHIOPRINE (IMURAN)

- Long-term therapy (2–4 mg/kg per day)
- Must be metabolized to 6-mercaptopurine to have an immunosuppressive effect
- Affects actively dividing cells preferentially
- Blocks synthesis of adenylic and guanylic acid necessary for DNA synthesis
- B-cell sensitivity exceeds that of T-suppressor cells

challenge and administration of drug. Administration of drug in relatively low dose prior to antigenic challenge can, in some situations, result in selective lysis of suppressor cells and augmentation of the subsequent immune response. High-dose cyclophosphamide inhibits both humoral and cell-mediated immune responses. Drug administration even days after immunization can ameliorate subsequent development of EAE and EAMG. The drug may also affect monocyte macrophages, resulting in anti-inflammatory effects. Cyclophosphamide effects are likely mediated by active metabolites produced by oxidases, mainly found in liver microsomes. Specific metabolites include phosphoramide mustard and acrolein; the latter compound induces toxic effects without apparent therapeutic benefits.

Azathioprine is a purine analogue, derived from the addition of an imidazole group to 6-mercaptopurine.[25] Azathioprine must be metabolized in the liver to 6-mercaptopurine in order to have immunosuppressive activity. Azathioprine blocks synthesis of adenylic and guanylic acid, necessary steps for DNA synthesis. Thus the drug is cell-cycle specific, in that it affects actively dividing cells. In vitro testing indicates some selectivity of azathioprine with regard to effects on lymphocyte function, with B-cell sensitivity exceeding that of T-suppressor cells; T-inducer/helper-cell function, including lymphokine release, is the most resistant, although DTH-mediated T-cell responses can be inhibited. In our experience in MS, T-cell-dependent Ig secretion was inhibited in azathioprine-treated patients with total white blood cell counts greater than 3000, without decrease in T-cell proliferation induced by exposure to stimuli (mitogens) or change in suppressor function. Azathioprine may also inhibit monocyte precursor proliferation, resulting in an anti-inflammatory effect.

Use of Cytotoxic Drugs for Neurologic Disease. Use of cytotoxic immunosuppressive drugs in human immune disease must take into account the mode of administration, duration of therapy, and toxicity of the drug. As discussed previously, immune-mediated disease within the CNS can involve both recruitment of systemic lymphocytes to the CNS and sustained intra–blood-brain barrier immune reactivity. The presumed concurrent presence of both mechanisms raises the issue of whether systemic immunosuppressive therapy or direct intrathecal therapies will be required to control CNS "autoimmune" disease. Both cyclophosphamide and azathioprine cross even the intact blood-brain barrier, thus making them suitable for systemic use. General guidelines for use of cytotoxic drugs for neurologic diseases are outlined below and in Tables 6–7 through 6–10. This area continues to be one of active clinical investigation; no single optimal treatment program including dosage, mode of administration, and duration of therapy, has yet been established. These drugs should be prescribed only by physicians proficient in their use.

The duration of therapy is a key issue both with regard to the long-term efficacy of an agent and its toxicity. Certain presumed immune-mediated diseases of the nervous system, such as postinfectious encephalomyelitis and, in most cases, GBS, are self-limited and thus therapy can be short term. In other conditions such as temporal arteritis and polymyositis, clinical experience dictates the need for longer-term therapy. In MG in the elderly, indefinite therapy is the accepted practice. In MS, the issue is unresolved, given the lack of an established effective agent, but experience with cyclophosphamide indicates that single-cycle, high-dose therapy is not effective long term, even in those who do initially respond. Treatment protocols in current use or under study using cyclophosphamide for neurologic disease (see Table 6–7) include chronic low-dose therapy (MG, polymyositis, neurologic manifestations of systemic vasculitis) and short-term intensive treatment for MS,[50] perhaps followed by intermittent "booster" therapy or retreatment when disease progression resumes. Azathioprine is used on a long-term basis, usually at dosages of 2 to 4 mg/kg per day, or in some cases titrated to produce white blood cell counts of less than 3000/mm.[34] With both cyclophosphamide and azathioprine, immune function should resume after cessation of therapy; other forms of short-term immunotherapy such as total lymphoid irradiation (TLI), however, may induce permanent impairment in overall immune function (see "Lymphoid Irradiation" p 195).

Toxic Effects. The toxic effects of these drugs are related to their effects on the DNA and replication properties of cells, both lymphoid and nonlymphoid. The major toxicities to be considered include (1) direct toxicity to cellular elements, (2) induction of chromosomal changes affecting reproduction, and (3) induction of cellular changes leading to neoplasia.[38,43]

Much of the available data regarding toxicity of cyclophosphamide is derived from relatively long experience in treatment of tumors and prevention of transplant rejection and from more recent experience in treatment of rheumatic disease. The agent's effects on rapidly dividing cells can result in bone marrow suppression, intestinal irritation, hair loss, and bladder epithelium damage, resulting in hemorrhagic cystitis. These effects are dose related, with cumulative drug dosage being a crucial factor. The dosages of cytotoxic agents required for immunosuppressive effects and those inducing toxicity, particularly hematopoietic depression, need not be linked. Metabolites of cyclophosphamide may be the actual mediators of some of the toxicities. Clinically, the drug effects may lag 8 to 12 days after a given dose, and thus drug dosages must be adjusted rapidly in response to changes in blood counts. Cyclophosphamide's interaction with other drugs can significantly influence toxicity as well as efficacy; the issue of drug interactions applies to most of the agents discussed in this chapter. Glucocorticoids may exert a protective effect on the hematotoxicity of cyclophosphamide, although animal data are conflicting. Allopurinol may enhance cyclophosphamide toxicity, perhaps by inhibiting liver microsomal enzymes required for drug metabolism.

Hemorrhagic cystitis usually occurs when the total drug dose is greater than 6 g/m² body surface area, and can occur within hours of a single large dose of cyclophosphamide. Maintenance of adequate hydration can prevent such episodes, though cyclophosphamide itself may impair water excretion.

Cyclophosphamide-induced infertility in male patients usually requires a total dose of 6 to 10 g, although 1 to 2 mg/kg per day for 2 months can reduce sperm counts. The effects are mainly due to loss of germinal epithelium of the seminiferous tubules; some Leydig cell dysfunction may also occur. Recovery from aspermia is unpredictable. In female patients, amenorrhea is noted in 50% of women receiving 40 to 120 mg/d of cyclophosphamide for 18 months;

normal pregnancies have occurred following cessation of treatment, however.

A teratogenic effect of cyclophosphamide is suggested but difficult to establish on the basis of human epidemiologic data, given the small number of pregnancies that have taken place and the short follow-up on such offspring. Reports do exist of malformations in human and animal offspring, especially with first-trimester therapy. The drug increases the frequency of chromosomal breaks.

Data on the carcinogenic effect of cyclophosphamide, particularly with regard to leukemias, lymphomas, and reticulum cell sarcomas, consist mainly of reports of single or small case numbers. Baltus and colleagues[4] reported a fourfold increase in malignancies (especially lymphoreticular) in rheumatoid arthritis patients treated with cyclophosphamide, and an apparent dose-dependent effect. Patients developing malignancy following cyclophosphamide, in whom other chemotherapeutic or radiation therapies have also been used, must be viewed separately since multimodal therapy seems to increase the risk of tumors. This issue is of specific importance in diseases of the nervous system in which either multiagents are used in sequence in the face of nonresponsiveness (e.g., MG, polymyositis, chronic inflammatory polyneuritis), or in diseases (e.g., MS) in which, at different times, different experimental protocols are being tested.

A wide range of other infrequently occurring toxicities are described with cyclophosphamide, including rare liver dysfunction and transient cerebral dysfunction.[27]

Azathioprine induces a series of reversible toxicities including bone marrow suppression, hypersensitivity reaction, intestinal complaints, meningitic reactions, and alopecia. Hepatotoxicity can occur. Data from renal allograft recipients indicates an increased risk of malignancy, especially lymphoreticular, and some epithelial tumors. Infertility is not as common a problem with azathioprine as with cyclophosphamide. Animal data do suggest that azathioprine can be teratogenic, but the risk in humans is apparently low. Azathioprine has been used to treat relapsing and progressive forms of MS for many years, with conflicting claims with regard to both efficacy and toxicity. All protocols have involved chronic oral therapy (dose range usually 2 to 4 mg/kg), sometimes instituted after a course of high-dose corticosteroids. The overall experience in MS has not suggested an increased risk of malignancy.[34]

A universal risk in patients receiving immunosuppressants, particularly the cytotoxic agents, is superinfection with bacterial, viral, and fungal agents. Recent experience with AIDS patients emphasizes the spectrum of infectious agents that can become activated in the immunocompromised host.

LYMPHOID IRRADIATION

Radiation of lymphoid tissues can induce long-lasting suppression of the immune system.[26] The immunosuppression likely reflects a number of different effects of this form of therapy on the immune system. As previously mentioned, lymphocyte interaction with antigen requires the involvement of antigen-presenting cells. These cells encompass the MHC class II-bearing adherent cells (i.e., monocytes and dendritic cells), and specialized cells within tissues (e.g., Langerhan cells of skin or glial cells within the CNS). Daily whole-body ultraviolet irradiation results in depletion of these cells with ensuing inefficient antigen presentation, without affecting most T- and B-lymphocyte functions. Ultraviolet irradiation has been shown to inhibit the development of acute EAE effectively in the mouse.

Total lymphoid irradiation was initially used as a treatment of Hodgkin's disease and other lymphomas. More recently, this therapy has been administered with promising results to patients with intractable rheumatoid arthritis and is now under investigation as a therapy in MS. Evaluation of rheumatoid arthritis patients, as well as previous studies of cancer patients receiving TLI, indicates that this therapy induces long-lasting depression of cell-mediated immunity. In the rheumatoid arthritis group, 2000 rads (20 Gy) delivered during 2 to 3 weeks to nodes above the diaphragm, and then equal amounts below the diaphragm, resulted in depression of lymphocyte counts for more than 1 year, depression of T-cell mitogen-induced proliferation, and probably an augmentation of suppressor-cell function. Total lymphoid irradiation likely also affects antigen presentation in the manner described for ultraviolet irradiation.

Clinical experience with TLI suggests a relative lack of toxicity, if used as the sole modality of treatment.[34] When combined with chemotherapy in the treatment of lymphomas, however, TLI was associated with an increased frequency of second malignancy. Whether patients with nonmalignant diseases receiving combined therapy will show such delayed toxicities remains unknown.

Biologic Response Modifiers

Biologic response modifiers modulate specific activities or properties of immune-mediating cells at usual dosages without inducing generalized cytotoxicity. Properties that may be either suppressed or amplified include specific intracellular activation pathways and release and binding of soluble factors. The biologic response modifiers can be either natural biologic agents themselves or synthesized agents.

The utility of neurotransmitter-neuropeptides (or their agonists or antagonists) in modifying immune reactivity in immune-mediated disease states is yet to be fully explored. The opiate-receptor antagonist naltrexone has been reported to inhibit EAE.

INTRACELLULAR-DIRECTED AGENTS

As discussed previously, intracellular cyclic nucleotide metabolism is central to T-cell activation. Pharmacologic agents acting via the purine salvage pathway exert significant effects on immune reaction.[20] For example, isoprinosine, an investigational drug in which inosine is complexed to p-acetomidobenzoic acid and NN-dimethyl-amino-Z-propanol, can induce T-lymphocyte functional changes similar to those observed with thymic hormones. The anti-viral effects claimed for isoprinosine may well act through immunomodulation. The effects of neurotransmitters and neuropeptides on lymphocyte function may also, to a large extent, act via cyclic nucleotide pathways.

CYCLOSPORINE

The fungal extract cyclosporine exerts profound immunosuppressive effects, with its most selective effect being inhibition of cytotoxic T-cell function (see Table 6–6).[21,23] This inhibition results from the drug's ability to inhibit transcription of mRNA for IL-2, a lymphokine usually required for T-cell proliferation. One study[21] demonstrated that cloned cytotoxic T-cell lines could respond to IL-2 in the presence of cyclosporine and that their effector activity was not inhibited if proliferation could occur via an IL-2 independent pathway. Others found that the drug decreased IL-1 and IL-2 secretion, with the latter dependent on the former. Production of other interleukins is also inhibited.[5] T-suppressor function is seemingly spared by cyclosporine. We found that MS patients with progressive disease treated with cyclosporine showed marked decreases in in vitro cytotoxic activity.[5] The activity was restored by addition of IL-2 to the cultures, indicating that their cytotoxic cells can respond to IL-2. The reduced suppressor levels observed in these patients were not restored after 3 to 6 months of therapy.

Cyclosporine exerts multiple other effects on cells, which may contribute to its role as a biologic response modifier. For example, cyclosporine is shown to bind to prolactin receptors,[7] which are present on lymphocytes and seem to overlap with the calmodulin-binding site. Inhibition of the calcium ionophore by cyclosporine could inhibit cell activation. Elevated prolactin levels do occur as a result of drug treatment, and prolactin itself directly affects lymphocyte function.

Toxicity data regarding cyclosporine were initially gathered from patients undergoing kidney or heart allografting. Data are now accumulated from clinical studies of a wide range of "autoimmune" diseases. Neurologic disorders in which cyclosporine has been evaluated include polymyositis, MG, MS (Table 6–8), and amyotrophic lateral sclerosis.[34,52] Use of cyclosporine for MS and other neurologic diseases remains investigational at this time and the benefit/risk ratio remains to be established.[34,52] The dose-limiting toxicity of cyclosporine is usually related to renal effects. Elevated creatinine values are almost universal as drug levels exceed 300 to 400 mg/mL. Prolonged high-dose therapy can result in irreversible renal damage. The development of hypertension as a result of cyclosporine A therapy seemingly is a consequence of reduced renal blood flow. Other toxicities include development of tremor and hirsutism. With regard to the latter, one notes the structural similarities of cyclosporine to phenytoin.

INTERFERONS

Converse to the above-mentioned considerations regarding immunosup-

Table 6–8 IMMUNOTHERAPY FOR MULTIPLE SCLEROSIS

RELAPSING DISEASE

Short-term therapy (days–weeks) to enhance recovery rate
  Corticosteroids   **ACTH** (+)[48]
    High dose—IV methylprednisone (+)[48]   Plasma exchange (+)[50]
    Low dose—prednisone 40–60 mg (not tested in clinical trials)
Long-term therapy (years) to reduce relapse frequency and cumulative disability
  Nonspecific immunosuppression   **Antigen-specific therapy**
    Azathioprine (+)[50]   Myelin basic protein (−)[50]
    Corticosteroids (−)[48]   Copolymer-1 (+)[34,50]
  Biologic response modifiers
    Interferon-alpha (+/−) or beta (+)[34]
    Interferon-gamma (−)[34]

PROGRESSIVE DISEASE

Long-term therapy (years) to reduce cumulative disability
  Nonspecific immunosuppression   **Biologic response modifiers**
    Cyclophosphamide[50]   Cyclosporine (+)[52]
    Chronic oral (+/−)
    Pulse IV ± "boosters" (+/−)
    Azathioprine ± corticosteroids (+/−)[34]
    Total lymphoid irradiation (+)[34]   **Antigen-specific therapy**
    Plasma exchange (+/−)[34]   Copolymer-1 (−)[34]

CURRENT RECOMMENDATIONS

Short term: ACTH or corticosteroids for disabling relapses
Long-term: Immunotherapy remains under clinical investigation; risk (toxicity): benefit ratio remains to be established for listed therapies.

Key: (+) = positive results in clinical trials; (−) = negative results in clinical trials.

pression, approaches exist to augment specific components of the immune response. Among the suspected human "autoimmune" diseases, such therapies have been particularly considered for MS, since data have been presented indicating that specific immune deficiencies exist in this patient group. These defects include reduced class II-restricted T cell cytotoxicity, reduced NK-cell function, and reduced IFN production by NK and lymphoid cells. The possibility of a persistent viral infection in MS cannot yet be excluded, and this possibility served as the basis for initial clinical therapeutic trials with IFNs in MS. These trials have included administration of systemic and/or intrathecal IFN-α and IFN-β.[33] A clinical trial with IFN-γ did not show efficacy in relapsing MS, although patients showed suppressed levels of pokeweed mitogen–induced IgG secretion in vitro. Preliminary trials of IFN-β suggest some clinical efficacy in relapsing MS; IFN-β is reported to down-regulate IFN-gamma-induced MHC class II antigen expression.[33] IFN-gamma administration has been shown to increase the frequency of disease exacerbations, perhaps providing indirect evidence of the autoimmune nature of the disease. Other immune potentiators such as levamisole and transfer factor either aggravated the disease or, at best, did not prove to be of benefit.

Specific Antigen- or Antibody-Directed Therapy

ANTIGEN-DIRECTED THERAPY

Therapeutic strategies in this area are aimed at either (1) actually eliminating a specific antigen from the individual, (2) inducing active suppressor mechanisms that will inhibit immune reactivity to antigen, or (3) eliminating or rendering unresponsive specific T and B cells sensitized to respond to the specific antigen. A study[47] of the chronic relapsing EAE model demonstrated that the MBP initially used subcutaneously to immunize the animals persisted in the skin for more than 1 year postinjection; amputation of the hind foot to remove antigenic deposits prevented subsequent episodes of clinical EAE. In addition, the amputee animals were shown to be resistant to development of EAE if specifically rechallenged with antigen, suggesting that locally present antigen can prevent the development of tolerance. This approach may apply to chronic human disease such as MS if the concept of antigenic mimicry is applicable to the disease pathogenesis. If exogenous agents (virus, bacteria) sharing antigenicity with CNS structures persist, perhaps eliminating them will affect the clinical disease.

The efficacy of administering specific antigens to induce resistance to development of disease upon subsequent exposure to the same antigens is illustrated by studies in EAE in which resistance can be achieved by intravenous administration of MBP in incomplete adjuvant or in saline, or by MBP inserted into liposomes or administered orally.[31,34,40] Attempts to use this strategy in MS are hampered by lack of convincing data regarding whether a specific "MS antigen" exists. Attempts to desensitize MS patients by subcutaneous injections of MBP did not benefit the clinical course of disease.[34] The synthetically produced compound copolymer-1, initially developed as an attempt to resemble MBP structurally, inhibits subsequent development of MBP-induced EAE when administered to animals. The effects of copolymer-1 on relapsing forms of MS are currently being evaluated. Copolymer-1-sensitized T-cell lines need not also be responsive to MBP and vice-versa, however.[34] A related experimental approach has used nonimmunogenic peptides resembling MBP to block the immune response by competing with MBP peptides at T-cell receptors in EAE.[54] This approach would be feasible in humans if the heterogeneity of T-cell receptors is as limited as it is in mouse EAE.

ANTIBODY-DIRECTED
THERAPY

In a number of human clinical disorders of suspected or established immune etiology, attempts have been made to remove systemic antibody nonselectively (plus other soluble factors — e.g., proteases, lymphokines) by use of plasmapheresis. The most convincing success is noted in disorders in which the humoral basis for the disease state is best established, such as MG or LES. In GBS, plasma exchange enhances the rate of disease recovery; whether this therapy reflects removal of a specific antibody or mediator of inflammation needs to be established.

If a putative, specific, disease-mediating antibody can be identified, then more selective approaches to controlling this immune response can be designed. The prototype model illustrating such approaches is EAMG. In EAMG, one can induce the clinical, electrophysiologic, and pathologic features of the disease by administration of mAbs directed against the AChR.[11] Even in EAMG, probably other cell types, particularly macrophages, are involved in the pathogenesis. One can show in EAMG that experimentally produced anti-id mAb injected prior to or up to 1 week after the immunization with AChR, even if not specifically directed against the antigen-binding site of the Ig molecule, interferes with the immune response, reducing anti-AChR antibody titers, and preventing the development of the disease. The anti-id used in these studies was directed at a site in the variable region of the anti-AChR-id at a distance from the antigen-binding site. Moreover, the target of the anti-id was expressed on only a small percentage of the anti-AChRs, whereas the reduction in titer involved the majority of the anti-AChR antibodies.

To be effective in the human disease, this type of effect would need to be produced months, and possibly years, after the initiation of the autoimmune response. In addition, one would have to ensure that the anti-id would not enhance, rather than reduce, the production of the corresponding id-bearing antibodies.

Similar strategies could be applied to antigen-specific T cells, in that antibodies recognizing determinants on the TcR unique to a given T-cell clonal population could be used (i.e., anticlonotypic antibody).[53] This treatment would be especially promising if the TcR usage in the autoimmune response were as limited as has been observed in EAE in inbred strains of mice and rats.[54]

Autoreactive Cell Immunotherapy

mAb THERAPY

The aim of this therapy is to use selective mAbs to remove or inactivate specific T cells that mediate an autoimmune process. The vastly expanded array of mAbs now available permit one to direct therapy toward all, or subsets, of T cells; T cells bearing antigens that appear only during the course of cell activation, MHC antigens; and soluble mediators and their receptors (e.g., IL-2). Substantial data are now available on the effectiveness of these mAbs in the treatment of experimental autoimmune neurologic disease. In both mice and rats, in vivo treatment of animals with anti–total-T-cell, anti–T-cell-helper, and anti–T-cell-receptor antibodies will abrogate development of EAE and EAMG.[54] Anti-MHC-class-II antibody also effectively inhibits these disorders, likely by interfering with cell-cell interaction between macrophages and lymphocytes, between subsets of lymphocytes, and between lymphocytes and either endothelial cells or target tissue cells. In the CNS, anti–MHC-class-II therapy can block lymphocyte trafficking across the blood-brain barrier and with interactions between lymphocytes and glial cells. Anti–MHC-class-II treatment may also induce suppressor cells. The polymorphic nature of this antigen may prove useful in the treatment of human disease. Treatment with a single anti-MHC antibody in a heterozygote may abrogate only those immune responses induced by antigens presented to T cells in conjunction with the particular MHC molecule recognized by the mAb's immune response induced by antigens complexed to other MHC class II allele would be preserved. Efforts are ongoing to treat autoimmune disease with mAbs directed against T-cell antigens, including activation antigen and T-cell receptors for IL-2.

Binding of mAb antibody to a cell need not mean destruction of the cell. Indeed, the resultant Ab-antigen complex may only be modulated off the cell surface, with regeneration of the antigen occurring quickly thereafter. Use of whole Ig-mAb can result in immune complex formation and sequestration of the cells in the reticuloendothelial system, rather than complement fixation and destruction of the T cell. An intriguing approach to enhance target cell lysis is to couple a toxin to the mAb (i.e., delivery of a "poison bullet").[49] This approach uses the mAb as a means to specifically seek out a precise target; only when the toxin-mAb conjugate is bound to the cell is the toxin able to enter the cell and induce cell injury. It has been difficult, however, to produce toxin conjugates that retain both specificity and toxicity in vivo.

Experience with mAb therapy in human "autoimmune" neurologic disease to date has been limited. The mAbs used have been generated in animals and a rapid immune response is generated against the mAb itself. Anti-CD4 mAb therapy, when administered to MS patients for several days, did not produce long-lasting immunosuppression. Use of this antibody has a potential advantage in that if the immune reactivity is suppressed by inactivating or removing CD4 cells, then perhaps the host will be unable to generate an immune response against the mAb even if it is of heterologous origin. An additional approach to avoid the problem of an immune response against the mAb is to generate chimeric mAbs comprised of human Ig constant regions and a specific variable region encoded by a variable region gene obtained from another species, determining the antibody specificity. As with the other immunosuppressant therapies, there is concern about suppression of "needed" immunity.

INTERFERENCE WITH LYMPHOCYTE-MONOCYTE MIGRATION

Autoimmune responses directed toward the CNS must involve migration of lymphocytes-monocytes through the blood-brain barrier to reach the target. Studies with cloned MBP-specific T-cell lines indicate that disease is most effectively transferred when the cells are injected systemically rather than directed intrathecally. Most of the cellular infiltrate within the CNS is comprised of cells recruited from the host. As therapeutic strategies, one might consider (1) altering migration pattern of cells, (2) manipulating the blood-brain barrier, and (3) affecting the recruitment of nonantigen-specific cells to the brain or their subsequent function.

Trafficking of lymphocytes is shown to depend on their surface glycoprotein properties. Whether altering the glycoprotein properties of the cells will alter disease-inducing capability needs to be determined. With regard to the second and third strategies, current studies are aimed at determining the therapeutic effectiveness of vasoactive amine agonists and antagonists (particularly alpha-adrenergic receptor antagonists, which alter blood-brain barrier permeability), and of inhibitors of the lymphocyte-secreted mediators, which can induce changes in blood-brain-barrier permeability. Heparin in low doses has been used to treat EAE, but studies of MS patients have not yet demonstrated efficacy.[34,50]

VACCINATION WITH "ALTERED" AUTOREACTIVE T-CELL LINES

As previously indicated, autoimmune disease-mediating T-helper cell lines (e.g., EAE, adjuvant arthritis), if exposed in vitro to radiation or hydrostatic pressure, not only will no longer be able to transfer disease but also will make the animal resistant to disease when untreated T-cell lines are subsequently injected. Such approaches are more difficult to employ in diseases such as MS, however, where an antigen-specific disease-mediating T-cell population has yet to be identified.

Inhibitors of Inflammation

The soluble factors released by lymphocytes and monocytes contribute significantly to the tissue injury associated with the inflammatory reaction that characterizes some of the autoimmune diseases, such as EAE and MS. At least two mechanisms of this tissue injury are potentially amenable to therapy. First is the release of prostaglandins and leukotrienes, products of the arachidonic-acid cascade, from macrophages. Inhibitors of the cyclo-oxygenase pathways are the mainstay of nonsteroidal anti-inflammatory therapy. Their role in EAE and MS is being explored. Colchicine, an inhibitor of macrophage function, is being studied in MS patients.[50] The second mechanism is the release of proteases from inflammatory cells and tissues. Experimental protease inhibitors such as poly-L-lysine, pepstatin, and ϵ-aminocaproic acid have been beneficial in EAE.

Many of these anti-inflammatory agents also have direct effects on lymphocyte function, however, so that one must be cautious in interpreting the basis of their observed clinical efficacy. In addition, conflicting actions may occur; indomethacin, an anti-inflammatory prostaglandin inhibitor, is claimed to exacerbate EAE and MS.

Corticosteroids

Corticosteroids, currently the most often used immune-directed therapy for neurologic disorders, are discussed last because of the multiple effects they exert. All the categories of effects mediated by immune-directed agents should be considered when discussing the effects of glucocorticoids. Each type of effect is dose dependent. Glucocorticoids exert effects on lymphocyte survival, cell trafficking, T-cell proliferation, soluble-mediator release, antibody production, NK-cell function, and suppressor-cell activity. They also affect the blood-brain barrier, edema, and inflammatory mediators. Their nonimmune effects include promoting conduction through demyelinated nerve. The non-neurologic side effects of glucocorticoids, however, complicate their use for management of chronic inflammatory or immune-mediated neurologic disorders. Nevertheless, they represent the most-accepted long-term therapy in polymyositis and temporal arteritis, both conditions that involve clear-cut tissue inflammation; and in MG, where their mode of action is unclear.

ACTH has frequently been used instead of glucocorticoids in the treatment of MS. Individuals vary markedly with regard to the adrenal glucocorticoid response to ACTH, perhaps accounting in part for variability in clinical efficacy of the treatment. Since ACTH may have effects other than via the adrenal glucocorticoid response, it is uncertain whether ACTH and glucocorticoids can be considered to be interchangeable therapies. Lymphocytes themselves contain mRNA for ACTH and can secrete ACTH particularly in response to IFN-γ or viral infections. The lymphocyte may be subject to the same controls as the classic endocrine organs. No good studies have shown whether ACTH is superior to corticosteroids.

A wide variety of treatment protocols have been devised to use corticosteroids and ACTH for neurologic disease. Several widely used approaches for treat-

Table 6–9 CORTICOSTEROIDS

SHORT-TERM THERAPY FOR MULTIPLE SCLEROSIS
High dose IV methylprednisolone: 1 g/d × 5 d
ACTH Gel: 40–80 U/d × 5 d then reduce by 20 U every 3 d
Lower dose oral prednisone therapy: 60–100 mg/d × 5–7 d, then taper over 30 d

LONG-TERM PREDNISONE THERAPY FOR MYASTHENIA GRAVIS
60–80 mg/d until improvement, then equivalent dose given on alternate days, then gradually reducing dose every 2 mo to determine minimum dose[37]

LONG-TERM PREDNISONE THERAPY FOR POLYMYOSITIS
60–100 mg/d until improvement, then slowly taper off 5 mg every 3 wk to 40 mg/d; may switch to alternate day equivalent dose

---

Table 6–11 IMMUNOTHERAPY FOR MYASTHENIA GRAVIS

SHORT-TERM THERAPY (days–weeks) to induce remission
Plasma exchange (+)[41]
Cyclophosphamide (+)[39]
Corticosteroids (+)[37]

LONG-TERM THERAPY (months–indefinite) to maintain clinical remission (see "Maintenance Therapy" below)

SURGICAL TREATMENT
Thymectomy (+)[6]

NONSPECIFIC IMMUNOSUPPRESSION
Slowly tapering doses of corticosteroids (+)
Azathioprine (+)[33]

CURRENT RECOMMENDATIONS
Acute relapse—optimize non-immune therapy (anticholinesterase), plasma exchange, initiate corticosteroids (see Table 6–7)
Maintenance therapy—corticosteroids tapered to low dose ± azathioprine; thymectomy early in disease course (when patient is clinically stable)

Key: (+) = positive results in clinical trials; (−) = negative results in clinical trials.

ment of MS relapse, MG, and polymyositis are outlined in Table 6–9. Current recommendations for using these protocols based on the recent literature are provided in Tables 6–8, 6–10, and 6–11. These tables attempt to place corticosteroid therapy in the context of the other immunopharmacologic approaches being taken to these disorders.

Table 6–10 IMMUNOTHERAPY FOR INFLAMMATORY DEMYELINATING POLYNEUROPATHY (IDPN)

ACUTE IDPN (Guillain-Barré Syndrome)
Short-term therapy (days–weeks) to enhance rate of recovery
Plasma exchange (+)[32]
Corticosteroids (+/−)[32]
No clinical trial available re: therapies to prevent initial deterioration

CHRONIC IDPN
Plasma exchange (+)[14]
Corticosteroids (+)
Human immunoglobulin (+)[15]
No clinical trial available re: therapies to prevent recurrence or progression

RECOMMENDATION:
Plasma exchange and/or corticosteroids to enhance recovery; long-term corticosteroids ± immunosuppression (azathioprine) may be needed to prevent recurrence or resumed progression.

SUMMARY

Several important neurologic disorders, including MG, inflammatory demyelinating polyneuropathy, polymyositis, and MS, are known or speculated to be mediated by the immune system. Current immunotherapy for neurologic disorders is based primarily on clinical experience with standard immunosuppressive agents used to treat systemic disorders and cancer. Corticosteroids and the cytotoxic agents azathioprine and cyclophosphamide, used alone or in combination, provide partially effective therapy for some patients with these immune-mediated neurologic disorders. Their use is limited by toxic effects, however, and by their relatively nonspecific effects on the immune system.

The array of agents capable of modulating immune reactivity continues to expand steadily as more is learned about the details of the immune system in health and disease. The intense effort now ongoing to generate reagents selective for specific components of the immune system raises the possibility of achieving the aim of immuno-pharmacology — effective therapy with acceptable levels of toxicity. New approaches that are used in clinical practice include plasmapheresis and infusion of human immunoglobulin. Removal of antibodies appears to be the mechanism by which plasmapheresis helps patients with GBS, chronic inflammatory demyelinating polyneuropathy (CIDPN), and MG. This approach has yielded mixed results in limited trials in MS. High-dose immunoglobulin therapy may help certain patients with CIDPN and MG by removing antibodies and suppressing humoral immunity.

Several new investigational approaches to immunotherapy appear promising but cannot be recommended for general use at this time. Cyclosporine, a relatively selective immunosuppressive agent that has revolutionized organ transplantation, has shown some positive effects in clinical trials for MS. Total lymphoid irradiation is also being used in trials for MS, but additional investigation of cyclosporine and TLI is required to determine their role in therapy. On the horizon are approaches based on new information about the molecular organization of the immune system. These strategies use biologic response modifiers, specific antibodies that eliminate offending antigens, biologic agents that interfere with the function of specific lymphocyte and monocyte populations, anti-inflammatory agents, and interferons that selectively augment parts of the immune system. Exploration of these leads in careful clinical trials, together with experimentation using established animal models of human immunologic diseases, promises to provide safer, more effective therapy for the future.

REFERENCES

1. Aiello FB, Maggiano, N, Larocca, LM, Piantelli, M, and Musiani, P: Inhibitory effect of Cyclosporin A on the OKT3-induced peripheral blood lymphocyte proliferation. Cell Immunol 97:131 – 139, 1986.

2. Antel, JP and Moumdjian, R: Paraneoplastic syndrome: A role for the immune system. J Neurol 236:1 – 3, 1989.

3. Bach, FH and Sachs, DH: Current concepts: Immunology. Transplantation immunology. N Engl J Med 317:489 – 492, 1987.

4. Baltus, JAM, Boersma, JW, Hartman, AP, and Vandenbroucke, JP: The occurrence of malignancies in patients with rheumatoid arthritis treated with cyclophosphamide: A controlled retrospective follow-up. Ann Rheum Dis 42:368 – 373, 1983.

5. Bania, MB, Antel, JP, Reder, AT, Nicholas, MK, and Arnason, BGW: Suppressor and cytolytic function in multiple sclerosis — Effect of Cyclosporine A and interleukin-2 (IL-2). J Clin Invest 78:582 – 586, 1986.

6. Buckingham, JM, Howard, FM, Bernatz, PE, Payne, WS, Harrison, EG, O'Brien, PC, and Weiland, LH: The value of thymectomy in myasthenia gravis: A computer-assisted matched study. Ann Surg 184:453 – 457, 1976.

7. Cardon, SB, Larson, DF, and Russel, DH: Rapid elevation of rat serum prolactin concentration by cyclosporine, a novel immunosuppressive drug. Biochem Biophys Res Commun 120:614 – 618, 1984.

8. Cohen, IR, Ben-Nun, A, Holoshitz, J, Maron, R, and Zerubavel, R: Vaccination against autoimmune disease using lines of autoimmune T lymphocyte. Immunology Today 4:227 – 230, 1983.

9. Cook, SD, Troiano, R, Zito, G, Lavenhar, M, Devereux, C, Hafstein, MP, Hernandez, E, Vidaver, R, and Dowling, PC: Effect of total lymphoid irradiation in chronic progressive multiple sclerosis. Lancet 1:1405 – 1409, 1986.

10. Dib, M, Vital, A, Vital, C, Georgescault, D, Baquey, A, and Bezian, J: The C57BL mice: An animal model for inflammatory demyelinating polyneuropathy. J Neurol Sci 81:101 – 111, 1987.

11. Drachman, DB: Myasthenia gravis: Biology and treatment. Annals of the New

York Academy of Sciences, New York, 1987, pp. 90–105.

12. Drachman, DB, de Silva, S, Ramsay, D, and Pestronk, A: Humoral pathogenesis of myasthenia gravis. In Drachman, DB (ed): Myasthenia Gravis: Biology and Treatment, New York Academy of Sciences, New York, 1987, pp 90–105.

13. Duijestijn, A and Hamann, A: Mechanisms and regulation of lymphocyte migration. Immunology Today 10:23–28, 1989.

14. Dyck, PJ, Daube, J, O'Brien, P, Pineda, A, Low, PA, Windebank, AJ, and Swanson, B: Plasma exchange in chronic inflammatory demyelinating polyradiculoneuropathy. N Engl J Med 314:461–465, 1986.

15. Faed, JM, Pollock, M, Taylor, PK, Nukada, H, and Hammond-Tooke, GD: High-dose intravenous human immunoglobulin in chronic inflammatory demyelinating polyneuropathy. Neurology 39:422–425, 1989.

16. Freedman, M and Antel, JP: Immunoregulatory circuits in multiple sclerosis: Is there a short? Ann Neurol 24:183–184, 1988.

17. Gerlier, D and Rabourdin-Combe, C: Antigen processing—From cell biology to molecular interactions. Immunology Today 10:3–5, 1989.

18. Goetz EJ, Sreedharan, SP, and Karkonen, WS: Pathogenic roles of neuroimmunologic mediators. Immunology and Allergy Clinics of North America 8(2):183–200, 1988.

19. Hadden, JW: Transmembrane signals in the activation of T lymphocytes by mitogenic antigens. Immunology Today 9:235–239, 1988.

20. Hadden, JW and Giner-Sorolla, A: Isoprinosine and NPT 15392: Modulators of lymphocyte and macrophage development and function. In Hersh, EM (ed): Augmenting Agents in Cancer Therapy. Raven Press, New York, 1981, pp 497–522.

21. Herold, KC, Lancki, DW, Moldwin, RL, and Fitch, FW: Immunosuppressive effects of cyclosporin on cloned T cells. J Immunol 136:1315–1321, 1986.

22. Johnston, RB: Current concepts: Immunology. Monocytes and macrophages. N Engl J Med 318:747–752, 1988.

23. Kahan, BD: Drug therapy: Cyclosporine. N Engl J Med 25:1725, 1989.

24. Kammer, GM: The adenylate cyclase-cAMP-protein kinase. A pathway and regulation of the immune response. Immunology Today 9:222–229, 1988.

25. Katz, P: Immunosuppressant therapy. Adv Intern Med 29:167–192, 1984.

26. Kotzin, BL, Strober, S, Engelman, EG, Calin, A, Hoppe, RT, Kansas, GS, Terrell, CP, and Kaplan, H: Treatment of intractable rheumatoid arthritis with total lymphoid irradiation. N Engl J Med 305:969–976, 1981.

27. Kovarsky, J: Clinical pharmacology and toxicology of cyclophosphamide: Emphasis on use in rheumatic diseases. Semin Arthritis Rheum 12:359–372, 1983.

28. Levich, JD, Parks, DE, and Weigle, WO: Tolerance induction in antigen-specific helper T cell clones and lines in vitro. J Immunol 135:873–878, 1985.

29. McCarron, RM, Spatz, M, Kempski, O, Hogan, RN, Muehl, L, and McFarlin, DE: Interactions between myelin basic protein-sensitized T lymphocytes and murine cerebral vascular endothelial cells. J Immunol 137:3428–3435, 1986.

30. McFarlin, DE: Immunogenetics in relation to neurologic disease. Immunology and Allergy Clinics of North America 8(2):201–212, 1988.

31. McKenna, RM, Carter, BG, and Sehon, AH: Studies on the mechanisms of suppression of experimental allergic encephalomyelitis induced by myelin basic protein-cell conjugates. Cell Immunol 88:251–259, 1984.

32. McKhann, GM: Guillain-Barré syndrome: Clinical and therapeutic observations. Ann Neurol 27(Suppl):S13–S16, 1990.

33. Martens, HG, Hertel, G, Reuther, P, Ricker, K: Effect of immunosuppressive drugs (azathioprine). Ann NY Acad Sci 377:691–699, 1981.

34. Myers, LW and Ellison, GW (eds): Rationale for immunomodulating therapies of multiple sclerosis. Neurology 38 (Suppl 2):1–89, 1988.

35. Nicholas, MK, Antel, JP, Stefansson, K,

and Arnason, BGW: Rejection of fetal neurocortical neural transplants by H-2 incompatible mice. J Immunol 139: 2275–2283, 1987.

36. Nossal, GJV: Current Concepts: Immunology. The basic components of the immune system. N Engl J Med 316:1320–1325, 1987.

37. Pascuzzi, RM, Coslett, HG, and Johns, TR: Long-term corticosteroid treatment of myasthenia gravis: Report of 116 patients. Ann Neurol 15:291–298, 1984.

38. Penn, I: Malignancies associated with immunosuppressive or cytotoxic therapy. Surgery 83:492–502, 1978.

39. Perez, M, Buot, W, Nercado-Danguilan, W, Bagabaldo, ZG, and Renales, LD: Stable remission in MG. Neurology (NY) 31:32–34, 1981.

40. Pesoa, SA, Hayosh, NS, and Swanborg, RH: Regulation of experimental allergic encephalomyelitis. J Neuroimmunology 7:131–135, 1984.

41. Pinching, AJ, Peters, DK, and Newson-Davis, J: Remission of myasthenia gravis following plasma-exchange. Lancet 2:1373–1376, 1976.

42. Ruijs, TCG, Olivier, A, Freedman, MS, and Antel, JP: Cultured human oligodendrocytes are susceptible to lysis by MHC class I-directed cytotoxic lymphocytes. J Neuroimmunol 27:89–97, 1990

43. Sieber, SM and Adamson, RH: Toxicity of antineoplasic agents in man: Chromosomal aberrations, antifertility effects, congenital malformations, and carcinogenic potential. Adv Cancer Res 22:57–155, 1975.

44. Sobel, RA, Blanchette, BW, Bahn, AK, and Colvin, RB: The immunopathology of experimental allergic encephalomyelitis. II. Endothelial cell Ia increases prior to inflammatory cell infiltration. J Immunol 132:2402–2407, 1984.

45. Strejan, GH, Gilbert, JJ, and St. Lewis, J: Suppression of chronic-relapsing experimental allergic encephalomyelitis in strain-13 guinea pigs by administration of liposome-associated myelin basic protein. J Neuroimmunology 7:27–41, 1984.

46. Sun, D, Quin, Y, Chluba, J, Epplen, JT, and Wekerle, H: Suppression of experimentally induced autoimmune encephalitis by cytotoxic T-T cell interactions. Nature 332:843–845, 1988.

47. Tabira, T, Itoyama, Y, and Kuroiwa, Y: Necessity of continuous antigenic stimulation by the locally retained antigens in chronic relapsing experimental allergic encephalomyelitis. J Neurol Sci 66:97–106, 1984.

48. Troiana, R, Cook, SD, and Dowling, PC: Steroid therapy in multiple sclerosis. Point of view. Arch Neurol 44:803–807, 1987.

49. Vietta, ES and Uhr, J: Immunotoxins. Annual Review of Immunology 3:197–212, 1985.

50. Weiner, HL and Hafler, DA: Immunotherapy of multiple sclerosis. Ann Neurol 23:211–222, 1988.

51. Wisniewski, HM and Bloom, BR: Primary demyelination as a nonspecific consequence of a cell-mediated immune reaction. J Exp Med 141–346, 1975.

52. Wolinsky, JS, et al (The Multiple Sclerosis Study Group): Efficacy and toxicity of cyclosporine in chronic progressive multiple sclerosis: A randomized, double-blinded, placebo-controlled clinical trial. Ann Neurol 27:591–605, 1990.

53. Wraith, DC, McDevitt, HO, Steinman, L, and Acha-Orbea, H: T cell recognition as the target for immune intervention in autoimmune disease. Cell 57:709–715, 1989.

54. Zamvil, SS, Mitchell, DJ, Moore, AC, Kitamura, K, Steinman, L, and Rothbard, JB: T-cell epitope of the autoantigen myelin basic protein that induces encephalomyelitis. Nature 324:258–260, 1986.

Chapter 7

PSYCHIATRIC DISORDERS

Joseph T. Coyle, M.D.

CLINICAL PSYCHOPHARMACOLOGY
NEUROLEPTICS
ANTIDEPRESSANTS
BENZODIAZEPINES

The founders of modern psychiatry, Kraepelin, Meynert, and Freud, emphasized the role that the brain played in the pathophysiology of major psychiatric disorders. Nevertheless, with the growing influence of psychodynamic theory in the 1930s and thereafter, psychologic concepts about the etiology of psychiatric disorders eclipsed biologically based ones in American psychiatry until recent years. The movement of the pendulum back to a more balanced and integrated conceptualization of psychopathology, epitomized by the biopsychosocial paradigm, has been driven to a considerable degree by advances in clinical and basic psychopharmacologic research accomplished during the past two decades.

The discovery of drugs that are efficacious in reducing symptoms, or even eliminating episodes, of several major psychiatric disorders prompted a more careful delineation of diagnostic entities responsive to specific psychotropic drugs and an intense search for the sites of therapeutic action and side effects of these medications. The recent development of recombinant genetic techniques for identifying DNA polymorphisms linked to genes responsible for heritable disorders, as well as the rapid advances in the use of molecular methods to identify genes encoding specific central nervous system (CNS) proteins, herald a new conceptual approach that will provide an exciting, clinically useful, and unifying strategy for understanding the pathobiology of a wide range of psychiatric disorders.[5,6,22] This approach promises to bring together the genetics of vulnerability for psychiatric disorders and characterization of the gene products responsible for these disorders, thereby leading to the development of more incisive methods for designing psychotherapeutic medications. Since current evidence suggests that penetrance of genes responsible for major psychiatric disorders is substantially less than 100%, the genetic advances should aid in identifying environmental factors that transform genetic risk to phenotypic expression.[6] Accordingly, rational approaches to mitigating these environmental factors, such as psychologic interventions, will also benefit from this new approach.

CLINICAL PSYCHOPHARMACOLOGY

Before considering specific classes of psychotropic drugs, it is important to review briefly the strategies that have permitted the identification of drugs with unique and specific psychotherapeutic effects.[4] The dawn of rational psychopharmacology came with the discovery in the early 1950s that chlorpromazine appeared to reduce psychotic symptoms in patients suffering from schizophrenia. Needless to say, this assertion was met with considerable skepticism because of the belief prevalent at the time that schizophrenia was the psychologic consequence of destructive early-life experiences. Thus, in this context, it was necessary to prove that the drug was effective in this disorder, for which no brain pathology had been identified and whose etiology remained obscure. Out of this conundrum evolved the double-blind, placebo-controlled study.[12] Double-blind refers to the fact that neither the patient nor the treating (or evaluating) physician knows whether the patient is receiving an active drug or a placebo. This strategy controls for the possibility that patients might experience reduction in symptoms as a consequence of the nonspecific effects of the therapeutic intervention. "Blindness" of the treating physician prevents conscious or unconscious biases with regard to the therapeutic impact of the drug. In these early studies, symptoms in patients were titrated with drugs, which allowed for the determination of the doses resulting in optimal therapeutic response.

These pioneering studies demonstrated that chlorpromazine significantly reduced the psychotic symptoms of patients suffering from schizophrenia, that it was clearly superior to placebo, and that this was not due to sedating side effects of chlorpromazine, since the sedative/anxiolytic phenobarbital was no more effective than placebo.[4,12,13] With the subsequent development of analogues of chlorpromazine, each was subjected to the same method of clinical analysis, often in comparison with chlorpromazine as the effective standard. These many studies led to the conclusion that certain analogues of chlorpromazine were effective, whereas others were not. In addition, all of the effective drugs were equally effective although they varied more than 100-fold in clinical potency. Finally, while extrapyramidal side effects and sedation were a common occurrence with these agents, these side effects did not correlate with the therapeutic action.

This clinical research strategy—the double-blind, placebo-controlled study—is now the golden standard to which virtually all drugs are subjected. Importantly, the structural activity relationships generated for each class of drugs, a fallout of these clinical studies, has facilitated the search for molecular sites of action of psychotropic drugs, including neuroleptics, antidepressants, and benzodiazepines. This information has permitted the development of correlations between the clinical efficacy and potency of a class of psychotropic medications and their interactions with specific brain parameters. For example, phenothiazines were found to inhibit adenosine triphosphate (ATPase)[1]; however, their ability to do this did not correspond with their clinical potency, suggesting that this action was likely unrelated to their therapeutic effects. In contrast, subsequent studies revealed a compelling correlation between antipsychotic potency and blockade of D-2 dopamine receptors, the likely site of action of neuroleptics.[14,45] The following discussion will rely heavily on such information in defining the mechanisms of action and side effects of commonly used psychotherapeutic drugs.

NEUROLEPTICS

Schizophrenia

Schizophrenia is a particularly malignant, chronic psychiatric disorder that typically has its age of symptomatic onset in late adolescence and young adulthood. While it appears to be equally represented in males and females, the onset of the syndrome often occurs at a somewhat earlier age in males.[34] Transcultural studies indicate that all races and cultures are affected by schizophrenia; its lifetime prevalence is approximately 1%.[36] Nevertheless, because of its chronic nature, schizophrenia accounts for a disproportionate number of users of residential as well as community psychiatric treatment facilities. Schizophrenia exhibits family aggregation, with the morbid risk in first-degree relatives of probands being approximately 10 times greater than that of the general population.[6] The concordance rate of nearly 50% in identical twins, as well as the increased risk for schizophrenia in offspring of schizophrenic parents who were adopted at birth, have provided compelling evidence that genetic factors play an important role in this disorder. Nevertheless, intrauterine viral infections, perinatal insults, and temporal lobe epilepsy (with a left-sided focus) point to environmental or epigenetic causes of schizophrenia.[22]

Table 7–1 lists a summary of the DSM-III-R diagnostic criteria for schizophrenia.[2] A useful way of categorizing the symptoms of this syndrome is to distinguish positive symptoms from the negative ones.[3] Positive symptoms include hallucinations, delusions, agitation, and thought disorder. These symptoms are often the most dramatic and bring the patient to the attention of the physician. The so-called negative symptoms, however, are the more disabling because they persist over time, often becoming more severe, whereas the positive symptoms wax and wane and can become less prominent in the aged schizophrenic. Negative symptoms include social withdrawal, social incompetence, and loss of drive. These negative symptoms appear to correlate with evidence of cortical atrophy and/or ventricular enlargement, as documented by tomographic scans of the brain.[54]

Table 7–1 SCHIZOPHRENIA: DIAGNOSTIC CRITERIA

1. Psychotic symptoms including bizarre delusions, auditory hallucinations, loosened associations, and inappropriate affect
2. Deterioration in the level of functioning
3. No underlying mood disturbance
4. Duration of at least 6 months

Source: Adapted from DSM-III-R.[2]

Most clinical studies suggest that the positive symptoms are most responsive to neuroleptic action, whereas the negative symptoms are minimally responsive or unresponsive.[54] This distinction may be important for several reasons. First, it reifies the evidence that neuroleptics are not a "cure" for schizophrenia; to the contrary, there is now evidence of a growing population of schizophrenics who remain incapacitated in spite of optimal treatment with neuroleptics. Second, this suggests that the site of therapeutic action of neuroleptics represents an ancillary, but not necessarily the causative, defect in schizophrenia.[29] And finally, it directs the physician's attention to the end point of effective symptomatic management of schizophrenics using neuroleptics.

Neuroleptic Site of Action

The propensity for neuroleptics to produce parkinsonian side effects pointed to the dopaminergic system as a potential site of action of these drugs. This connection was strengthened by the demonstration that reserpine, a drug that depletes the brain of biogenic amines by irreversibly inhibiting their vesicular storage process, also exhibits antipsychotic efficacy. Carlsson and Lindquist[10] first proposed that neuroleptics might act by blocking the brain's receptors for dopamine. However, confirmation was delayed for nearly a decade until methods for receptor characterization were developed.

The first dopamine receptor (now designated D-1) was identified because its transduction mechanism is linked to adenylate cyclase. The D-1 receptor could be distinguished from beta receptors due to the low intrinsic activity of epinephrine, high intrinsic activity of dopamine, and insensitivity to propranolol but marked inhibition by phenothiazine neuroleptics.[30] The D-1 recognition site is now known to be intercollated in the neuron membrane and, when activated by dopamine, binds Gs protein that subsequently activates adenylate cyclase on the internal surface of the neuron membrane. Thus, cyclic adenosine monophosphate serves as the intracellular second messenger that accounts for the physiologic effects of activation of this receptor. Curiously, the clinically potent butyrophenone neuroleptics, such as haloperidol, exhibited only weak inhibition of the D-1 receptor, indicating that this receptor was unlikely to mediate the antipsychotic action of neuroleptics.

Using [^{3}H]haloperidol as a ligand, Creese and associates[14] were able to demonstrate a recognition site (D-2) to which it bound with high affinity. Bound [^{3}H]haloperidol was displaced by dopamine and other dopamine receptor agonists. As shown in Figure 7–1, there was a remarkably high correlation between the clinical potency of

neuroleptics, regardless of chemical structure, and their ability to compete at the receptor recognition site labeled by [^{3}H]haloperidol. Current evidence suggests that this D-2 receptor is linked to a potassium channel, which mediates its inhibitory neurophysiologic effects, and also to G_1 protein.[46] Recent studies indicate that the D-1 receptors have approximately a fourfold greater density than D-2 receptors. Both dopamine receptors are differentially expressed on neurons in regions of the brain receiving dopaminergic innervation. There is some suggestion of cooperative as well as antagonistic interactions between the two receptors; however, maximal expression of behaviors mediated by the dopamine system involves activation of both D-1 and D-2 receptors. Recent molecular cloning ex-

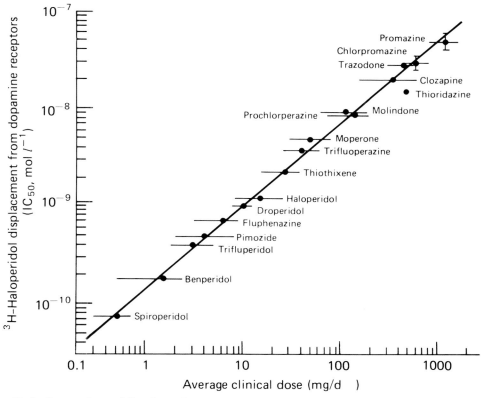

Figure 7–1. Comparison of the clinical potencies of neuroleptic drugs. The drugs have the ability to displace ^{3}H-haloperidol from the D_2 dopamine receptor sites in membranes prepared from bovine caudate nucleus. (From Seeman et al.[45] Reprinted with permission from NATURE vol. 261, pp 717–720. Copyright © 1976 Macmillan Magazines Ltd.)

periments indicate that there is a third dopamine receptor (D-3) that is expressed primarily in limbic areas of the brain.[48] The D-3 receptor has probably been identified previously as a subtype of the D-2 receptor. It is of great interest because it is localized to areas in the brain that are important in emotional control.

Since there is compelling evidence that the mechanism of antipsychotic action of neuroleptics can be ascribed to their ability to block D-2 receptors, the role of these receptors in the pathophysiology of schizophrenia and related psychotic disorders, as well as in neuroleptic-induced neurologic side effects, has been an issue of intense interest. It is generally agreed that blockade of D-2 receptors in the caudate-putamen accounts for extrapyramidal side effects associated with these drugs (see p 211), whereas blockade of D-2 receptors in the frontal cortex, hippocampus, and limbic system may account for their antipsychotic effects. An intriguing hypothesis is that dysregulation of dopamine receptors may be the proximate cause of the positive symptoms of schizophrenia. In support of this hypothesis, several postmortem studies have revealed an increase in the number of D-2 receptors in the forebrain in schizophrenics.[46] Furthermore, a recent study, exploiting positron emission tomography (PET), has revealed a considerable increase in density of the D-2 receptor in the caudate-putamen of untreated schizophrenics,[56] although this finding has been contested.[19] The discovery of the D-3 receptor opens new areas of research into the pathogenesis and treatment of schizophrenia.[48]

Clinical Use of Neuroleptics

The primary indication for neuroleptic treatment is the management of the positive symptoms of schizophrenia. In addition, neuroleptics can be useful in the symptomatic management of psychotic symptoms that occur in mania and in major depressive disorders, although neuroleptics are usually prescribed in combination with a more specific pharmacologic intervention for these latter disorders, such as lithium for mania and antidepressants for major depressive disorder. In the case of schizophrenia, neuroleptics are used in two contexts: the acute management of a psychotic episode as a prophylaxis to prevent recurrence of, or at least attenuate, positive symptoms of the disorder. These two strategies need to be considered separately.[13]

The therapeutic potency of neuroleptics has been computed against the standard, chlorpromazine. For ease of discussion, dosages will be presented in terms of chlorpromazine equivalents (Table 7–2). This does not imply, however, that chlorpromazine is the recommended drug; to the contrary, the more potent neuroleptics are generally preferred because of fewer associated side effects such as sedation and orthostatic hypotension. The goal of management of an acute psychotic episode is to reduce the psychotic symptoms rapidly with minimal side effects. Typically, the

Table 7–2 COMPARATIVE POTENCY OF NEUROLEPTICS

Neuroleptic	Dose Equivalent (mg)*
Phenothiazine	
Chlorpromazine	100
Thioridazine	100
Perphenazine	10
Trifluoperazine	5
Fluphenazine	2
Thioxanthines	
Chlorprothixene	100
Thiothixene	3
Butyrephenone	
Haloperidol	2
Indolone	
Molindone	10
Dibenzoxazepine	
Loxapine	15

*Values are presented in terms of milligrams of orally administered drug equivalent to 100 mg of chlorpromazine.

acutely psychotic adult patient would be started on 200 to 500 mg of chlorpromazine equivalents, administered in divided doses by mouth. The dose would then be increased in approximately 100- to 200-mg increments every few days, titrating the symptom response against dose. The time course and absolute dose required for resolution of symptoms in the acutely psychotic schizophrenic varies among individuals and may range from 800 mg to more than 2000 mg of chlorpromazine equivalents per day. Improvement in overall behavior, such as decreased agitation and seclusiveness and increased attention to activities of daily living, heralds resolution of the psychotic episode. Reduction of the intrapsychic symptoms, such as delusions and auditory hallucinations, often lags behind the behavioral improvement, although the patient is apparently less preoccupied with the psychotic experiences. As the acute psychotic episode resolves, many patients become more sensitive to the sedating side effects of neuroleptics. At this point, dosage reduction may be considered, which should proceed slowly and incrementally with careful monitoring for recurrence or exacerbation of psychotic symptoms.

Maintenance or prophylactic treatment with neuroleptics should be restricted to patients for whom there is clear evidence that the disorder is chronic, because of the risk for developing tardive dyskinesia with long-term neuroleptic treatment. The goal of prophylactic treatment is to prescribe the minimal amount of neuroleptic that effectively controls symptoms. Typically, the daily dose ranges between 200 to 500 mg of chlorpromazine equivalents, although some patients may require substantially higher doses. Dosage needs may fluctuate over time, depending upon life stresses, which can exacerbate symptoms. In fact, recent studies indicate that certain forms of family therapy and psychologic interventions that alleviate emotional stress for the schizophrenic patient may significantly reduce maintenance neuroleptic

requirements.[18,26] Other studies suggest that selected schizophrenic patients, when closely monitored, can tolerate periods without neuroleptics, which reduces lifetime neuroleptic exposure.

Maintenance treatment with neuroleptics is often complicated by lack of patient compliance because of apathy, suspiciousness, or difficulty in comprehending the treatment regimen. When compliance is a significant problem, long-acting neuroleptics (decanoate esters of the potent neuroleptics fluphenazine or haloperidol) can be administered by intramuscular injection once every 2 to 4 weeks.[17] Thus, the treating physician can be confident that the patient is receiving steady blood levels of neuroleptic as long as he or she returns for periodic treatment. Most studies indicate that this approach reduces the relapse rate in patients suffering from chronic schizophrenia. The half-life for relapse of schizophrenic patients who have placebo substituted for neuroleptic is approximately 6 months, whereas the half-life for those receiving neuroleptic is three to five times longer.

Acute Neuroleptic Side Effects

The same D-2 receptor that appears to account for the antipsychotic effects of neuroleptics also mediates the action of dopamine in the basal ganglia and in the pituitary. Thus, neurologic and neuroendocrine side effects are a frequent and predictable complication of neuroleptic treatment. Clinicians are paying increasing attention to these side effects because (1) they are a major source of patient reluctance to comply with treatment,[53] (2) they can be stigmatizing and thereby interfere with reintegration of patients into their social setting, and (3) they can, on occasion, have medically serious, if not fatal, consequences.

The three most common acute neurologic side effects associated with neuroleptic treatment are parkinsonian symptoms, dystonic reactions, and akathisia.[13] Parkinsonian symptoms include tremor, bradykinesia, and rigidity as well as the associated signs of masked facies, stooped posture, and drooling. The prevalence of parkinsonian side effects increases with age. Dystonic reactions typically present as episodic or persistent cramping of muscles, especially near the midline, and include oculogyric crisis, opisthotonos, torticollis, and pharyngeal/lingual spasm. Notably, dystonic symptoms can wax and wane and may transiently disappear when the patient is stressed or distracted. Their bizarre appearance and variability often lead to the misimpression that they are "hysterical" in nature because of the underlying psychiatric disorder. Severe forms of dystonic posturing coupled with akinesia may be misdiagnosed as catatonia. Dystonic reactions occur more frequently in younger patients.

Akathisia represents an inner sense of restlessness that may be manifest in a mild form as fidgetiness, and in severe forms, as ceaseless agitation. Unfortunately, akathisia may be misinterpreted as recrudescence of the psychosis, prompting larger doses of neuroleptics, thereby exacerbating the symptoms. Many patients can distinguish the peripheral manifestations of akathisia from the psychic symptoms of their underlying disorder. The safest avenue is to assume that any striking motoric symptoms in a patient receiving neuroleptics represent a drug side effect and are not simply a manifestation of the underlying psychopathology.

Considerable evidence indicates that the striatal dopaminergic afferents exert a tonic inhibitory influence mediated by D-2 receptors over striatal neurons, especially the cholinergic interneurons. Accordingly, blockade of D-2 receptors results in a disinhibition of striatal cholinergic neurons, thereby causing an excessive stimulation of their postsynaptic muscarinic receptors. Consistent with this synaptic relationship, the motoric consequences of

D-2 receptor blockade can be mimicked to a certain extent in experimental animals by administration of centrally active muscarinic acetylcholine-receptor agonists. Drugs that block muscarinic cholinergic receptors have been used effectively since the days of Charcot to treat the extrapyramidal symptoms induced by impaired dopaminergic function. These classic antiparkinsonian, anticholinergic medications are available in a number of different structures, including tropines, phenothiazines, and even antihistamine structures, although it is now clear that their ability to block M-1 muscarinic receptors correlates highly with their efficacy in treating extrapyramidal side effects.

Nevertheless, the ability of antiparkinsonian, anticholinergic drugs to reverse the neurologic side effects of neuroleptics is not uniform. Dystonic reactions and rigidity appear to be the most responsive, whereas bradykinesia, and especially akathisia, are much less responsive. Recent studies have disclosed a compartmentalization of synaptic circuitry of the afferent and intrinsic neurons within the caudate-putamen, in which a cholinergic-rich matrix surrounds patches ("striasomes") that are relatively deficient in cholinergic innervation. Whereas the matrix appears to be preferentially innervated by motor-sensory afferents, the striasomes receive input primarily from frontal-limbic areas.[23] This segregation of striatal circuitry may contribute to differences in the responsiveness of the neuroleptic-induced extrapyramidal side effects to anticholinergic drugs.

Tardive Dyskinesia

A potentially irreversible neurologic complication of long-term neuroleptic treatment is tardive dyskinesia.[29] This disorder is characterized by pulsive movements of the tongue, facial grimacing, and vacuous chewing in its mild form, but can proceed to choreoathetotic movements of the extremities and lordotic posture. The prevalence of this disorder among neuroleptic-treated patients varies from 2% to 5% in outpatient programs to as high as 40% among chronically institutionalized patients. The true prevalence of this side effect may be underestimated because neuroleptic administration can suppress the symptoms. Risk factors for tardive dyskinesia include total dose exposure, age, preexisting organic brain disorder, female sex, and underlying affective disorder.

The etiology of this side effect remains obscure. Interestingly, there are reports of similar movement disorders in chronic schizophrenic patients prior to the introduction of neuroleptics, although the prevalence appears to be much higher now. Chronic pharmacologic blockade of neurotransmitter receptors results in up-regulation and the development of supersensitivity. This mechanism has been proposed as the cause of tardive dyskinesia, with the chronic blockade of the dopamine D-2 receptor resulting in the development of irreversible supersensitivity.[11] This hypothesis is consistent with the clinical observations that reduction in neuroleptic dose often exacerbates and increase of dose attenuates symptoms, and that anticholinergic drugs generally increase symptoms. However, irreversible up-regulation of D-2 receptors has not been observed in experimental animals chronically administered neuroleptics, and postmortem studies have not demonstrated differences in the density of D-2 receptors in the caudate-putamen of neuroleptic-treated patients with or without tardive dyskinesia. Recent findings in nonhuman primates suggest an alternative mechanism in which tardive dyskinesia is associated with a loss of striato-pallidal-nigral GABAergic (gamma-amino-butyric acid) projections analogous to Huntington's disease.[24]

Consistent with the complex and diverse structures of neuroleptics, individual neuroleptics cause a variety of other neurologic, autonomic, and endocrine side effects. These reflect ancil-

Table 7–3 SIDE EFFECTS OF NEUROLEPTICS

Neurologic
  Acute
    Parkinsonism
    Dystonic reactions
    Akathisia
    Dyskinesia

  Delayed
    Tardive dyskinesia
  Idiosyncratic
    Neuroleptic malignant syndrome

Autonomic
  Orthostatic hypotension
  Blurred vision
  Impotence

Endocrine
  Galactorrhea
  Hyperprolactinemia
  Suppression of growth hormone

lary receptor interactions of the drugs, including blockade of muscarinic, alpha-adrenergic, and histamine receptors. (See Table 7–3 for a partial list of these side effects.)

Neuroleptic Malignant Syndrome

An uncommon, but by no means rare, complication of neuroleptic treatment of particular relevance to neurologists is the neuroleptic malignant syndrome (NMS).[32] Although fewer than 50 case reports describing the syndrome appeared in the world literature during the first 20 years of neuroleptic usage, recent studies suggest that symptomatic manifestations of NMS may affect approximately 1% of patients treated with neuroleptics.[40] This apparent increase in prevalence may reflect greater diagnostic sensitivity as well as more aggressive use of high-potency neuroleptics. Neurologists should be especially sensitive to this complication because they are likely to be consulted in the evaluation of patients presenting with the cardinal symptoms of NMS: profound rigidity, fever of unknown origin, delirium, and rhabdomyolysis. Furthermore, with the increasing use of neuroleptics to treat purely neurologic disorders and evidence that this syndrome may be precipitated by abrupt withdrawal of antiparkinsonian agents in patients with Parkinson's syndrome, it is now evident that NMS is a complication not unique to psychiatric patients.

While the debate remains about the pathophysiology of NMS, the most parsimonious explanation is that it represents a severe extrapyramidal syndrome resulting from insufficient stimulation of dopamine receptors, typically precipitated by treatment with high-potency neuroleptics. While it shares many features with malignant hyperthermia, most studies suggest that patients suffering from NMS do not exhibit the same muscular metabolic defect that is responsible for malignant hyperthermia. Certain risk factors such as extreme heat, dehydration, and acute increase in neuroleptic dosage may predispose for development of NMS. Such interactions best explain the observation that many patients who have developed NMS do not exhibit a recurrence of symptoms when subsequently challenged with the offending neuroleptic.

The profound rigidity, which on occasion may resemble catatonic waxy flexibility, results in the generation of excessive heat through adenosine triphosphate (ATP) hydrolysis in the striate muscles, causing rhabdomyolysis. Thus, the hyperthermia does not appear to be a consequence of central temperature dyscontrol per se, as the affected patients are often quite diaphoretic. In addition, dystonia of the oral-pharyngeal region interferes with efficient clearance of secretions, which can cause complicating aspiration pneumonia. Hyperthermia and dehydration due to diaphoresis and impaired oral intake contribute to cardiovascular instability; rhabdomyolysis can cause renal damage. A peculiar and poorly understood feature of the disorder is that symptoms can persist for days to weeks after the last administration of neuroleptics. The fatality rate has been estimated to be 20%.

The medically acute and uncommon occurrence of NMS has precluded carefully controlled studies of its management.[25] Nevertheless, review of published reports suggests that the following treatment principles may be reasonable. First, anticholinergic antiparkinsonian drugs should be avoided because they interfere with diaphoresis and thereby exacerbate the hyperthermia. Rather, dantrolene, a drug that directly interferes with myosin-induced ATP hydrolysis and, therefore, heat production, appears to be an effective agent for rapidly reducing the hyperthermia and reversing the rhabdomyolysis. However, it should be remembered that some patients may have developed complicating infections due to aspiration, which may cause fever for other reasons. Nevertheless, dantrolene is ineffective in treating the rigidity, delirium, and oral dystonias. Several reports suggest that bromocriptine, administered in increasing doses to titrate patients' symptoms, is most effective for reversing these latter symptoms. While some have suggested that bromocriptine is the primary drug of choice, the delay in attaining the optimal dose may result in unnecessary persistence of hyperthermia and rhabdomyolysis, which could be rapidly controlled with dantrolene. Finally, once the patient has responded to bromocriptine treatment, the dose should be tapered gradually and cautiously, with attention paid to possible recurrence of the NMS symptoms.

Other Uses of Neuroleptics

While neuroleptics are generally considered in the context of their antipsychotic effects, they actually have broader application in neurology in the treatment of a variety of disorders involving presumptive excessive stimulation of D-2 receptors. Nevertheless, it should be emphasized at the outset that in spite of their designation as "major tranquilizers," they should not be prescribed as sedatives or anxiolytics because more effective drugs with fewer untoward side effects (such as the benzodiazepines) are available. However, low doses of high-potency neuroleptics such as haloperidol and pimozide have proved useful in reducing tics in Tourette's syndrome, the dyskinetic movements in Huntington's disease, and hemiballismus.

ANTIDEPRESSANTS

Depression

Major depressive disorder (MDD) is the most common serious psychiatric disorder. Epidemiologic studies indicate that up to 15% of the population will experience an episode of MDD during their lifetime. In addition, 1% of the population suffers from manic depressive illness, in which episodes of major depression interspersed with episodes of mania or hypomania occur periodically. Because of the protean symptoms of a major depressive disorder, in which depressed mood is only one of the manifestations, the diagnosis of MDD is regrettably often missed by primary physicians, and even psychiatrists. Of importance to neurologists is that MDD may be an accompanying complication of brain damage, especially left-sided strokes; may coexist in Parkinson's syndrome, Alzheimer's disease, and multiple sclerosis; and can be precipitated by a variety of drugs used to treat cardiovascular disorders. Notably, untreated MDD presents a significant risk for suicide, thereby representing a potentially fatal psychiatric disorder.

The accurate diagnosis of MDD has been greatly assisted by the development of validated diagnostic criteria with the explicit inclusion and exclusion items as described in Table 7−4. A less severe form of depression, but one that may persist for longer periods of time than MDD, is dysthymia. In some patients, a rather persistent dysthymic disorder is punctuated by episodes of MDD.

Three distinct drug groups play an important role in the management of affective disorders: tricyclic antidepressants (TCA) and their newer analogues, monoamine oxidase (MAO) inhibitors, and lithium. While the molecular sites of action of each of these three classes are quite distinct, there is now compelling evidence that they all affect central aminergic neurotransmission. The findings that drugs that interfere with central aminergic neurotransmission can precipitate depression, that structural damage to the left frontal cortical aminergic afferents causes a depressive syndrome, and that biogenic amine metabolism and neuroendocrine function are often altered in MDD suggest that disruption in cortical aminergic neurotransmission is involved in the pathophysiology of MDD.

Table 7−4 MAJOR DEPRESSIVE DISORDER: DIAGNOSTIC CRITERIA

1. Five of the following symptoms:
   a. Depressed mood
   b. Anhedonia
   c. Weight change
   d. Sleep disorder
   e. Psychomotor agitation or retardation
   f. Loss of energy
   g. Feelings of worthlessness
   h. Impaired concentration
   i. Suicidal thinking
2. Not a response to grief or an organic cause
3. Not associated with schizophrenia

Source: Adapted from DSM-III-R.[2]

Tricyclic Antidepressants

The primary mechanism for inactivation of biogenic amine neurotransmitters is their removal from the synaptic cleft by transport back into the presynaptic terminal.[21] These transport processes, which are driven by the sodium gradient maintained across the neuron membrane, are distinct for the given neurotransmitter released by the neuron, for example, dopamine, norepinephrine, and serotonin. More than a quarter of a century ago, Axelrod demonstrated that TCA inhibited the uptake process for norepinephrine, thereby prolonging the action of the neurotransmitter in the synaptic cleft. Subsequent studies have fleshed out these original observations and have demonstrated that tertiary amine TCAs tend to be potent inhibitors of the serotonin transport process, whereas secondary amine TCAs are more effective as inhibitors of the norepinephrine transport process. Neither group demonstrates much potency for the dopamine carrier, although some experimental antidepressants, known to be clinically effective, do inhibit dopamine transport.

The marked potency of the TCA in inhibiting either the norepinephrine or serotonin transport processes have recommended them as ligands to label these carriers.[4,21] Indeed, [3H]desimethylimipramine binds in a reversible, saturable, and high-affinity manner to a site closely linked to the norepinephrine carrier. Similarly, [3H]imipramine, a potent inhibitor of the serotonin transport process, is an effective radioligand that labels a site on the serotonin carrier. Whether these agents label putative "antidepressant receptors" remains moot; nevertheless, the [3H]TCAs proved to be clinically useful presynaptic probes for the noradrenergic and serotonergic systems. For example, several reports describe significant reductions in the specific binding of [3H]imipramine in the cerebral cortex of individuals who died from suicide and in platelets in individuals suffering from MDD.

The TCAs interact with a number of different neurotransmitter receptors, which contribute to the spectrum of their side effects (Table 7-5). As a group, these drugs are relatively potent antagonists of muscarinic acetylcho-

line receptors. Blockade of these receptors accounts for important peripheral parasympathetic side effects. To variable degrees, TCAs also block alpha-1 adrenergic receptors, which accounts for their propensity to cause orthostatic hypotension. Histamine-1 receptor blockade appears to correlate with the sedating side effects of the drugs. Finally, as a group, the TCAs exhibit a quinidinelike membrane-stabilizing effect in the heart that substantially alters cardiac conduction at blood levels in excess of 500 ng/mL. Indeed, these cardiotoxic effects of TCAs make them the most common cause of fatal overdose for psychotropic medications.

A major advance in the rational use of the TCA has been the definition of serum values associated with therapeutic response. Pharmacokinetic studies have revealed considerable variation in the steady-state serum levels attained among adults given the same dosage of TCA. Optimal symptomatic response in MDD generally occurs with serum levels in excess of 50 ng/mL of the parent TCA and active metabolites. With nortriptyline, serum levels in excess of 180 ng/mL interfere with therapeutic response. In the case of the other TCA, side effects generally become counterproductive with serum levels much in excess of 250 ng/mL, effectively defining a therapeutic "window." Accordingly, clinicians are increasingly relying upon serum TCA measurements to optimize treatment, especially for patients who exhibit poor therapeutic response on standard doses.[51]

Treatment response to TCA is generally gradual in onset, even at optimal

Table 7-5 SIDE EFFECTS OF TRICYCLIC ANTIDEPRESSANTS

Receptor	Symptoms	Affinity
Muscarinic	Dry mouth, constipation, tachycardia, urinary retention	A > Dx > P > I > N > Des
Alpha-1	Orthostatic hypotension	Dx = A > I > N > Des > P
Histamine-1	Sedation	Dx > A > I > N > P > Des

Key: A = amitriptyline; N = nortriptyline; I = imipramine; Des = desipramine; Dx = doxepin; P = protriptyline.

serum levels, taking place during 3 to 6 weeks.[4] Vegetative symptoms often exhibit the earliest change, with improvement in appetite, sleep pattern, and activity preceding changes in mood and the cognitive symptoms. For this reason, the patient may be a poor barometer of response, as the persistent cognitive symptoms may prevent his or her appreciation of these early improvements. In fact, this early period of partial response may be most hazardous for the suicidal patient as it can activate the patient, thereby facilitating suicidal actions.

MAO Inhibitors

The MAO inhibitors were the first type of effective antidepressants developed. Although early controlled studies indicated that they were clearly more effective than placebo in treating depression, their use was eclipsed by the TCA because of the perceived greater efficacy of the latter drugs, as well as the risk for hypertensive crisis associated with MAO inhibitors. Nevertheless, during the past decade, there has been a resurgence of interest in the clinical use of MAO inhibitors, since they appear to be as effective as TCA when given in proper doses. Notably, some patients appear to be uniquely responsive to MAO inhibitors.[42] The hypertensive side effect can be avoided through judicious dietary proscriptions.[43]

The two commonly prescribed MAO inhibitors in the United Sates are phenelzine and tranylcypromine. They act as suicide substrate inhibitors, thereby irreversibly inhibiting the enzyme. In other words, as the enzyme catabolizes the drug, it is converted to a highly reactive intermediate that covalently binds to the active site of MAO. Thus, recovery of MAO activity after discontinuing the drug requires the synthesis of new enzyme molecules.

Monoamine oxidase resides on the outer surface of the mitochondrion and plays a critical role in catabolyzing free or unprotected catecholamines and se-rotonin within the nerve terminal. Thus, inhibition of MAO results in increased levels of intraneuron catecholamines and serotonin and augmented release of these neurotransmitters upon nerve terminal depolarization. Two isozymes of MAO have been identified: MAO_A and MAO_B, which are encoded by different genes. MAO_A acts preferentially upon norepinephrine and serotonin, whereas MAO_B acts more broadly on phenethylamines. Consistent with their localization on mitochondria, these two enzymes are widely but unevenly distributed throughout the tissues of the body and the brain.[55]

Monoamine oxidase serves an important role in the gut and in the liver, as a catabolic barrier to phenethylamines in food products. The content of phenethylamines is particularly high in aged foods, wherein protein undergoes proteolysis and nonenzymatic decarboxylation of phenylalanine, tryosine, and tryptophan to generate phenethylamine, tryamine, and tryptamine, respectively. Under normal circumstances, these substances are efficiently deaminated by MAO in the gut and liver. Patients receiving MAO inhibitors have this enzymatic barrier inactivated; thus, dietary amines gain ready access to the general circulation, where they exert amphetaminelike action, acutely releasing norepinephrine from peripheral sympathetics, thereby increasing both blood pressure and heart rate.[43]

Recent studies indicate at MAO inhibitors are as effective in treating MDD as TCAs when used in appropriate doses. Like the TCA, the therapeutic response to treatment with MAO inhibitors is generally delayed in onset with improvement occurring during a several-week period. Studies with phenelzine indicate that optimal clinical effects are observed with doses in excess of 60 mg/d, which results in inhibition of platelet MAO activity by greater than 80%. These comparative studies also suggest that phenelzine has greater anxiolytic effects than TCAs. For this reason, MAO inhibitors may be the drug of choice in treating certain atypical forms of depression, which are characterized by prominent anxiety, phobias, and "neurotic" symptoms. Quitkin and his colleagues[42] have also delineated a subgroup of MAO inhibitor–responsive, depressed individuals that have been designated "hystoroid dysphorics," who are characterized by unusual sensitivity to rejection, mood lability, weight fluctuations, and craving for chocolate.

Antidepressants and Panic Disorder

Panic disorder is a relatively common and rather chronic disorder that can be quite socially disabling, but is responsive to pharmacologic management. The disorder is characterized by abrupt episodes of sympathetic discharge and hyperventilation resulting in tachycardia, palpitations, and other autonomic symptoms that cause feelings of panic, derealization, and impending doom in affected individuals. These dramatic episodes may bring the patient to the attention of neurologists because of the patient's concern that an undiagnosed medical condition is causing the symptoms. The patients often develop anticipatory anxiety, fear the recurrence of the symptoms, and link the episode to the particular circumstances when they experienced panic attacks, such as driving an automobile, speaking in public, or walking in open spaces. As a consequence, the affected individual will increasingly avoid such circumstances and may ultimately become housebound.

While panic disorder is clearly distinguishable from the affective disorders, there nevertheless appears to be some pathophysiologic relationship, as panic disorder and affective disorder have been found to aggregate in families. In this regard, it is interesting to note that the most effective medications for treating panic disorder are the TCAs and the MAO inhibitors.[31] In contrast, while benzodiazepines, the most commonly prescribed anxiolytics, may assist in allaying anticipatory anxiety, they are not very effective in preventing the panic attacks themselves, with the possible exception of alprazolam and clonazepam.[47,49] However, increasing concern about the high risk for dependency and the need for escalating doses of alprazolam has tempered interest in its use as a primary treatment of panic disorder.[20]

Lithium

Lithium is a unique psychotropic medication because it is not an organic compound but rather an inorganic salt. The serendipitous discovery of the psychotropic properties of lithium salt by Cade[9] resulted from his search for an agent that might counteract the presumed endogenous toxin responsible for mania in manic depressive illness (MDI) (Table 7–6). He observed that lithium salt had a calming influence on guinea pigs and, as a result, examined its efficacy in patients suffering from mania. His preliminary description of the antimanic properties of lithium salt, however, did not lead to wide usage of the agent for nearly 20 years. Most physicians were chary of its toxic properties, since lithium salts caused a number of deaths in the 1930s, when it had been used as a salt substitute in pa-

Table 7–6 MANIC SYNDROME: DIAGNOSTIC CRITERIA

1. A distinct period of abnormally and persistently elevated, expansive, or irritable mood
2. At least three symptoms:
    a. Grandiosity
    b. Decreased sleep
    c. Pressured speech
    d. Racing thoughts
    e. Distractibility
    f. Agitation
    g. Improvident or reckless behavior
3. Impairment in functioning
4. Mood-congruent hallucinations or delusions
5. Absence of schizohrenia or organic cause

Source: Adapted from DSM-III-R.[2]

tients suffering from hypertension. In the early 60s, however, the Danish psychiatrist Schou[44] amassed compelling longitudinal clinical data demonstrating that treatment with lithium salt virtually eliminated episodes of mania and depression in individuals suffering from MDI. Subsequent studies demonstrated that approximately 80% of patients suffering from MDI exhibit a positive response to treatment with lithium salt, with a reduction in both the frequency and severity of affective episodes.

In the clinical setting, lithium is used for the acute treatment of mania but more importantly as prophylaxes in patients with MDI to eliminate or reduce the incidence and severity of subsequent episodes of depression and mania.[41] Thus, lithium must be viewed not simply as an "antimanic" drug but rather as a mood-stabilizing agent, a contention supported by studies on its dampening effects on diurnal mood variation in asymptomatic individuals with MDI.

While lithium is the drug of choice in the treatment of mania, it is rarely used alone because of the delayed onset of therapeutic action. Typically, high-potency neuroleptics are administered symptomatically to treat the agitation and psychotic features of mania until the lithium becomes effective, which may require at least 1 week. It should be noted that concurrent lithium administration may exacerbate the extrapyramidal side effects of neuroleptics. The therapeutic serum level for lithium in acute manic episodes ranges from 1.0 to 1.5 mEq/L. For preventive therapy after the episode has resolved, serum levels should be maintained in the range of 0.6 to 1.0 mEq/L, although optimal values vary among individuals.

The molecular mechanisms responsible for the therapeutic effects of lithium remain obscure. While lithium ion enters neurons through sodium and potassium channels, it is not an efficient substrate for the sodium potassium ATPase; as a consequence, it accumulates intraneuronally where it affects the ex-

citability of neurons. Until recently, it has been difficult to relate these general electrophysiologic properties of lithium to its more specific effects on affective disorders. However, synaptic neurochemical and electrophysiologic studies have provided evidence that lithium ions enhance serotonergic neuron transmission, a system that has been implicated in the pathophysiology of affective disorders.[8] These observations led to the proposal[16] that the addition of lithium may result in an improved response in patients treated with TCAs. In fact, this strategy, known as "lithium augmentation," has proved to be effective in many patients suffering from MDD, who incompletely respond to TCA treatment.

A third possible mechanism of therapeutic action of lithium concerns its ability to inhibit myo-inositol-1-phosphatase, a critical enzyme in the metabolic pathway involved in phosphoinositide turnover.[7] This enzyme is rather specifically sensitive to the lithium ion at intracellular concentrations that are relevant to clinical situations. The phosphatidylinositol (PI) pathway is part of a system involved in postreceptor-signal transduction, especially those systems activated by protein kinases and responsive to calcium and diacylglycerol. The PI system is linked to responses mediated by acetylcholine muscarinic, alpha-adrenergic, serotonin, and glutamate receptor responses. Nevertheless, the association between this action and the mood-stabilizing effects of lithium salts remains unclear.

SIDE EFFECTS

The side effects of lithium (Table 7–7) can be divided into two major categories: those associated with therapeutic levels and those resulting from toxic levels of the drug. With the initiation of treatment with lithium salts, many patients experience nausea and diarrhea. This problem seems to correspond to changing blood levels of lithium and resolves when steady-state levels are

Table 7–7 SIDE EFFECTS OF LITHIUM

Within therapeutic range (≤1.5 mEq/L)
  Nausea, vomiting, diarrhea (initial)
  Vasopressin-insensitive diabetes insipidus
    (inability to concentrate urine)
  Goiter
  Intentional tremor
Above therapeutic range (≥1.5 mEq/L)
  Gross tremor, ataxia, myoclonus, confusion,
    obtundation, coma

achieved. Since lithium interferes with receptor–adenylate-cyclase coupling, it exhibits high propensity for causing vasopressin-insensitive diabetes insipidus.[33] The severity of this problem varies among patients and can be progressive. The inability to concentrate urine and the large volume of urine output can be hazardous in situations in which the availability of water is limited. Interference with thyroid-stimulating hormone receptor–mediated responses is associated with the development of nontoxic goiter in some patients.[35] Most patients on therapeutic levels of lithium exhibit a modest intentional tremor.

Blood levels of lithium in excess of 1.5 mEq/L are associated with progressive impairment of neurologic functions. It is important to keep in mind that the ratio between therapeutic and toxic doses of lithium salts is relatively narrow. Furthermore, abrupt reduction in fluid intake, restriction of sodium intake, or the addition of thiazide diuretics or analgetics that act as prostaglandin-synthesis inhibitors can produce electrolyte disturbances and cause lithium retention, resulting in toxicity in the absence of a change in the dose of lithium salts.[28]

BENZODIAZEPINES

While benzodiazepines are among the frequently prescribed psychotropic medications, their use for purely psychiatric indications is rather limited. Benzodiazepines are commonly used to reduce anxiety, which may be related to situational life stress or can arise out of neurotic conflicts. There is considerable variation among individuals with regard to their basal level of anxiety (trait anxiety) as well as their ability to tolerate anxiety-provoking circumstances (state anxiety). The benzodiazepines have supplanted previously used anxiolytics such as the barbiturates and glutethimide, which have a poor toxic-to-therapeutic ratio and a greater liability for physical dependence. A substantial number of benzodiazepines are available for prescription use, which differ with regard to potency, metabolic characteristics, and half-lives, but which all appear to act through a common mechanism.

Receptor-ligand binding techniques,[38] patch-clamping electrophysiologic studies, immunochemical studies,[15] and recent molecular biologic strategies[5] have clarified the mechanism of action of the benzodiazepines and related sedative/anticonvulsants of the barbiturate class. The GABA receptor is a macromolecular complex consisting of a binding site for GABA, an ionophore for chloride, and a modulatory site to which benzodiazepines bind.[50] In ligand-binding analyses, GABA enhances the affinity of benzodiazepines to their receptor recognition site, thereby confirming an allosteric interaction between the two sites within the macromolecular receptor complex. Conversely, patch-clamping studies, in which the physiologic characteristics of individual GABA receptors can be monitored, demonstrate that benzodiazepines enhance the potency of GABA with regard to chloride fluxes through the ionophore. In contrast, the barbiturates directly increase the chloride flux in the absence of receptor agonists.[38] Furthermore, barbiturates appear to interact with a more broadly distributed population of chloride ionophores linked to inhibitory receptors. Consistent with this observation, in vitro receptor autoradiographic studies have revealed a more restricted distribution of benzodiazepine receptors than GABA receptors, suggesting that the former sites are found on a subpopulation of GABA inhibitory receptors.[52] Notably, the regions of highest benzodiazepine receptor density include the cerebral cortex, hippocampus, and limbic system, whereas the density in midbrain and brainstem structures is quite low.

While the molecular sites of action of benzodiazepines in the CNS have been well characterized, the neuron circuits that mediate the various therapeutic effects remain less clearly defined. It is presumed that activation of cortical receptors contributes to the sedating effects of benzodiazepines and their anticonvulsant action. Intracerebral injection studies suggest that the amygdala may play a key role in the anxiolytic action. Microinjection of benzodiazepines in this region results in striking anxiolytic effects in various animal paradigms, associated with decreased turnover of norepinephrine and decreased release of corticotropin releasing factor, a neuropeptide system with activity that is highly correlated with anxiety. Finally, the benzodiazepine receptors associated with GABA receptors in the spinal cord mediate the muscle-relaxant effects of these drugs.

While overdoses of benzodiazepines alone are associated with a low risk of respiratory depression and death, when benzodiazepines are taken in combination with ethanol or barbiturates, the toxic effects of the latter agents can be markedly potentiated. The positive interactions between barbiturates, which act at the chloride ionophore, and benzodiazepines can be readily understood by their cooperative molecular sites of action. Recent studies suggest that an important action of ethanol involves an enhancement of GABAergic neurotransmission at the receptor level. Again, the mechanisms of these positive interactions are apparent.

From a pharmacologic perspective, benzodiazepines can be viewed as having "agonist" properties. Benzodiazepine analogues have been synthesized that exhibit specific antagonistic properties and thereby reverse the action of benzodiazepines.[27] These agents, although currently not available in the United States, have been used in clinical situations to reverse the effects of benzodiazepine overdose. As pure antagonists, they have negligible effects in the absence of a benzodiazepine receptor agonist. Another class of benzodiazepine compounds have been synthesized that are "inverse agonists." In this case, they produce neurophysiologic and behavioral effects that are the opposite of benzodiazepines in the sense that they interfere with GABAergic neurotransmission. On a behavioral level, they increase arousal, have proconvulsant actions, and have been reported to reverse the acute effects of ethanol.

In spite of the clinical superiority of benzodiazepines over existing sedatives/anxiolytics, medical experience dictates cautious use of them to treat anxiety symptoms in patients. First, while they can be quite helpful in reducing stress-related anxiety in patients, the chronically anxious patient is at risk for dependency due to prolonged use. Furthermore, while reductions of severe anxiety may be quite helpful, especially in the context of acutely stressful situations, when the anxiety is recurrent and appears to be related to neurotic conflicts, the persistent use of benzodiazepines may deter the patient from dealing more directly with these conflicts through psychologic treatment. Of course, such anxiety should be distinguished from panic disorder, which is neither particularly responsive to benzodiazepines nor clearly related to psychologic conflicts. Second, it is now clear that chronic administration of benzodiazepines can result in both psychologic and physiologic dependence. In the case of the longer-acting benzodiazepines, acute withdrawal can result in delayed recurrence of anxiety symptoms, jitteriness, insomnia, and on occasion, seizures. Recent studies suggest that the short-acting benzodiazepines such as alprazolam, when administered continuously, are associated with a marked propensity for seizures and profound anxiety symptoms upon acute withdrawal.[37] Withdrawal from substantial doses of alprazolam (greater than 6 mg/d) may require several weeks to months and can be facilitated by coadministration of carbamazepine or substitution of a long-acting benzodiazepine.

CONCLUSION

Fundamental neuropsychopharmacologic research carried out during the past decade has clarified the molecular sites of action of the major classes of psychotropic medications. These advances have contributed substantively to our understanding of their mechanisms of action at the neuron and subcellular level, and of many of their centrally mediated side effects. Thus, with an increased appreciation of pharmacodynamics as well, these agents can be used in a much more rational and specific fashion.

Identification of the sites of action of the psychotropic medications and the appreciation of their disorder-specific therapeutic effects have led to the hypothesis that disruption in the normal function of the processes related to these sites of action might be etiologically responsible for the disorders. Some studies have lent credence to this belief, such as the demonstration of an elevation in the number of dopamine D-2 receptors in the caudate and putamen in the brains of schizophrenic patients and the reduction in [^{3}H]imipramine-binding sites in the cerebral cortex of individuals who have committed suicide.

With the exploitation of molecular approaches to clone and map the genes encoding the sites of action of psychotropic medication, there will be increasing opportunities to determine whether they are linked to genes that may be responsible for a broad range of psychiatric disorders for which there is evidence of hereditary vulnerability. In this regard, recombinant genetic studies have demonstrated a restriction fragment length polymorphism (RFLP) that is closely linked to the risk for MDI in an extended pedigree of the Old World Amish. Notably, this RFLP is localized to chromosome 11 in close proximity to the gene encoding for tyrosine hydroxylase, the initial and rate-limiting step in this synthesis pathway for catecholamines. Thus, as we look to the future, molecular approaches in psychopharmacology may dovetail with the genetic approaches in psychiatric research to clarify the pathophysiology of a broad range of major mental disorders.

REFERENCES

1. Akera, T and Brody, TM: The interaction between chlorpromazine free radicals and microsomal sodium- and potassium-activated adenosin triphosphatase from rat brain. Mol Pharmacol 5:605–614, 1969.
2. American Psychiatric Association: Diagnostic and Statistical Manual of Mental Disorders, ed 3, revised. American Psychiatric Press, Washington, DC, 1987.
3. Andreasen, NC and Olsen, S: Negative versus positive schizophrenia: Definition and validation. Arch Gen Psychiatry 39:789–794, 1982.
4. Baldessarini, RJ: Chemotherapy in Psychiatry: Principles and Practice. Harvard University Press, Boston, 1985.
5. Barnard, EA, Darlisom, MG, and Seeburg, P: Molecular biology of the GABA$_A$ receptor: The receptor/channel superfamily. Trends in Neuroscience 10: 502–508, 1987.
6. Baron, M: Genetics of schizophrenia: Familial patterns and mode of inheritance. Biol Psychiatry 21:1051–1066, 1986.
7. Berridge, MJ, Downes, CP, and Hanley, MR: Lithium amplified agonist dependent phosphatidylinositol responses in brain and salivary glands. Biochem J 206:587–595, 1982.
8. Blier, P, DeMontigny, C, and Tardis, D: Short-term lithium treatment enhances

responsiveness of postsynaptic 5-HT$_{1A}$ receptors without altering 5-HT autoreceptor sensitivity. Synapse 1:225–232, 1987.

9. Cade, JFJ: Lithium salts in the treatment of psychotic excitement. Med J Aust 36:349–352, 1949,

10. Carlsson, A, and Lindquist, M: Effect of chlorpramazine or haloperidol on formation of 3-methoxytyramine and normetanephrine in mouse brain. Acta Pharmacol 20:140–144, 1963.

11. Clow, A, Theodorou, A, Jenner, P, et al: Cerebral dopamine dysfunction in rats following withdrawal from one year of continuous neuroleptic administration. Eur J Pharmacol 63:145–151, 1980.

12. Cole, JO, Goldberg, SC, and Davis, JM: Drugs in the Treatment of Psychosis: Controlled Studies. In Solmon, P (ed): Psychiatric Drugs. New York, Grune & Stratton, 1966.

13. Coyle, JT: The clinical uses of antipsychotic medications. Med Clin North Am 66:993–1009, 1982.

14. Creese, I, Burt, DR, and Snyder SH: Dopamine receptor binding predicts clinical and pharmacologic potencies of antischizophrenic drugs. Science 192:481–483, 1976.

15. deBlas, A, Vitorica, J, and Friedrich, P: Localization of the GABA$_A$ receptor in rat brain with a monoclonal antibody to the 57,000 Mr peptide of the GABA$_A$ receptor/benzodiazepine receptor/CL$^-$ channel complex. J Neurosci 8:602–614, 1988.

16. DeMontigny, C, Cournoyer, G, Morissette, R, Langlois, R, and Caille, G: Lithium carbonate addition in tricyclic antidepressant resistant unipolar depression. Arch Gen Psych 40:1327–1334, 1983.

17. DeVito, RA, Brink, L, Sloan, C., et al: Fluphenazine decanoate versus oral antipsychotics. A comparison of their effectiveness in the treatment of schizophrenia as measured by a reduction in hospital readmissions. J Clin Psychiatry 39:26–31, 1978.

18. Falloon, IRH: Family Management of Schizophrenia. Johns Hopkins University Press, Baltimore, 1985.

19. Farde, L, Hall, H, Ehrin, E, and Sedval,

G: Quantitative analysis of D$_2$ receptor binding in the living human brain by PET. Science 231:258–261, 1986.

20. Fyer, HJ, Liebowitz, JR, Gorman, JM, et al: Discontinuation of alprazolam treatment in panic patients. Am J Psychiatry 144:303–308, 1987.

21. Goodman, WK and Charney, DS: Therapeutic applications and mechanism of action of monoamine oxidase inhibitor and heterocyclic antidepressant drugs. J Clin Psychiatry 46:6–22, 1985.

22. Gottesman, II and Shields, J: Schizophrenia: The Epigenetic Puzzle. New York, Cambridge University Press, 1982.

23. Graybiel, AM, Baughman, RW, and Eckenstein, F: Cholinergic neuropil of the striatum observes striosomal boundaries. Nature 323:625–628, 1986.

24. Gunne, L-M, Haggstrom, J-E, and Sjoquist, B: Association with persistent neuroleptic induced dyskinesia of regional changes in brain GABA synthesis. Nature 309:347–349, 1984.

25. Guze, BH and Baxter, LR: Current concepts: Neuroleptic malignant syndrome. N Engl J Med 313:163–166, 1985.

26. Hogarty, GE, Schooler, NR, Ulrich, RS, Mussare, F, Ferro, P, and Herron, E: Fluphenazine and social therapy in the after care of schizophrenic patients: Relapse analysis of a two-year control trial. Arch Gen Psychiatry 36:1283–1294, 1979.

27. Hunkeler, W, Moler, H, Pieri, L, et al: Selective antagonists of benzodiazepines. Nature 290:514–516, 1981.

28. Jefferson, JW, Griest, JH, and Baudhuin, M: Lithium: Interactions with other drugs. Journal of Clinical Psychopharmacology 1:124–134, 1981.

29. Jeste, DV and Wyatt, RJ: Understanding and Treating Tardive Dyskinesia. Guilford Press, New York, 1982.

30. Kebabian, JW, Petzold, GL, and Greengard, P: Dopamine-sensitive adenylate cyclase in caudate nucleus of rat brain and its similarity to the "dopamine receptor." Proc Natl Acad Sci USA 69:2145–2149, 1972.

31. Klein, DF, Ross, DC, and Cohen, P:

Panic and avoidance in agoraphobia: Application of path analysis to treatment studies? Arch Gen Psychiatry 44:377–385, 1987.

32. Levenson, JL: Neuroleptic malignant syndrome. Am J Psychiatry 142:1137–1145, 1985.

33. Lokkegaard, A, Andersen, NS, and Henriksen, E: Renal function in 153 manic-depressant patients treated with lithium for more than 5 years. Acta Psychiatr Scand 71:347–355, 1985.

34. Loranger, AW: Sex difference in age of onset of schizophrenia. Arch Gen Psychiatry 41:157–161, 1984.

35. Myers, DH, Carter, RA, Burns, BH, et al: A prospective study of the effects of lithium on thyroid function and on the prevalence of antithyroid antibodies. Psychol Med 15:55–61, 1985.

36. Myers, JK, Weissman, MN, Tischler, GL, et al: Six month prevalence of psychiatry disorders in three communities. Arch Gen Psychiatry 41:959–967, 1984.

37. Noyes, R, Garvey, MJ, Cook, BL, and Perry, PJ: Benzodiazepine withdrawal: A review of the evidence. J Clin Psychiatry, in press.

38. Olsen, RW: Drug interactions of the GABA receptor-ionophore complex. Annu Rev Pharmacol Toxicol 22:245–277, 1982.

39. Pearlson, G and Coyle, JT: The dopamine hypothesis in schizophrenia. In Coyle, JT and Enna, SJ (eds): Neuroleptics: Neurochemical, Behavioral and Clinical Perspectives. Raven Press, New York, 1983, pp 297–324.

40. Pope, HG, Keck, PE, and McElroy, SL: Frequency and presentation of neuroleptic malignant syndrome in a large psychiatric hospital. Am J Psychiatry 143:1227–1233, 1986.

41. Prien, RS, Kupfer, DJ, Mansky, PA, et al: Drug therapy in the prevention of occurrences in unipolar and bipolar affective disorders. Arch Gen Psychiatry 41:1096–1104, 1984.

42. Quitkin, F, Rifkin, A, and Klein, DF: Monoamine oxidase inhibitors: Review of antidepressant effectiveness. Arch Gen Psychiatry 35:749–760, 1979.

43. Rabkin, J, Quitkin, R, Harrison, W, et al: Adverse reactions to monoamine oxidase inhibitors. J Clin Psychopharmacol 4:270–278, 1984.

44. Schou, M: Lithium in psychiatric therapy and prophylaxis. J Psychiatr Res 6:67–95, 1968.

45. Seeman, P, Lee, T, Chao-Wong, M, et al: Antipsychotic drug doses and neuroleptic/dopamine receptors. Nature 261:717–720, 1976.

46. Seeman, P: Dopamine receptors and dopamine hypothesis of schizophrenia. Synapse 1:133–152, 1987.

47. Sheehan, DV, Coleman, JH, Greenblatt, DJ, et al: Some biochemical correlates of panic attacks with agoraphobia and their response to a new treatment. Journal of Clinical Psychopharmacology 4:66–75, 1984.

48. Sokoloff, P, Giros, B, Martres, M-P, Bouthenet, M-L, and Schwartz, J-C: Molecular cloning and characterization of a novel dopamine receptor (D_3) as a target for neuroleptics. Nature 347:146–148, 1990.

49. Spier, SA, Tesar, GE, Rosenbaum, JF, et al: Treatment of panic disorder and agoraphobia with clonazepam. J Clin Psychiatry 47:238–242, 1986.

50. Tallman, JF and Gallagher, DW: The GABAergic system: A locus of benzodiazepine action. Annu Rev Neurosci 8:21–44, 1985.

51. Task Force on the Use of Laboratory Tests in Psychiatry: Tricyclic antidepressants—Blood level measurements and clinical outcome. Am J Psychiatry 142:155–162, 1985.

52. Unnerstall, JR, Kuhar, MJ, Niehoff, DL, and Palacios, JM: Benzodiazepine receptors are coupled to a subpopulation of gamma-amino butyric acid (GABA) receptors: Evidence from quantitative autoradiographic study. J Pharmacol Exp Ther 218:797–804, 1981.

53. Van Patten, T: Why do schizophrenic patients refuse to take their drugs? Arch Gen Psychiatry 31:67–71, 1974.

54. Weinberger, DR, Bigelow, LD, Kleinman, JE, et al: Cerebral ventricular enlargement in chronic schizophrenia: An association with poor response to treatment. Arch Gen Psychiatry 37:11–13, 1980.

55. Westlund, KN, Denney, RM, Kochersperger, LM, Rose, RM, and Abell, CW: Distinct monoamine oxidase A and B populations in primate brain. Science 230:181–183, 1985.

56. Wong, DF, Wagner, HN, Tune, LE, et al: Positron emission tomography reveals elevated D_2 receptors in drug-naive schizophrenics. Science 234:1558–1563, 1986.

Chapter 8

COGNITIVE DISORDERS

Michael V. Johnston, M.D.

MEMORY DISORDERS
DEMENTIA
THERAPY FOR DEMENTIA
COGNITIVE DISORDERS IN YOUNG
PEOPLE

Therapy for cognitive disorders is an emerging area of neuropharmacology primarily because of the increasing number of individuals with age-related memory disorders and dementia.[62,67,135,142,143] Several other cognitive disorders, including learning disabilities, mental retardation, attention deficit disorder, and amnesia following traumatic brain injuries are also prevalent in younger individuals. There is considerable investigative interest in finding safe, effective therapies to improve cognitive efficiency and to reverse degenerative processes that attack the brain's cognitive systems.

Improved understanding of the molecular lesions in dementing brain illnesses, together with the identification of cognition-enhancing compounds in preclinical models, suggests that rational therapy for certain types of cognitive disorders holds substantial promise. Because of the large number of patients affected, development of active therapies would have a substantial impact even if their effects are modest. A 20% to 30% improvement in cognitive function would prolong independent living and reduce care needs in many patients.

Despite the paucity of therapies with clearly documented effectiveness, sev-eral drugs are approved by the US Food and Drug Administration (FDA) to improve cognition. Several other compounds have been reported to enhance cognition in animal models and in young people with dyslexia and amnesia. Others, such as tetrahydroaminoacridine (THA, or tacrine), have stimulated public and professional interest as possible treatments for Alzheimer's disease (AD). The neurologist, psychiatrist, and other physicians are likely to become increasingly familiar with this relatively new area of therapy. This chapter discusses the rationales for these therapies and critically assesses their efficacy.

MEMORY DISORDERS

One of the brain's most important cognitive functions is memory, the ability to store and recall information or skills that have been learned. The rationale for pharmacologic therapy for memory disorders is based on the premise that certain biochemical and structural systems in the brain have specialized roles in memory that can be enhanced by drugs. This hypothesis is supported by a limited amount of neuroanatomic, clinicopathologic, and pharmacologic evidence, which will be reviewed briefly. Before this information is presented, however, it would be useful to outline the clinical settings in which memory disorders occur and their relationship to each other.

Major Syndromes with Memory Loss

Amnesia, delirium, dementia, and memory disorder of aging describe distinct clinical syndromes that include memory loss as a major feature. *Amnesia*, or relatively isolated memory loss, is a troubling, sometimes debilitating problem, but reasoning and social function are usually much better preserved than in dementia. Amnesic patients (e.g., from head injury or hypoxic-ischemic damage to the mesial temporal structures) typically are unable to form new memories but may have good recall of past events. In contrast to isolated amnesia, *delirium* describes a more global state of mental confusion with a reduced level of attention and consciousness.[101] It is produced by a diverse group of toxic, metabolic, and other disorders and is often reversible. In contrast to amnesia and delirium, *dementia* is a progressive disorder that disrupts memory, reasoning, and social functioning relentlessly. Demented patients generally remain clearheaded for some time and they usually are not delirious or confused until late in the course of disease, unless they are exposed to certain drugs or metabolic derangement. Although sometimes resembling early dementia, *memory disorder of aging* is a more benign disorder of recent memory, which shows little progression. Many elderly people find this problem embarrassing or frightening and seek help for it. The rest of this section focuses on the organization of systems important for understanding primary disorders of memory; the section that follows discusses the more pervasive disorders associated with dementia.

Organization of Memory

Memory can be classified according to its duration, its content, and the modality by which it is stored (e.g., visual or auditory). The temporal classification separates relatively evanescent memory registration, which stores information for brief periods, from long-term memory registration, which stores it for hours or longer. A process of "consolidation" is thought to convert short-term memories into long-term or permanent ones (Table 8–1). Memory can

Table 8–1 ORGANIZATION OF MEMORY

Type of Memory	Example	Brain Region
MODALITY*		
Vision	Familiar faces	Visual cortex
Hearing	Music	Auditory cortex
Touch	Stereognosis	Parietal cortex
Taste	Taste	Limbic cortex
Smell	Smell	Limbic cortex
CONTENT*		
Declarative	Facts, names	Sensory cortex
Accessible through language	Episodes	Thalamus
		Hippocampus
		Basal forebrain
		Amygdala
Procedural	Playing the piano	Motor cortex
Remembered through motor activity	Assembling puzzle	Thalamus
	Tying knots	Basal ganglia
		?Basal forebrain
		?Amygdala
TIME*		
Short-term	New phone numbers	Probably similar for each
Long-term	Own birthday	

*These are the three most common conceptual frameworks for describing memories.

also be classified according to whether the stored information is recalled as a fact or episode (declarative memory) on one hand or as a skill or procedure (procedural memory).[157] These two types of memory are stored using circuitry connecting somewhat different regions of the brain.[111]

Experiments in subhuman primates have shown that the hippocampus and other mesial temporal structures are essential for storage of declarative memories in the cerebral cortex. Activation of the amygdala and basal forebrain regions are also important for memory storage. Participation of these areas appears to enhance the storage process, possibly by preparing the cortex to accept the information into storage. The neuronal pathways containing acetylcholine projecting from the basal forebrain into the cortex, as well as catecholamine and serotonergic pathways from the brainstem, contribute to this process (Fig. 8–1). Participation of the amygdala accounts, in part, for the prominent role that emotional state and context play in determining how readily memories are stored and recalled.[119]

Drug-Induced Memory Loss

From a therapeutic standpoint, memory disorders produced by drugs are important to recognize because they may

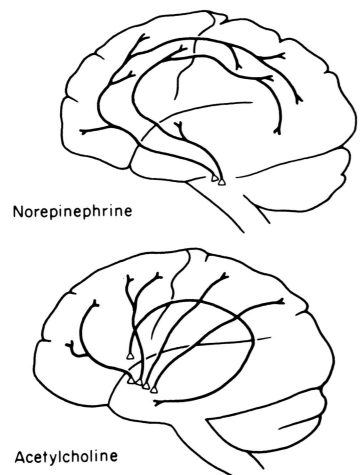

Norepinephrine

Acetylcholine

Figure 8–1. Diffuse neuronal projections from the brainstem into the cerebral cortex that are involved in attention, memory, and other functions. Noradrenergic axons are projected from the locus ceruleus of the pons. Other projections not shown extend into the hypothalamus, other limbic areas, and spinal cord. Cholinergic axons are projected from the basal forebrain into the neocortex and hippocampus.

imitate disease and are often reversible. Drug-induced memory disorders also provide insights into the basic mechanisms of memory. Certain drugs, especially benzodiazepines and anticholinergics, are an important cause of memory dysfunction in clinical practice.[141,163] Benzodiazepines prescribed for sedation for medical and surgical procedures commonly produce relatively selective amnesia even in young people. For example, lorazepam (Ativan) is used to produce amnesia for procedures such as endoscopy and cancer chemotherapy. Triazolam (Halcion), a triazolobenzodiazepine hypnotic agent, has also been reported to produce episodes resembling transient global amnesia in certain individuals.

These clinical observations have been extended into studies of the effects of benzodiazepines on memory in normal human subjects.[163] Benzodiazepines disrupts attention, vigilance, and memory for information requiring processing effort, but access to knowledge already memorized remains intact. Pharmacologic experiments suggest that benzodiazepines may act in part by decreasing acetylcholine release from the basal forebrain cholinergic system.

Muscarinic acetylcholine blocking agents have a prominent amnestic effect, which was the basis for using scopolamine as an amnestic hypnotic agent for obstetrics. Drachman and Leavitt[44] administered scopolamine to normal college students and compared the deficits it produced in memory to the memory disorder associated with aging. They tested standard digit span, superspan digit recall, free recall for words, category retrieval, and the Wechsler Adult Intelligence scale. Administration of 1 mg of scopolamine subcutaneously produced deficits in each of these abilities that were quite similar to the spectrum for aged subjects. Another study[150] reported that the muscarinic agonist arecoline enhances serial learning in young human subjects. Older patients with age-related memory decline are more sensitive to scopolamine and other cholinergic blockers

than younger individuals. When certain elderly subjects are given scopolamine (e.g., to prevent motion sickness), they may become so cognitively impaired that it is difficult to distinguish their behavior from that of demented patients. Both anticholinergic and benzodiazepine drugs (and possibly others) may cause pseudodementia and/or delirium in elderly individuals, so that doses must often be reduced for them.[69a]

Acute or subacute toxic metabolic disorders such as hypoxemia, alcohol withdrawal, hypothyroidism, and other metabolic disorders are also important potentially treatable causes of cognitive dysfunction, including delirium and amnesia. Like drugs, their presence may exaggerate modest cognitive decline in older individuals and tip the balance toward confusion and total dependence on others. Manifestations of these disorders are usually associated with more confusion and delirium than in primary dementia but the clinical presentation may be indistinguishable.

Roles of Neurotransmitters in Memory

Evidence that drugs such as muscarinic antagonists cause memory loss stimulated interest in the neurochemical basis of human memory disorders.[44,163] A variety of neurotransmitter systems play a role in brain circuits serving memory. The neurochemical abnormality that has been proposed most commonly to contribute to age-related memory changes is a decline in the cortical machinery for muscarinic, cholinergic neurotransmission.[4,30,44] This hypothesis is based on the effects of muscarinic blocking drugs and agonists in humans and investigations in animal models.[163] Although it is undoubtedly simplistic, the cholinergic hypothesis has played an important role in the development of thinking about therapy for memory disorders. The cholinergic hypothesis is described here in detail, and the role of other neurotransmitters, such as excitatory amino acids (EAAs), is described in the following section on dementia.

CHOLINERGIC INNERVATION OF THE CEREBRAL CORTEX

The cholinergic innervation of the cerebral cortex is derived predominantly from subcortical projections.[92,109] The organization of the basal forebrain cholinergic projection to the cerebral cortex and features of cholinergic synaptic function are shown in Figures 8–1 and 8–2. Four cholinergic cell groups in the basal forebrain (the medial septum, the vertical and horizontal limb of the diagonal band of Broca, and nucleus basalis of Meynert) project axons into the hippocampus and cerebral cortex. These cholinergic cell bodies have been grouped and named Ch1 through Ch4. Cholinergic cell bodies in the medial septal nucleus and the vertical limb of the diagonal band provide the major cholinergic innervation into the hippocampus, whereas those of the horizontal limb of the diagonal band provide cholinergic axons to olfactory structures. The cerebral cortex receives the vast majority of its cholinergic input from the Ch4 region of the nucleus basalis. The cortical cholinergic innervation is distributed diffusely throughout cortical layers; laminar differences in density are found in different subregions of cortex. The vast majority of the cholinergic innervation to the cerebral cortex in primates comes from the basal forebrain projection.[109] These basal forebrain nuclei receive substantial input from the hypothalamus and components of the limbic system. In physiologic studies, electrical activity in the nucleus basalis has been shown to increase after monkeys are rewarded with juice for successful performance of a motor task.

The basal forebrain cholinergic projection appears to play a role in integrating cognitive, vegetative, and motivationally relevant information.[28] Evidence during the past decade (since

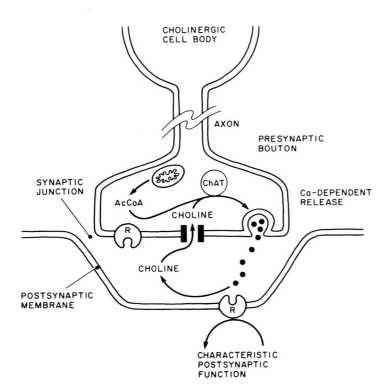

Figure 8–2. A cholinergic synapse in the cerebral cortex. Acetylcholine (*black dots*) is synthesized by choline acetyltransferase (ChAT) from choline and acetylcoenzyme A (AcCoA) produced in mitochondria. Choline is recycled by uptake into the presynaptic terminal after acetylcholine is degraded in the synapse by acetylcholinesterase. Acetylcholine alters postsynaptic neuronal activity through interaction with receptor activated channel and second-messenger activity. (Drawn by Dr. Michael McKinney.)

the recognition of this system's importance) continues to suggest that a strong relationship exists between the disruption of function in nucleus basalis neurons and memory loss.[61] Experiments in which the glutamate analogue neurotoxin ibotenic acid was used to damage the nucleus basalis of squirrel monkeys demonstrated that this lesion produced severe and enduring learning and memory deficits in several visual memory tasks.[86] Decker and colleagues[38] demonstrated changes in high-affinity choline uptake into cholinergic nerve endings in the hippocampus and the cortex as a result of training on a spatial memory task. This result suggests that the cholinergic pathways may be activated by the training.

BIOCHEMICAL MACHINERY OF
THE CHOLINERGIC SYNAPSE

The biochemical machinery of the cholinergic synapse, which has been the object of therapeutic interest, is shown in Figure 8–2.[11] Acetylcholine is synthesized from acetylcoenzyme A (AcCoA) and choline by choline actyltransferase (ChAT). The usual brain concentrations of choline (30 μmol/L) and AcCoA (2 to 20 μmol/L) are usually below those needed to saturate ChAT. Experimental elevation of brain choline or AcCoA can alter the rate of acetylcholine turnover. Choline is able to pass easily across the blood-brain barrier via a facilitated diffusion system in the capillary endothelial cell. Brain choline concentrations tend to be higher than those in the plasma, possibly related to the fact that the brain neurons can synthesize choline by sequential methylation of the phospholipid phosphatidylethanolamine or ethanolamine plasmalogens. Choline can then be formed by hydrolysis of the resulting phospholipids.[10]

The other major source of intraneuronal choline is the uptake of choline from the synaptic cleft into cholinergic axons after it is formed by hydrolysis of acetylcholine by acetylcholinesterase (AChE). Both high-affinity and low-affinity uptake systems for choline have been characterized. Dietary choline administered to rats has been reported to raise brain acetylcholine concentrations.[11,88,173,183] The high-affinity system may be saturated at low plasma concentrations; the low-affinity mechanism is the most likely to mediate the increase in tissue choline occurring after plasma choline rises. Experimental evidence also suggests that the extent to which a cholinergic neuron synthesizes more acetylcholine when provided with additional choline is related to its physiologic activity. These observations have led to a number of trials of dietary choline or a phospholipid source, phosphatidylcholine (lecithin), to increase acetylcholine production.

Acetylcholine released from cholinergic nerve endings may act at both muscarinic and nicotinic receptors. Muscarinic receptors appear to predominate in the brain and are of greatest importance for cognitive function. Presynaptic muscarinic receptors (so-called M_2 receptors) appear to provide a feedback inhibition of acetylcholine release, since muscarinic blockers such as scopolamine and atropine enhance acetylcholine release. The electrophysiologic actions of acetylcholine appear to be mediated by both second-messenger systems and ionic channels. Muscarinic-stimulated phosphoinositide turnover has recently been studied and may mediate important actions of acetylcholine with respect to memory. The molecular action of acetylcholine in memory processes is not precisely understood. A number of physiologic studies have suggested that it may augment excitatory responses induced by other excitatory transmitters. Acetylcholine pathways may regulate receptivity to memory storage in localized regions of the cerebral cortex.

Acetylcholinesterase enzyme activity responsible for hydrolysis of acetylcholine released into the synapse is found predominantly associated with presynaptic nerve terminals. Lesions of the basal forebrain in animals lead to a marked depletion in AChE activity in cortex. Inhibition of AChE activity substantially enhances the effect of acetylcholine and this strategy has been exploited to attempt to treat AD.

NEUROTRANSMITTER DYSFUNCTION IN AGE-RELATED MEMORY LOSS

Studies in aged animals showed a decrease in the maximal velocity of sodium-dependent high-affinity uptake of choline into presynaptic nerve terminals; acetylcholine synthesis may also be diminished.[38,39] At least two experimental studies in aged rodents showed a substantial decrease in acetylcholine synthesis in the whole brain and hippocampus.[39] A similar effect was noted in human temporal cortex biopsy specimens.[59] In contrast to AD, however, in which major reductions in cortical ChAT activity are found, no reproducible change has been identified in aging.[4] Several studies have reported decreases in binding of muscarinic antagonists to the cerebral cortex of elderly humans and rodents compared to younger individuals. Microiontophoretic studies of acetylcholine responsiveness also suggest that the postsynaptic muscarinic response is diminished.[4]

A recent, interesting report[53] showed that in aged rodents, the basal forebrain cholinergic projective cell bodies are smaller than in younger controls, though their number is normal. The animals also had memory defects demonstrable using a water maze paradigm. A continuous infusion of the protein nerve growth factor, which stimulates cholinergic neuron metabolism, appeared to increase the size of the basal forebrain cholinergic neurons visualized by immunocytochemistry for ChAT and also improved performance in the water maze.

This evidence points to the appearance of several age-related abnormalities in the metabolic neurotransmitter function of cholinergic neurons and to the responsiveness of postsynaptic receptors to acetylcholine. Aging is not thought to be associated with death of cholinergic neurons and therefore might be expected to be responsive to an appropriate therapy. Other, possibly equally important biochemical lesions may also be important in memory loss of aging.[2] A deficit in the metabolism of norepinephrine neurons has been reported in patients with Wernicke-Korsakoff syndrome.[106]

Therapy for Memory Disorders

Therapy for a memory disorder begins with a careful evaluation for reversible medical, metabolic, or pharmacologic causes (e.g., hypoxemia, hypothyroidism). Drugs such as benzodiazepines and anticholinergics should be used sparingly in elderly patients who are predisposed to this problem.[69a] For patients whose memory disorder is related to delirium, small doses of a neuroleptic drug such as haloperidol (Haldol) may help.

Although there appears to be a rationale for enhancing cholinergic function in memory disorder of aging, attempts to treat the disorder by augmenting production of acetylcholine by administration of choline or lecithin have not produced much improvement.[4,35,84,89] The use of physostigmine to inhibit breakdown of acetylcholine has been reported to produce short-term memory improvement in normal subjects and improvement in amnesia due to herpes encephalitis.[125,126] Several other approaches have been tried with mixed success.[90,106,118] One report indicated some success using clonidine, an alpha-2 adrenergic agonist to improve memory in patients with Wernicke-Korsakoff syndrome.[106] Nevertheless, it seems reasonable that more effective agents might be developed to activate cholinergic synapses.[4]

DEMENTIA

Types of Dementia

Dementia, as defined by a National Institutes of Health (NIHI) panel, is a progressive, pervasive disorder characterized by loss of memory and intellectual abilities affecting social or occupational functioning, and with one of the following findings: decline in abstract thinking or judgment, related cortical signs such as aphasia, or personality change.[107] Senile dementia of the Alzheimer's type accounts for more than half of the cases of dementia in older persons (Table 8–2)[143,172] and accounts for about half of admissions to nursing homes in the United States. According to the NIH criteria, a definite diagnosis of Alzheimer's disease (AD) should be made only on the basis of a neuropathologic diagnosis. The NIH statement also suggests criteria for diagnoses of *probable* AD and *possible* AD. It is important to exclude reversible causes of pseudodementia such as depression, sedative drugs, vitamin deficiency, or hypothyroidism.

Vascular, multi-infarct dementia is the second most common cause of dementia (see Table 8–2). Multi-infarct dementia is caused by multiple areas of cortical infarction in patients with other forms of cardiovascular disease, including hypertension and atherosclerosis. Detection of patients with multi-infarct dementia can be improved using the ischemic score reported by Hachinski.[72,172] Using this clinical rating, patients attaining seven points or more for a combination of signs and symptoms are likely to have either multi-infarct dementia or a vascular component to their mental impairment. Another form of vascular dementia, senile dementia of the Binswagner type, is associated with prominent white matter lesions.[136] A radiologic lesion in white matter (leukoariosis) is believed to reflect ischemic periventricular leukoencephalopathy. Cognitive dysfunction in this disorder appears to result from cortical disconnection.

In addition to AD and multiple infarctions, dementia in adults is also caused by less frequent disorders such as Pick's disease and progressive supranuclear palsy as well as endocrine disorders, vitamin deficiencies, alcoholism, brain tumor, Parkinson's disease, subdural hematoma, and head trauma. Infectious causes such as acquired immune deficiency syndrome encephalopathy, syphilis, and progressive multifocal leukoencephalopathy are becoming more common causes in younger people. In children, metabolic diseases such as ceroid lipofuscinosis, Wilson's disease, metachromatic leukodystrophy, and adrenoleukodystrophy or idiopathic disorders such as Rett syndrome are prominent causes of the relatively small number of cases of dementia.

Accurate diagnosis of these diverse disorders in living patients is not always possible.[71,172] Using careful clinical criteria with imaging and laboratory data, however, several organized longitudinal studies[83,107,172] report a diagnostic accuracy of more than 80% compared to pathologic diagnoses. Nevertheless, in clinical practice, accuracy may be lower than 80%, and patients who suffer from more than one condition, such as multi-infarct dementia and AD, are sometimes difficult to classify.

Table 8–2 CAUSES OF DEMENTIA

Diagnosis	Rochester (n = 178)	Ontario (n = 65)
AD	60%	58%
Multi-infarct	8%	9%
Mixed	10%	15%
Other	22%	18%

The study from Rochester, Minnesota,[143] reported autopsy diagnoses on persons older than age 29 who developed dementia from 1960 to 1964. The study from Western Ontario[172] followed 65 patients longitudinally.

Synaptic Abnormalities in AD

DEFECTS IN CHOLINERGIC SYSTEMS

In AD, the axodendritic connections within the cerebral cortex degenerate progressively, accompanied to a somewhat lesser degree by loss of large neurons. As the synaptic fabric of the cortex becomes disrupted, the neuropathologic hallmarks of this condition, neurofibrillary tangles, granulovacuolar degeneration, and neuritic plaques, appear. There is a close association between the density of neuritic plaques and the severity of dementia. Silver-staining neurites surrounding the amyloid core of the plaque represent the wreckage of destroyed neuron circuitry.[46]

Loss of the cholinergic innervation of the cerebral cortex emanating from the basal forebrain is an early prominent part of this destruction of the brain's neuropil.[28,180] There is a close coordination between the loss of ChAT activity, severity of dementia, and plaque density (Fig. 8–3).[9,108] Loss of ChAT activity is highest (−70% to −90% of control) in areas such as temporal and parietal cortex, which are most severely affected morphologically in AD. The activity

of AChE associated with cholinergic axons is also severely diminished in AD, and AChE staining is seen in degenerating neurites. Loss of ChAT reflects progressive destruction and disease in cholinergic synaptic terminals. Although loss of cholinergic perikarya in the nucleus basalis is a common finding in advanced AD, some studies have reported that neuron number is preserved with shrinkage in perikaryal size.[122] This observation suggests that the disruption in function of synaptic terminals is greater than the loss of cholinergic cell bodies and may antedate cell body loss.

Loss of acetylcholine synthetic capacity and a reduction in the ability of cortex to take up radioactive choline into pinched-off synaptic terminals has been found in cortical biopsy specimens of patients with relatively early AD. One study[59] found that the in vitro estimate of acetylcholine synthesis determined

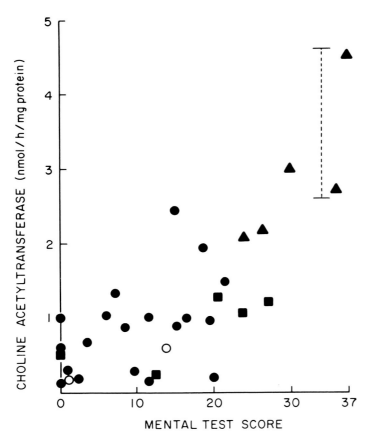

Figure 8–3. Relationship between postmortem ChAT in temporal cortex (Brodmann area 21) and performance (within 6 months of death) in a simple memory and information test of mental ability. Key to symbols: triangles = depression; filled circles = Alzheimer's disease; squares = Parkinson's disease; open circles = combined Parkinson's and Alzheimer's disease. Line and bars represent mean and standard deviation for an age-matched normal group (with test score arbitrarily set between 30 and 37). (Adapted from Perry,[124] p 67.)

Figure 8–4. Correlation between acetylcholine synthesis and cognitive impairment in patients with early-onset Alzheimer's disease. An in vitro estimate of acetylcholine synthesis in vivo was significantly correlated (Spearman's coefficient of correlations, −0.63; $P < 0.007$) with a rating of cognitive impairment on a scale from 0 to 9 (absent to severe). The control value of 6.6 ± 1.2 is the mean rate of acetycholine synthesis in 22 samples of apparently normal neocortex removed to allow access to tumors and treated like samples from the patients with Alzheimer's disease. This is believed to be a good indicator of the value for normal tissue. (From Francis, et al,[59] p 8, with permission.)

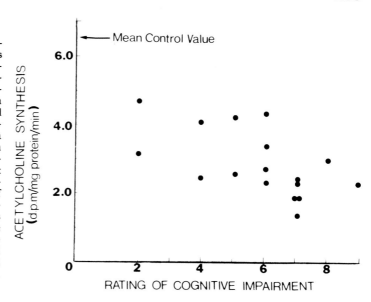

in cortical biopsy specimens was significantly correlated with the rating of cognitive impairment in AD patients (Fig. 8–4). These results suggest that the deficits in presynaptic cholinergic systems are relatively early changes in the development of clinical features of AD.

In contrast to the severe decrease in biochemical markers for cholinergic nerve terminals, little change has been found in muscarinic receptors in the postmortem AD brain. When agonist displacement studies have been used to separate binding to predominantly postsynaptic (M_1) muscarinic acetylcholine receptors, little decrease in density has been found. The M_2 type, localized predominantly on presynaptic muscarinic receptors, may be reduced. A reduction in nicotinic acetylcholine receptors has also been found in cortex from patients with AD. The potential therapeutic importance of this observation is uncertain.

SEROTONIN DEFICITS

Deficits have been found in levels of serotonin (5-hydroxytryptamine,5-HT) and in 5-HT uptake into serotonin nerve terminals in cerebral cortex from AD patients.[12] Some studies have also reported a reduction in the metabolite 5-hydroxyindoleacetic acid. A reduc-

tion of approximately 50% in serotonin binding has also been found in AD cortex. Both the HT_1 and HT_2 serotonin receptor subtypes are reduced, but loss of binding to the HT_2 subtype appears to predominate. Some of the 5-HT_2 receptor loss defined by these techniques may be located on damaged cholinergic nerve terminals. A considerable amount may also reflect a postsynaptic defect. Bowen and Davison[12] have hypothesized that the 5-HT_2 receptors lost in AD are localized to pyramidal neurons bearing tangles in the cerebral cortex, rather than the raphe serotonergic projection to cortex. Unlike the change in biochemical markers for cholinergic nerve terminals, there does not appear to be a quantitative relationship between either the presynaptic or postsynaptic deficits in the serotonin markers and other markers and disease severity. While the serotonergic changes may well be relevant to cognitive loss, much remains to be learned about the therapeutic relevance of this observation.

CATECHOLAMINE DEFICITS

Many postmortem specimens from patients with AD have a reduction in biochemical markers for the noradrenergic projection from the pons into the cerebral cortex.[137] Some studies suggest that there is a greater reduction in cortical norepinephrine concentrations in younger patients with AD than in older patients. One group[59] found a 64% reduction in endogenous cortical norepinephrine in cortical biopsy specimens from patients younger than 80 years of age with AD, and a 50% increase in the norepinephrine metabolite 3-methoxy-4-hydroxyphenylglycol (3-MHPG). This metabolite change is not reflected in cerebrospinal fluid (CSF). In contrast, biopsied patients aged 80 and older had a reduction in endogenous norepinephrine of 38% and no significant change in MHPG. The relative importance of the noradrenergic loss in the memory dysfunction found in AD is not clear. The researchers[59] suggested that since younger patients had a compensatory increase in norepinephrine turnover, they might not benefit from therapy with drugs to augment noradrenergic impulse flow. Despite the loss of presynaptic noradrenergic markers, the density of postsynaptic receptors for alpha-1, alpha-2, and beta subtypes in the hippocampus and in temporal cortex is reportedly normal.

In contrast to the norepinephrine projection, there does not appear to be a significant reduction in dopamine concentrations in the cerebral cortex of patients with Alzheimer's dementia. Some studies, however, have reported low concentrations of the endogenous dopamine metabolite homovanillic acid (HVA) in CSF, and low concentrations of dopamine and HVA in the caudate, putamen, amygdala, and hypothalamus.[96,97,152] Behavior studies in rhesus monkeys indicate that dopamine depletion in circumscribed areas of association cortex produces impaired spatial memory performance almost as severe as that caused by ablation of the same area.[16] Dopamine replacement therapy repairs the deficit. This observation may be relevant to cognitive disorders in patients with Parkinson's disease, but there is little evidence that this mechanism is relevant to treatment of AD.

AMINO-ACID NEUROTRANSMITTER ABNORMALITIES

Amino acid neurotransmitters are extremely important in cortical function for both inhibitory (e.g., gamma-aminoutyric acid, or GABA) and excitatory (e.g., L-glutamate) neuron function. Excitatory amino acid neurotransmitters (e.g., glutamate) play an important role in memory storage in the hippocampus and cerebral cortex. GABAergic inhibitory neurons are predominantly intrinsic interneurons in the cerebral cortex. Many large pyramidal neurons appear to be glutamatergic. Early studies[13] showed the biochemical enzymatic marker for GABAergic neurons, glutamate decarboxylase (GAD), to be reduced in the brains of demented patients with a prolonged period of anoxia before death. In patients who died rapidly, GAD was not decreased although there was a profound deficit in ChAT activity. This, along with the observation that small interneurons are relatively preserved in AD, led to the consensus that GABAergic neurons are relatively spared in Alzheimer's dementia. However, other researchers[75] demonstrated a 70% loss of uptake of tritiated GABA into nerve terminals in the cortex and hippocampus in AD. This is compatible with previous reports that immunoreactivity for GAD is found in neuritic plaques in aged primate brains.[46] Also, the neuropeptide somatostatin, which is co-localized with GAD in some neurons, has been found to be decreased in AD brains.[31,166] These findings suggest that disruption of GABAergic neuron terminals could surpass the loss of cell bodies. $GABA_A$ receptor binding has also been reported to be reduced by up to 50% in hippocampal pyramidal cell layer in AD,[187] while $GABA_B$ receptors are reduced significantly in outer layers of the cerebral cortex.

Excitatory neurotransmitter pathways also appear to be disrupted in AD.[87,187] Sodium-dependent binding of tritiated 3H-D-aspartate to presynaptic EAA uptake sites on nerve terminals is reduced in the temporal cortex. Glutamate-like immunoreactivity has been found in neurons containing neurofibrillary tangles in 50% to 70% of CA1/CA2 pyramidal cells of AD hippocampus. Glutamate (but not aspartate or several free amino acids) measured in CSF was correlated with measures of cognitive impairment in one study.[152]

Postsynaptic receptors for glutamate measured in vitro by autoradiography using 3H-glutamate to measure binding to N-methyl-D-aspartate (NMDA) sensitive sites are reported to be reduced in AD cerebral cortex and hippocampus by 50% to 85%.[68,69] Glutamate receptors of the NMDA type are coupled to an ion channel, which can be labeled using the dissociative anesthetic (phencyclidine) receptor site; these binding sites are also reduced in AD. These observations suggest the presence of a major disruption in excitatory synaptic function in AD. It has also been suggested that excessive excitation mediated by these pathways could play a role in progressive neuron degeneration in AD. Excessive excitation of the NMDA receptor induces calcium overload and metabolic derangements associated with metabolic or "oxidative stress," in which oxygen free radicals are generated. In neuron culture systems, antioxidant compounds may reverse effects of EAA neurotoxicity.

Excitatory amino acid neurotransmitter systems, especially the channel containing the NMDA/dissociative anesthetic site, have been implicated in learning and memory, and the associated electrical phenomenon of long-term potentiation in the hippocampus. Degenerative changes in EAA pathways involved in learning may be important in the pathogenesis of dementia.

NEUROPEPTIDE DEFICITS

Several abnormalities in brain neuropeptides have been reported in AD. The peptide neurotransmitters and modulators, including cholecystokinin, neuropeptide Y, and somatostatin, are found in relatively high concentrations in the cerebral cortex, while vasoactive intestinal peptide, substance P, corticotropin releasing factor (CRF), adrenocorticotropic hormone, and dynorphin are found in smaller concentrations. These peptides are localized predominantly in interneurons, especially in cortical layers 2, 3, and 6. Major reductions in somatostatin were reported in most cortical areas of postmortem specimens with AD.[31]

Reinikainen and associates[133] found a 42% decrease in somatostatin immunoreactivity in frontal cortex, a 28% decrease in temporal cortex and a 42% decrease in parietal cortex in AD. They reported a correlation between decreases in ChAT activity and somatostatin in some brain areas and found reductions in CSF somatostatin that correlated with psychologic test scores. Severely demented patients showed lower somatostatinlike immunoreactivity than moderately demented individuals, but this difference was not statistically significant. Other researchers[166] found low CSF somatostatin levels in patients with AD, correlating with somatostatin levels in AD cortex. They also found that CSF levels correlated with performance and neuropsychologic testing but bore no relationship to the duration of AD. CSF somatostatin levels correlated with the overall cerebral glucose utilization rates, especially in the posterior parietal lobe. In contrast, other studies[31] did not suggest a relationship between reduction in cortical somatostatinlike immunoreactivity and severity of dementia, suggesting that this peptide may not play a role in the memory loss in AD. Both somatostatin and neuropeptide Y have been identified in the degenerating neurites in senile plaques. Several immunocytochemical studies have shown abnormalities in somatostatin- and neuropeptide Y–containing neurons in Alzheimer's dementia.[6]

Concentrations of CRF-like immunoreactivity are also reduced in Alzheimer's cortex;[40] the change is significantly correlated with the decrements in ChAT activity. There are reciprocal increases in CRF receptor binding in affected cortical areas. Several studies have reported no change in the substance-P levels. Similarly, vasoactive intestinal peptide, which is found in intrinsic cortical neurons, and cholecystokinin have generally been reported to be unaltered in AD.[46]

In contrast to the reductions reported in somatostatin and CRF, the concentration of immunoreactive galanin has been reported to be elevated twofold in a study of nucleus basalis in AD brain and postmortem controls.[6] Galanin is co-localized with acetylcholine in the large cholinergic neurons in the nucleus basalis and in interneurons there. In the same study, the ChAT activity and serotonin concentration were reduced in AD nucleus basalis but the concentrations of other peptides and neurotransmitters were unchanged. Galanin inhibits acetylcholine release and produces cognitive deficits in animals, and could contribute to cognitive deficits in AD.

Other Neurochemical Abnormalities in AD

MEMBRANE PHOSPHOLIPIDS

Phospholipids are the most abundant membrane lipid, and they serve as major structural elements in neuron membranes. Abnormalities in membrane phospholipid metabolism have been suggested to play a role in degenerative changes in AD.[22,110] The major phospholipids are phosphoglycerides, which contain two fatty-acid molecules esterified to the first and second hydroxyl groups of glycerol. The third hydroxyl group of glycerol forms an ester with phosphoric acid, which is esterified to a polar alcohol group to form compounds such as phosphatidylethanolamine (PE) and phosphatidylcholine (PC), phosphatidylserine or phosphati-

dylinositol (PI). The phospholipids are arranged in membranes with hydrophobic nonpolar tails oriented inward and the polar hydrophilic phosphoric-acid derivative ends oriented outward toward the surface of the membrane (see Chapter 1, Fig. 1–2).

Wurtman has linked the "cholinergic hypothesis" of AD with an abnormality in phospholipid metabolism, suggesting that depletion of membrane phosphatidylcholine in cholinergic neurons may play a role in their selective degeneration in AD.[10,183,184] Choline for acetylcholine synthesis in cholinergic nerve terminals can be derived from facilitated transport from the blood across the blood-brain barrier from reuptake into cholinergic nerve terminals or from breakdown of membrane PC. It has been estimated that PC represents 80% of membrane-bound choline, making it a potential cellular reservoir for free choline. Electrical stimulation of brain slices causes release of acetylcholine and a decline in levels of membrane PC, which can be replenished by adding choline. This observation suggests that during states of high activity, cholinergic neurons might maintain their rate of choline conversion to acetylcholine at the expense of structural membrane PC, resulting eventually in cholinergic neuron destruction. This work led to the hypothesis that cholinergic neurons are vulnerable in AD in part because they are the only cell type that uses PC both as a structural component of the membrane and as a reservoir for acetylcholine synthesis. This hypothesis is supported by evidence that degradation of PC provides choline for acetylcholine synthesis in a human neuron cell line and that choline supports the survival of human neurons in culture.

Abnormalities in PC metabolism have been reported in AD brain.[45] A nuclear magnetic resonance (NMR) spectroscopy study[110] of brain samples obtained at autopsy from seven patients with AD and nine control subjects showed a significant reduction in the concentrations of the phosphomonoesters phosphoethanolamine and phosphocholine, and a significant increase in the phosphodiesters glycerophosphoethanolamine and glycerophosphocholine (GPC). Another group[3] suggested that the relatively increased GPC in Alzheimer brain may reflect a decreased degradation of GPC to glycerol phosphate and choline. The phospholipase that catalyzes PC hydrolysis to release free choline is reported to be reduced in brains of patients with AD to an extent comparable to the reduction in ChAT.[93,94] Other researchers[127,128] also reported an abnormality in phospholipid metabolism, using phosphorous 31 NMR in a patient with AD. They found decreased levels of PC, PE, and cholesterol in 17 AD brains, using high-performance liquid chromatography. Their studies suggested an increase in PC synthesis early in AD. Although these observations suggest that phospholipid metabolism may be abnormal in AD, the nature of the abnormal regulatory steps remains unclear. Phosphorus 31 NMR spectroscopy may be useful to study these compounds in living patients and assess their response to therapeutic trials.

Another potential role of phospholipids in neurotransmitter dysfunction underlying disorders of learning and memory is their role in PI turnover. The diminished responsiveness of neurons in aged brain to acetylcholine (see p 231) has been hypothesized to be related to decreased PI turnover. Phospholipids involved in this neurotransmitter-stimulated second-messenger activity may play a role in learning and memory. These abilities might be disturbed by a disruption of phospholipid metabolism. Breakdown of phosphatidylinositol 4,5-bisphosphate (PIP_2) in response to activation of glutamate or cholinergic muscarinic receptors leads to formation of inositol 1,4,5-triphosphate (IP_3) and diacylglycerol. Diacylglycerol activates protein kinase C, which may play a role in learning and memory by phosphorylating specific proteins in the cerebral cortex. Dysfunction in this important second-messenger pathway is a potential locus of metabolic derangements in phospholipid metabolism. One study[160] found considerably less PI in anterior temporal cortex samples from Alzheimer patients than in controls. The concentration of PI 4-phosphate and PIP_2 were also somewhat lower in AD cortex, but not to a statistically significant degree.

CYTOSKELETAL PATHOLOGY

Neurofibrillary tangles, which reflect a disruption in the organization and physiology of the neuron cytoskeleton, are a hallmark of AD.[66] Normal cytoskeletal function is essential for transport of materials within the neuron. Neurofibrillary tangles are composed largely of paired helical filaments, which are unlike any other normal cytoskeletal element.[145] They are found predominantly in the pyramidal neurons of the cerebral cortex and hippocampus. A remarkable feature of the proteins in neurofibrillary tangles is their relative insolubility in most of the agents that dissolve neurofilaments and other normal cytoskeletal components. Paired helical filaments and neurofibrillary tangles in AD have some features of normal neurofilaments and some that are antigenically unique. Amyloid accumulation is also a cardinal feature of AD.[145] Amyloid fibrils, composed of a 4-kilodalton beta amyloid (A4) protein, are found in cerebral blood vessels and in senile plaques in the disease.[138] The A4 protein is a fragment of a larger precursor called beta-APP (pre-A4) which is coded for by DNA on human chromosome 21. Some studies suggest that deposition of beta amyloid in an amorphous "preamyloid" form may be a very early feature of both AD and of young adult brain in Down's syndrome. These abnormalities undoubtedly reflect an important pathogenic mechanism in the evolution of neuron pathology in AD, but results so far have not suggested a plausible therapeutic approach.

DISORDERS OF
ENERGY METABOLISM

Primary energy failure may also be an important mechanism for cognitive dysfunction in dementia. Hypoxemia produces a prominent, relatively selective decrement in memory in both man and animals.[62,65,139] Alzheimer's disease is associated with reductions in energy metabolism most prominent in the posterior parietal regions of the cerebral cortex. These disturbances have been identified using positron emission tomography (PET) and the 2-deoxyglucose method.[77,83] Bowen and associates'[113] early metabolic studies of postmortem Alzheimer brain also identified abnormalities in glucose metabolism. Reductions were found in the activity of soluble hexosekinase as well as of three other glycolytic enzymes, aldolase, phosphohexoseisomerase, and phosphoglyceromutase. Reduced activity of succinate dehydrogenase activity also suggested defective mitochondrial function. Reductions in hexoseisomerase and aldolase have also been identified in biopsy specimens.[147–149]

In contrast to the reductions in energy metabolism noted in in vivo PET studies, examination of biopsied cerebral cortex in vitro demonstrated an increase in the oxidation of U-14-C glucose to $14\text{-}CO_2$. Recent studies also indicate that glucose metabolism is increased and mitochondrial activity is decreased in cultured skin fibroblasts from patients with AD.[149] More detailed studies of in vitro oxygen uptake by homogenates of fresh biopsy samples of neocortex from patients with dementia and neurosurgical controls indicated that maximal respiratory rates were similar in AD and control patients. However, under conditions of adenosine diphosphate depletion producing submaximal metabolic activity, oxygen uptake rates were significantly elevated in the dementia group. These observations suggested the possibility that mitochondrial function is partially uncoupled in the cortex in AD. The

relationship of these subtle in vitro changes to the in vivo reductions in glucose metabolism is presently unclear. It is possible that the metabolic changes observed under conditions of submaximal respiration might reflect a functionally important defect that contributes to neuron damage.

A defect in energy metabolism simulating chronic hypoxia could contribute to certain aspects of the neuron degeneration in AD.[8] In support of this idea, a team led by Gibson[65] found that acetylcholine production and U-14-C-glucose incorporation into amino acids were reduced more by hypoxia in aged animals than in younger ones. This observation would be compatible with the hypothesis that age-related changes might enhance the expression of a genetic, metabolic defect. A progressive metabolic defect might make it more difficult for neurons to deal with both oxidative stress and calcium overload, which trigger the arachidonic acid cascade and cause generation of free radicals. A report that the calcium antagonist nimodipine improved learning in aged rabbits could be consistent with this hypothesis.[42] If excessive EAA activity and calcium overload are operative mechanisms contributing to AD, a defect in energy metabolism might enhance their toxicity. A metabolic contribution to the pathogenesis of dementia deserves careful examination for developing potential therapies.

Abnormalities in Vascular Dementia and Other Dementing Disorders

Specific lesions in neurotransmitter circuitry and other neurochemical abnormalities in other forms of dementia have received much less attention than changes in AD. Early studies by Bowen and associates[13] of postmortem tissue from demented patients compared biologic changes in AD with those in mixed senile and vascular dementia. These observations indicated many similarities between the two groups with respect to changes in ChAT and AChE activity, and other neurochemical changes. Further exploration and comparison with AD of synaptic and metabolic changes in vascular forms of dementia would be worthwhile because of the possibility that abnormalities in oxygen utilization contribute to neuropathology in both conditions.

A few neurochemical studies of rare forms of dementia such as Pick's disease and progressive supranuclear palsy (PSP) have been reported. Neurochemical deficits in both dopaminergic and cholinergic systems have been reported in PSP.[58]

THERAPY FOR DEMENTIA

Approach to Assessment

Numerous challenges face the clinician wishing to test the effect of drugs in patients with dementia and other cognitive disorders. In most cases, the field has not reached a consensus about the best clinical rating scales, the most appropriate refined tests of cognitive functions, and other features of study design.[71,119] Often beneficial effects in tests of narrow areas of cognition or behavior may not carry over into functionally important areas and may have little practical benefit on clinically significant patient performance. On the other hand, focused testing instruments provide more mechanistic information than is available from more general behavior rating scales.

RATING SCALES AND OTHER OUTCOME MEASURES

Critical evaluation of the importance of the conclusions in the literature requires a careful determination of the dependent variables being measured, along with their limitations.[116] Tests reported in the literature to examine effects of cognition-enhancing drugs include screening tests for orientation and cognition such as the Mini Mental State Examination,[57] ratings of mood or depression such as the Hamilton Depression scale, disability rating scales, activities of daily living, and behavior ratings of social and self-care skills.[116] Detailed neuropsychologic assessments may be comprehensive or focused on one aspect such as verbal or visual spatial memory. Typically portions of several tests are chosen by investigators and combined to measure a broad field of skills (e.g., digit span, naming, language fluency, paired associate memory). Objective laboratory tests are also being used to test effects of cognition-enhancing drugs, but they have not been reported widely. These tests include measurement of cerebral blood flow and glucose metabolic rate using PET and quantitative electroencephalography. These approaches are attractive because they might allow rapid quantitation of effects that in the long term would lead to behavior changes.

An example of a popular clinical assessment tool combining behavior, cognitive, affective, and somatic measures is the Sandoz Clinical Assessment Geriatric scale.[73] This rating scale uses 18 different items plus an overall impression of the patient rated on a seven-point scale. A factor analysis of this scale in more than 500 patients suggests that it measures five factors relatively independently: cognitive dysfunction, interpersonal relationships, apathy, affect, and somatic dysfunction. The analysis suggested that changes in apathy occurred concomitantly with changes in cognitive dysfunction and did not tend to correlate with depression alone. This type of scale is likely to reflect an overall improvement in patient functioning.

PATIENT SELECTION

A careful diagnostic evaluation is important because of the complex array of disorders that may produce dementia.[175] Appropriate staging of patients into homogeneous groups is also extremely important. Several testing scales are sensitive to floor or ceiling effects and are not able to distinguish changes in very mild or very severe cases. Also, careful choice of patients in appropriate stages is needed to test effects of drugs intended to slow or reverse the underlying degenerative changes in dementia as opposed to simply improving function. For example, a therapy that may promote neuron survival during the early, degenerative stages of dementia may be ineffective once a certain threshold of neuron degeneration has been reached. Similarly, therapy intended to improve synaptic efficiency using neurotransmitter replacement may have some effect only if a sufficient mass of the appropriate synaptic machinery remains intact.

Symptomatic Treatment of Behavior Problems

The strategies used to attempt to treat dementia are shown in Table 8–3. Apathy, depression, delusions, confusion, emotional outbursts, sleep disturbances, and a variety of other problems accompany AD and other cognitive disorders. These are often treated empirically and there has been relatively little clinical investigation to delineate and classify these problems or to evaluate rational therapy for them. Some therapies in use, such as ergoloid mesylates, appear to have some effect on these behavior problems. In the past, ampheta-

Table 8–3 POTENTIAL THERAPIES FOR DEMENTIA

Symptomatic therapy
Neurotransmitter therapy
  Cholinergic
    Cholinergic precursors
    Acetylcholinesterase inhibition
    Postsynaptic cholinergic agonists
    Benzodiazepine antagonists
  Adrenergic
  Neuropeptide
Cognition activation therapy
  "Metabolic activators"
  Vasodilators
  Nootropic compounds
Neuroprotective therapies

mines have been tried as stimulants and antidepressants for some patients, but careful study has shown that these drugs have no effect on improving either memory or behavior symptoms.[67,96,135] Neuroleptic drugs such as haloperidol or thioridazine are used commonly to control emotional outbursts, restlessness, and insomnia, and may be particularly useful for delirium. Thioridazine is used frequently and may be superior to benzodiazepines for controlling anxiety and agitation. Benzodiazepines should be used sparingly because they degrade memory at ordinary doses. The actions and use of drugs for behavior disorders and depression were discussed in Chapter 7.

Cholinergic Augmentation Therapy

This has been the most prominent strategy pursued in clinical studies.[11,30,44,124,142] Although attempts to enhance cholinergic neurotransmission in humans have not produced dramatic improvement in AD and memory disorders of aging, several positive studies have stimulated continued interest in this approach. Combinations of precursor therapy to enhance the capacity for acetylcholine production by inhibition of acetylcholine breakdown with anticholinesterase drugs have produced the most consistent, albeit modest, responses (see Tables 8–4 and 8–5). Direct infusion of cholinergic agonists into the brain has also produced some limited positive effects on mood and behavior.

CHOLINERGIC PRECURSOR THERAPY

Because acetylcholine synthesis may be enhanced by loading presynaptic terminals with choline,[183] choline chloride was administered to patients with AD and other neurologic disorders in a series of clinical studies in the late 1970s and early 1980s.[35,84,87,89] Studies of oral choline therapy in patients with

Table 8–4 ACETYLCHOLINESTERASE INHIBITOR THERAPY

Drug	Investigators	Patients	Design	Measurement	Result
Physostigmine 0.8 mg SC	Peters and Levin, 1977[126]	Amnesia, herpes encephalitis	Randomized DBCO placebo	Memory, selective reminding test	Enhanced long-term storage and retrieval
Physostigmine 1 mg IV	Davis, et al, 1978[36]	Normal male subjects	SB, randomized, placebo	Short-term and long-term memory; digit span memory scanning task, retrieval from memory	Enhanced storage retrieval of information from long-term memory
Physostigmine 1 mg SC	Smith and Swash, 1979[153]	Biopsy-proven severe AD, age 55	Randomizd, DBCO, placebo	Raven's colored matrices; word memory	Reduced inappropriate recall (intrusions)
Physostigmine 1 mg qid × 1 mo	Caltagirone, et al, 1982[19]	8 AD <65 years old	Open trial	Mental deterioration battery	Behavior improved; overall no change
Physostigmine 0.125–0.5 mg IV	Davis and Mohs, 1982[33]	10 AD 50–68 years old	Randomized, DBCO, placebo	Famous faces, digit span; pictures	Improved storage into long-term memory
Physostigmine PO 2–2.5 mg/d plus lecithin 10.8 g/d	Thal, et al, 1983[169]	8 early AD	Open and DBCO, placebo	12 trial, free recall task	Decrease in inaccurate recalls correlated to decrease in CSF acetyl-cholinesterase activity
Physostigmine 0.5 mg q2h increased to 4 mg q2h plus lecithin 3.6 g 3 times/d	Thal and Fuld, 1983[168]	12 AD patients	Open trial Responders in DBCO placebo	Buschke and Fuld reminding task	8 patients improved on both trials
Physostigmine 0.01 – .02 mg/kg SC plus lecithin	Wettstein, 1983[177]	8 AD, 3 mild 3 moderate, 2 severe	DBCO	Selective reminding, naming plus drawing, digit span	No change
Physostigmine 0.5–3 mg PO plus 7.2 g oral lecithin	Peters and Levin, 1977[126]	9 patients, 54–79 years old mild–moderate AD; 1 with benign memory disturbance	Open	Selective reminding, digit span 12 trial, 12 item selective reminding tests	Short-term and long-term improvement in long-term recall and storage
Physostigmine	Beller, et al, 1985[7]	8 moderate AD 58–83 years old	Multiple DBCO, placebo	Buschke scale of selective reminding; Sandoz Clinical Assessment	Dose-related verbal memory improvement

(continued)

243

TABLE 8–4—Continued

Drug	Investigators	Patients	Design	Measurement	Result
Physostigmine 0–2 mg/d q 2 × 3–5 d	Mohs, et al, 1985[115]	12 AD, 52–76 years old	Dose finding Randomized, DBCO, placebo	Alzheimer assessment scale	3 improved; 4 marginally improved
Physostigmine 0.004–0.13 mg/kg IM plus lecithin PO	Schwartz and Kohlstaedt, 1986[144]	11 AD, 61–83 years old	Placebo controlled, DBCO placebo	Buschke-Fuld selective reminding word list	Improved memory correlated with severity; 4 patients had behavior improvement
Physostigmine 13 mg/d orally	Stern, et al, 1988[159]	AD	DBCO placebo	Selective reminding test; neuropsychologic battery	Improved on Wechsler Adult Intelligence Scale revised digit symbol subtest; no change in selective reminding test; improvement sustained during 1 yr
THA IV	Summers, et al, 1981[162]	Alzheimer-like dementia	Open testing 1, 6, and 24 h postinfusion	Orientation test; names learning test; clinical staging	6/12 improved memory; 9/12 improved globally
THA oral 15–200 mg/d plus lecithin	Summers, et al, 1986[161]	17 moderate to severe AD	Open Randomized DBCO placebo Long term	Global assessment, orientation test, name learning test, Alzheimer deficit scale	14/17 patients improved in recent memory and orientation; long-term global severity improved at 1 yr; functional improvement
THA 30 mg plus lecithin 6.0 g	Kaye, et al, 1982[95]	10 AD 51–71 years old	4 trials; lecithin ± placebo and THA ± placebo	Serial learning, Buschke recall, free word recall	Milder group had enhanced performance
THA 100 mg/d plus lecithin 4.7 g/d	Gauthier, et al (Canadian Multicenter Trial), 1990[63]	46 AD; intermediate stage; mean age 67 years old: 39 completed	Titration to maximal tolerated dose; DBCO	Mini Mental State; Hierarchic dementia scale, Rapid Disability Rating II, Reisberg Behavior scale	No clinical benefit; Mini Mental showed small significant increase

Key: AD = Alzheimer's disease; DBCO = double-blind crossover; CSF = cerebrospinal fluid; PC = placebo controlled; SB = single blind; THA = tetrahydroaminoacridine; ("tacrine").

TABLE 8–5 MUSCARINIC AGONIST THERAPY

Drug	Investigators	Patients	Design	Measurement	Result
Arecoline 4 mg SC plus oral choline 10 g/d	Sitaram, et al, 1978[150]	Normal college students	Randomized SB, placebo	Categorized serial learning list of words	Improvement inversely related to baseline performance
Bethanechol chloride, intracerebroventricular infusion 0.22–0.33 mg/d; 12 weeks drug vs. placebo	Harbaugh, 1987[74]	12 AD 55–82 years old (10 biopsies, AD; 1 Pick; 1 nondiagnostic)	Open and randomized, DBCO with placebo	Wechsler Adult Intelligence Scale subtests; Wechsler memory scale; Buschke-Fuld selective reminding; word fluency; Boston naming; Mini Mental State	Significant improvement, drug vs. placebo: no clear improvement in activities of daily living
Bethanechol (intracerebroventricular) 1) 0.35 mg/d in 4-wk periods by intracerebroventricular route 2) Escalating dose to 1.75 mg/d	Penn, et al, 1988[123]	11 AD; mean age = 64.9 y	Randomized DBCO with placebo Open escalating dose	Mini Mental State; controlled oral word association; Benton's serial selective reminding; activities of daily living; daily patient behavior report; reaction time; alertness; language comprehension; picture naming	1) No difference 2) Improvement related to escalating dose in serial digit learning, behavior scales; higher doses (1.05 mg/d) improved behavior but Mini Mental State, reaction time, and activities of daily living worse

(continued)

TABLE 8–5—*Continued*

Drug	Investigators	Patients	Design	Measurement	Result
Bethanechol 0.1 mg/kg SC plus methylscopolamine	Davous and Lamour, 1985[37]	16 AD, age 46–80	8 nonrandom assigned to either saline or bethanechol plus methyl-scopolamine	Reaction time	Shorten reaction time 15 min but not 30 min later
RS-86, 18-wk period; up to 3.0 mg orally	Wettstein and Spiegel, 1984[178]	AD	PC dose finding study DBCO during 6-wk periods at 0.75 mg qid in 6 patients	Mini Mental State, word and picture recognition, visuomotor tasks, list learning	Improved picture recognition, picture matching, visuomotor task (high dropout rate)
RS-86, 0.5–5 mg/kg/per day	Bruno, et al, 1986[17]	8 AD, mild to moderate	Double blind, PC	Tests of verbal and pictorial memory; dichotic listening and reaction time	No consistent change
RS-86, up to 4 mg	Foster, et al, 1989[58]	10 patients with progressive supranuclear palsy	9 week PC, DBCO	Selective reminding, visual spatial memory	No improvement

Key: AD = Alzheimer's disease; DBCO = double-blind crossover; PC = placebo controlled; SB = single blind.

tardive dyskinesia suggest that this strategy may enhance central cholinergic activity under certain circumstances,[71] but administration of up to 16 mg of choline chloride per day was not effective in improving cognitive disorders in AD.[4] Administration of the choline precursor deanol also had little effect.[51,54,103]

Lecithin (phosphatidylcholine, PC) has also been used to provide choline for the synthesis of acetylcholine.[14,15,21,43,47,48,102] Choline chloride produces an unpleasant fishy odor in patients because of a breakdown product in the gastrointestinal tract. When given as PC, little odor is produced and reasonably high levels of choline in the blood can be produced during 6 to 8 hours. Relatively pure PC must be used to produce these levels, however. Most commercially available lecithin may contain as little as 15% of PC, with the remainder representing related phosphatide compounds. Lecithin is normally contained in the diet in eggs or soybeans, but this is an inefficient way of increasing lecithin consumption. Approximately half the PC ingested is absorbed across the gastrointestinal tract undegraded. A dose of 9 grams of 8% pure PC has been reported to increase plasma choline levels approximately twofold (to approximately 16 nmol/mg) within 2 hours and the level is maintained for approximately 4 hours. A dose of 9 g of PC given twice, 4 hours apart, may produce peak levels almost four times higher than normal plasma choline levels. In the form of relatively pure PC, lecithin appears to be a well-tolerated method, superior to oral choline chloride, for producing a sustained increase in plasma choline levels.

Although lecithin administration appears helpful for patients with tardive dyskinesia, who may have relatively intact cholinergic nerve endings, controlled and open studies[14,21,35,43,47,48,54,102] have not shown this therapy alone to be helpful for symptomatic improvement of patients with age-related cognitive disorders or AD. Lecithin was also used in a 6-month, randomized, double-blind trial in patients with early AD to determine whether it would prevent disease progression.[82] This trial was based on the hypothesis described previously, that autodestruction of cholinergic neuron membranes might result from consumption of phospholipids to produce choline. In this trial, lecithin alone had no important therapeutic effect on this early-onset group. As outlined in the next section, however several studies have detected a possible enhancing effect of lecithin on memory improvement produced by anticholinesterase therapies.

AChE INHIBITION THERAPY

Several randomized, double-blind trials suggest that physostigmine, a rapidly acting AChE inhibitor, produces a small, transient, but measurable improvement in memory in patients with AD (see Table 8–4).* A single injection may also enhance storage and retrieval of information from long-term memory in normal subjects. Another report indicates that physostigmine enhances retrieval from long-term memory in normal subjects. Another report indicates that physostigmine enhances retrieval from long-term memory in patients with amnesia.[126] Davis and Mohs[33] found that intravenous physostigmine improves long-term memory storage in Alzheimer's patients in a randomized, double-blind, crossover, placebo-controlled trial using famous-faces, digit-span, and picture-recognition tests. Thal and associates[169] found an improvement in the selective reminding test in 12 Alzheimer's patients when oral physostigmine was combined with oral lecithin. Schwartz and Kohlstaedt[144] also reported improvement from intramuscular physostigmine and oral lecithin on the selective reminding test in patients with AD.

---

*References 20, 33, 34, 36, 117, 125, 151, 153, 168, 169.

Assessment of the effects of physostigmine is difficult, however, because of its narrow therapeutic window; high or low doses may be ineffective.[129] Many studies of physostigmine have been criticized because the optimal dose was not determined for each patient. This factor was taken into consideration in a study by Stern and colleagues,[159] which examined the response of patients to different daily doses of oral physostigmine using a selective reminding test. An optimal dose per day was determined in nine patients, with a mode of 13 mg/d, which was used in a subsequent double-blind crossover study. The other 13 patients were given the highest dose tolerated. The selective reminding test and a full neuropsychologic battery were given during the drug and placebo periods. As a group, the 22 patients improved significantly on the Wechsler Adult Intelligence Scale, a digit symbol subtest, and a shape cancellation test. Nine patients showed improved performance on the selective reminding test during physostigmine therapy, nine showed no response, and four performed better during placebo treatment. The dose did not help in predicting the response in the crossover study, and only two of the nine showed improvement on the best dose. Also, dementia severity did not predict crossover response. The authors suggested that physostigmine had no pronounced effect on memory in AD and had no greater benefits in mildly than in moderately demented patients. They did note that the digit symbol and shape cancellation tests appeared to be more sensitive than memory tests to the effect of oral physostigmine.

With few exceptions,[177] most of the clinical research on physostigmine suggests that it produces modest temporary improvement. Stern's group,[159] however, found that the effects of oral physostigmine were sustained during 1 year in some individuals. Trials using physostigmine may well underestimate the value of anticholinesterase therapy because of the drug's short half-life and potential for troublesome systemic side

effects at effective doses. Studies have not demonstrated an improvement in activities of daily living.

In contrast, a long-acting anticholinesterase drug, THA, has been reported to improve memory and general functioning in AD patients. A study of 12 patients[162] reported transient improvement after intravenous THA; a follow-up study[161] reported improvement with a combination of oral THA plus lecithin in 17 patients. In an open phase of the study, improvement occurred in the subjects' performance on a global assessment scale, an orientation test, and a name-learning test. During a second phase, subjects served as their own controls in a double-blind, placebo-controlled, crossover study in which the order of administration of the drug and placebo was randomly assigned. Fourteen subjects completed the second phase of the THA trial and improved on the global assessment scale, orientation test, and the name-learning test. Twelve subjects who entered phase 3 for long-term administration of oral THA reported symptomatic improvements during a 1-year period with no serious side effects. This report stimulated considerable interest, and THA is undergoing continued clinical investigation. The original study design has drawn a number of criticisms, however, about the inclusion criteria for patients and the rating scales used to assess their improvement. In a larger, multicenter double-blind crossover trial of 46 AD patients given up to 100 mg/d of THA plus 4.7 g/d of lecithin, no clinical benefit was found,[63] although there was a significant improvement in the Mini Mental State test. THA is currently being considered for approval by the US FDA for treatment of dementia.

POSTSYNAPTIC CHOLINERGIC AGONIST THERAPY

Strategies that attempt to enhance production of acetylcholine molecules or prevent their destruction might be limited by the destructive effect of AD on cholinergic nerve terminals. As already noted, however, muscarinic acetylcholine receptors on postsynaptic neurons have been reported to be preserved. Muscarinic agonists have been administered in clinical trials to stimulate them (see Table 8–5). A potential limitation of this approach is that all muscarinic receptors would be stimulated at the same time, and the normal spatial and temporal modulation of acetylcholine provided by the biochemical machinery within the presynaptic nerve terminals will be lost. Nevertheless, this strategy has received considerable attention.[18–20,150]

Just as muscarinic blockade degrades memory in younger people, some evidence suggests that muscarinic agonists may produce a small improvement. Sitaram and associates[150] administered subcutaneous arecoline and oral choline to normal college students in a randomized, single-blind, placebo-controlled study and demonstrated an improvement in their ability to learn a serial list of words. The improvement appeared to be inversely correlated to each subject's baseline performance, suggesting that the chemotherapy helped poor learners more than better learners. Arecoline is a natural alkaloid acting at muscarinic receptors, but it also has a significant nicotinic action. The contribution of nicotinic receptor stimulation is uncertain, although there is some evidence that they may play a marginal role in cognition.[179] However, RS-86, another muscarinic agonist, did not help AD patients in a controlled trial.[17,18] RS-86 also failed to improve memory in patients with progressive supranuclear palsy, who also have a deficit in cholinergic systems in the brain.[58]

Bethanechol, a stable choline ester that is resistant to cholinesterase activity and lacks significant action at nicotinic receptors, has been reported to augment memory in patients when given subcutaneously. At least two trials of direct intracerebral ventricular administration of bethanechol in AD patients have been reported. In Harbaugh's study,[74] neuropsychologic testing showed small but significant improvement compared with placebo and baseline, but the improvement in activities of daily living was less striking (see Table 8–5). A group led by Penn[123] performed a study of intracerebroventricular bethanechol in two parts: (1) a randomized, double-blind, crossover study with placebo at a fixed daily dose and (2) an escalating dose study. They found no difference in the Mini Mental State Examination or other neuropsychologic testing in the first part. In the escalating dose phase, however, there were improvements in the serial digit learning and behavior scales. At higher doses, they noted improved behavior but reduced performance on the Mini Mental State, reaction-time, and activities-of-daily-living tests.

EXPERIMENTAL BENZODIAZEPINE ANTAGONISTS

Another approach to therapy that has received attention in clinical studies involves enhancing the activity of remaining cholinergic neurons by disinhibiting them. Some pharmacologic evidence suggests that activity of cholinergic neurons, acetylcholine release, and high-affinity choline uptake may be under the control of the inhibitory amino acid GABA and benzodiazepine receptors.[141] As noted previously, benzodiazepine drugs are a common clinical cause of reversible memory loss. In experimental studies, injection of GABA agonists into the basal forebrain of rats decreases acetylcholine release.[14] Anatomic evidence suggests that GABA terminals in the basal forebrain may synapse on cholinergic cell bodies, and the density of benzodiazepine-binding sites in the basal forebrain is relatively high. Benzodiazepines and related beta-carboline compounds with agonist activity have been shown to induce amnesia. In contrast, antagonist beta-carboline compounds such as ZK93426 are able to attenuate the disruptive effects of scopolamine in a passive avoidance test in mice. The compound has also been reported to improve memory performance in these animals. In one double-blind, placebo-controlled study, ZK93426 improved performance in a logic reasoning and picture differences test in young human volunteers.[141] This group of drugs might provide a new approach toward enhancing the activity of cholinergic neurons relatively selectively.

The cholinergic hypothesis of memory dysfunction in AD has generated a large amount of clinical research, but no therapy has emerged that is clearly beneficial. The modest effects of the presynaptic and postsynaptic cholinergic therapies is disappointing but does not destroy the foundation of the hypothesis. The few positive results provide a basis for further work to improve the function of cholinergic neurons and promote their survival.

Therapies Directed Toward Other Neurotransmitter Targets

Several clinical studies have examined the effects of drugs that act on other neurotransmitter-specific synaptic targets, but results have generally not been strikingly successful (Table 8–6). Based on a potential role of dopaminergic catecholamine pathways in cortical function, at least three studies[91,97,100] have examined the effects of L-dopa on patients with dementia and found no effect. The alpha-2 adrenergic agonist clonidine has been reported[16] to improve spatial working memory in aged monkeys and has also been reported[106] to improve memory in patients with amnesia from Korsakoff's syndrome, although a recent double-blind, placebo-controlled trial in eight patients with AD showed no effect.[114]

Therapeutic trials of several neuropeptides have aroused interest. The neuropeptide vasopressin has been implicated in learning and memory in animals, and several studies have reported small statistical improvements in memory in limited patient groups (see Table 8–6).[99] This does not appear to be an effective strategy, however. Adrenocorticotropic hormone (ACTH) and its analogue amino acids 4-10 and 4-9 (ORG 2766) have been shown to have an effect on memory in animals but only small effects have been found in humans.[154] It has been suggested that ACTH may act in animals more to increase motivation than to enhance memory.

Reports that opioid compounds may interfere with memory led to several small investigations of the antagonist naloxone. Although one report[134] demonstrated a positive response in seven AD patients, a subsequent controlled and blinded study[80] did not confirm this result. Other potential directions for synaptic neurotransmitter chemotherapy could include the serotonin system, which appears to be heavily disrupted in AD.[12,13]

None of the other neurotransmitter therapies appears to have potential for clinical utility in the foreseeable future. Their demonstrated effect is far less than the very modest effects produced by cholinergic manipulation. Although the present state of neurotransmitter enhancement therapy for AD is primitive, interest is high, as new observations about the pathophysiology of the disease emerge. Several trials are underway to enhance other neurotransmitter systems, including EAA pathways. It is likely that this clinical investigative activity also will spill over into attempts to treat other cognitive disorders such as multi-infarct dementia and posttraumatic amnesia.

"Cognition-Activating" Drugs

The most fashionable current rationales for therapy of cognitive disorders are based on information about specific lesions in neurotransmitter systems. The most widely used drugs, however, are thought to be "cognition activators," which do not have well-defined mechanisms of action (Table 8–7).[67]

Table 8–6 THERAPIES DIRECTED TO NONCHOLINERGIC SYNAPTIC TARGETS

Drugs	Investigators	Patients	Result
NEUROTRANSMITTERS			
L-dopa	Lewis, et al, 1978[100]	14 dementia	Improved communication, intellectual function
L-dopa	Johnson, et al, 1978[91]	5 dementia	No effect
L-dopa	Kristensen, et al, 1977[97]	18 demented treated 6 mo	No effect
Memantine (dopaminergic agent)	Fleishhacker, et al, 1986[55]	20 AD	No change
Clonidine	McEntee and Mair, 1980[106]	8 Korsakoff's syndrome	Improved memory, in contrast to amphetamine and methylsergide
Clonidine	Mohs, et al, 1989[114]	8 AD	No effect at doses that produce side effects
NEUROPEPTIDE AGENTS			
Vasopressin nasal spray	Oliverso, et al, 1978[118]	4 amnesia, alcohol and trauma	Improved memory
Desmopressin	Jenkins, et al, 1981[90]	5 posttraumatic amnesia	No change
Vasopressin	Weingartner, et al, 1981[174]	Dementia	Statistical improvement
Vasopressin	Anderson, et al, 1979[1]	3 Lesch-Nyhan patients	Improved passive avoidance learning
Vasopressin	Peabody, et al, 1986[121]	14 AD patients	Less depression, no cognitive scale change
ACTH	deWied and van Ree, 1982[41]	Aging	Improvement in amnesia, cognitive disturbances in aging
ACTH 4-10	Ferris, et al, 1976[52]	24 older patients, memory loss, aging	No change, verbal memory; slight change, visual memory
ACTH 4-9 (Org 2766)	Soininen, et al, 1985[154]	77 AD patients	No effect
Naloxone	Reisberg, et al, 1983[134]	7 AD patients	Positive
Naloxone	Steiger, et al, 1985[158]	AD	No effect
Naloxone	Henderson, et al, 1989[80]	54 AD, DBCO, PC, 1–30 mg	No effect

Key: ACTH = adrenocorticotropic hormone; AD = Alzheimer's disease; DBCO = double-blind crossover; PC = placebo controlled.

The first therapies for dementia were aimed at improving cerebral blood flow, based on the theory that cerebral atherosclerosis caused a range of confusional and dementing disorders in the elderly. This led to the development of potentially vasoactive drugs including ergoloid mesylates and papaverine. Now it is recognized that reduced cerebral blood flow in patients with dementia is related predominantly to a reduction in demand and in cerebral glucose metabolic rate. Attempts to increase blood flow are not thought to be helpful even if

Table 8–7 "COGNITION-ACTIVATING" COMPOUNDS

Drugs	Investigators	Patients	Result
VASOACTIVE/METABOLISM-ENHANCING			
Ergoloid mesylates (approved for use in dementia)	McDonald, 1979[105] Holister and Yesavage, 1984[85] Kopelman and Lishman, 1986[96]	30 studies in AD and mixed dementia	Consistent modest improvement
Nafronyl (naftidrofuryl)	Thompson, et al, 1990[170] Gerin, 1974[64]	80 patients in DBCO study Elderly confused patients	No effect Inconsistent improvement
Pyritinol (vitamin B_6 derivative)	Cook and James, 1981[26] Tazaki, et al, 1980[167] Herrmann, et al, 1986[81]	Elderly, cerebrovascular disorders	Electroencephalogram improvement; equivocal changes in deterioration of cognitive function
Papaverine	Cook and James, 1981[25] Yesavage, et al, 1979[186]	Mixed dementia	Several studies report modest improvement but consensus is no practical improvement
Cyclandelate	Westreich, et al, 1975[176] Davie, et al, 1978[29] Cook and James, 1981[25]	Mixed dementia	Inconsistent or no improvement
Isoxsuprine	Yesavage, et al, 1979[186]	Mixed dementia	No practical benefit
Cinnarizine	Cook and James, 1981[26] Passerl, 1978[120]	"Chronic ischemia," dementia	Controlled double-blind studies showing benefit and lack of benefit
OTHER COMPOUNDS			
Nicotinic acid	Cook and James, 1981[26]	Dementia	No double-blind studies; positive anecdotes
NOOTROPIC DRUGS			
Piracetam	Friedman, et al, 1981[60] Ezzat, et al, 1985[49] Growden, et al, 1986[70] Tallal, et al, 1986[165]	Dementia, amnesia, AD	Positive and negative double-blind controlled studies of AD; verbal memory better; positive reports in dyslexia and postelectroshock amnesia
Pramiracetam	Poschel et al, 1983[131]		
4-aminopyridine	Goodnick and Gershon[67]	AD patients	Improvement

Key: AD = Alzheimer's disease; DBCO = double-blind crossover.

it were possible. Vasodilation in multi-infarct dementia also would not be useful.

Despite this change in perspective, several of the vasoactive drugs appear to have some beneficial clinical effects. The explanation for these effects is unknown and does not appear to involve cerebral blood flow. There is some evidence that these compounds may enhance neuron metabolism in relatively nonspecific ways, which would have the effect of augmenting production of important molecules such as AcCoA for acetcylcholine. Because of their uncertain mechanism, they are referred to as vasoactive/metabolism-enhancing compounds.

VASOACTIVE/METABOLISM-ENHANCING DRUGS

Ergoloid Mesylates. Ergoloid mesylates (Hydergine) is approved by the US FDA for treatment of dementia. It is also approved in several other countries. A mixture of hydrogenated ergot alkaloids including dihydroergocristine mesylate and dihydroergocryptine mesylate, it has been reported to have activity to block alpha-adrenergic receptors. It may have several other synaptic effects, including agonist actions of serotonin and dopamine receptors. Ergoloid mesylates may also have a direct effect on cerebral metabolism.

Several studies have reported improved functioning in demented patients given ergoloid mesylates (see Table 8–7). Most studies report modest but statistically significant effects; a few patients are said to be markedly improved. Improvements, often measured using the Sandoz Clinical Assessment Geriatric scale, have been more in the behavior realm than in cognitive function, however. Most studies have been limited to 3 months but it has been reported[85] that some patients continue to respond during 6 months. Improvements in various studies from 11% to 20% have been reported in ratings of self-care, emotional lability, recent memory, orientation, mental alertness,

confusion, and mood depression. A recent placebo-controlled, double-blind trial in 80 patients, however, found no benefit of ergoloid mesylates.[170]

The commonly recommended dose is 1 mg three times a day, but doses up to 12 mg have been used in some studies. The drug may produce hypertension or headache but is generally well tolerated. The mean half-life of unchanged drug in plasma is approximately 4 hours. Despite the fact that a clearcut therapeutic rationale is lacking, some experts suggest that a trial of ergoloid mesylates may be worthwhile in many patients since little other therapy is available.

Vasodilators. Several other drugs approved by the Food and Drug Administration as vasodilators for peripheral-vascular disease have been studied in demented patients with poor results (see Table 8–7). Naftidrofuryl has been used in Europe for elderly confused patients but improvement is inconsistent.[27] Cinnarizine is a vasodilating and calcium antagonist compound prescribed in Europe for vertigo and dementia related to chronic ischemia. Several double-blind studies have been performed showing some benefit, but others showed none.[26,120] Papaverine, cyclandelate, and isoxsuprine have also been studied in dementia based on their vasodilator effects, but no beneficial effect was found. Papaverine has been reported to produce improvement in psychologic test scores in six of nine double-blind control studies, but only one study claimed practical clinical benefit.[25,186]

A vitamin B_6 derivative, pyritinol, has also been studied with mixed results in elderly patients with dementia related to cerebrovascular diseases.[81] Vasodilator drugs may have an effect on energy metabolism. Pentoxifylline, a vasodilator that may improve memory in animals, reportedly acts to increase adenosine triphosphate and inhibit phosphodiesterase.[26]

The potential impact of these drugs on multi-infarct dementia has not been separated from effects on a population with mixed AD, vascular dementia, and other causes.[120] In general, studies of "vasodilator" drugs have suffered from inadequate patient classification and poor experimental design.

Other Compounds. Several other miscellaneous drugs have been used for dementia but also have no convincing evidence to support their use. Nicotinic acid, which may act as a vasodilator, and the local anesthetic procaine have been recommended anecdotally[26] both for mixed dementia and memory loss of healthy older subjects. Another potentially interesting drug that has received little study is 4-aminopyridine, which may alter calcium influx and enhance neurotransmitter release and/or stimulate neurotransmitter synthesis. One brief study found that 4-aminopyridine improved memory in 14 AD patients during a 6-week period.[67]

NOOTROPIC DRUGS:
PIRACETAM AND
ITS ANALOGUES

The word "nootropic" was coined to describe a class of drugs that selectively improve cognitive efficiency without other psychoactive features. The precise boundaries of this classification are vague, and several types of drugs with apparent cognition-enhancing activity, including ergoloid mesylates, might fit into this group. The experimental prototype drug, piracetam (2-oxo-1-pyrrolidineacetamide, Nootropil) has been used in Europe but is not approved in the United States. Piracetam shows little significant toxicity in animal studies and has been used in clinical investigations in children and adults without apparent side effects.

In animal experiments, piracetam improves learning acquisition, habituation, and retrieval in normal rodents.[62] It has also been shown to block amnesia produced by hypoxia and electroconvulsive shock and to antagonize scopolamine-induced memory disruption.[139,140] Piracetam was the first in a

series of related compounds including pramiracetam, aniracetam, oxiracetam, and etiracetam, which have similar pharmacologic profiles. The mechanisms for piracetam's robust effects in animal experiments are unknown. Although it resembles the structure of GABA, piracetam does not modify GABA levels in the brain. One group of researchers[185] found that piracetam decreased acetylcholine levels by 32% in the hippocampus of naive rats, suggesting that it increased acetylcholine turnover. Others[5] reported a marked improvement in memory in rats given a combination of choline and piracetam. They also found that piracetam reduced endogenous acetylcholine in the hippocampus, and suggested that piracetam was able to augment acetylcholine turnover and enhance use of additional choline.

In Europe, piracetam is used to treat cognitive disorders.[113] It is rapidly absorbed orally, reaching peak plasma levels after abut 30 minutes and has a half-life of approximately 5 hours.[164] Villardita and colleagues[171] reported that 1600 mg/d of oxiracetam in 40 outpatients with mild-to-moderate dementia produced significant improvement on the Mini Mental State Examination, an auditory continuous performance task, word fluency,and instrumental activities of daily living. They reported no side effects. Some investigators[50] reported improvement in some patients on choline plus piracetam. Bartus and co-workers[4,5] reported that the responders had higher baseline levels of red-cell choline than nonresponders. Growdon and associates[70] administered piracetam alone or in combination with PC to 18 patients with AD and measured the effects of treatment on a broad range of cognitive functions. They used double-blind, crossover protocols, and the replication study used a higher dose of piracetam with and without PC given concurrently. Blood choline levels rose significantly during piracetam and PC administration but the treatment did not affect cognition in the AD group as a whole or in any single patient. The patients in the study, however, had mild-to-moderate dementia and tended to be younger than many Alzheimer patients, with a mean age of 64 (none older than 75 years of age). This difference may have explained differences from previous results.

Therefore, nootropic drugs have shown especially promising results in preclinical studies but there is as yet little clearcut evidence that they are effective in AD patients.[77] This strategy may be useful for other related cognitive disorders such as dyslexia, however (see later discussion). An effect on amnesia produced by electroshock has also been reported. Ezzat and colleagues[49] used the Wechsler Memory test to compare two groups of depressed patients given electroshock therapy. They found that intravenous piracetam was able to prevent memory loss in the treated group.

Neuroprotection: Strategies for Promoting Neuron Survival or Restoring Neuron Function

Most of the pharmacologic strategies attempted for cognitive disorders, such as replacing neurotransmitters, have focused on repairing important symptomatic cognitive deficits with chemicals. Another approach is to attempt to retard or reverse the fundamental process responsible for neuron degeneration. Definitive therapy for AD and other degenerative disorders will be based on information about the underlying biochemical defects, but several experimental strategies are currently being developed to attempt to arrest the degenerative process.[32,61]

NERVE GROWTH FACTOR

One strategy would use neurotrophic factors to promote neuron survival.[130] Nerve growth factor (NGF) is one protein of interest because it appears to promote survival of developing or injured cholinergic forebrain neurons.[76,98] Cholinergic neurons retrogradely transport labelled NGF injected into the cortex. There is a close relationship during development between expression of messenger RNA for NGF and the expression of the acetylcholine synthetic enzyme ChAT.[104,112] NGF acts as a survival factor, and several investigators have hypothesized that administration of NGF (or molecules that imitate it) at the NGF receptor, which is highly localized to basal forebrain neurons, might slow the degenerative process.[130] Recently, one study[53] showed in aged rats that impairments in learning and memory could be reversed by constant infusions of NGF into the brain. These infusions of NGF were also associated with an enlargement of basal forebrain cholinergic neurons, which become shrunken in aged animals.

GM1 GANGLIOSIDE

Another growth factor–like substance is GM1 ganglioside. Gangliosides in the brain are complex lipids associated with developing synapse. Parenteral administration of GM1 ganglioside is capable of preventing neuron degeneration in several animal models.[56,155] Parenterally administered GM1 ganglioside also has been shown to prevent retrograde degeneration of cholinergic neurons in the rat basal forebrain resulting from damage to the cerebral cortex and underlying hippocampus.[155] Florian and associates[56] demonstrated that a reduction in acetylcholine release from the cerebral cortex induced by unilateral lesions of the nucleus basalis could be prevented by administration of GM1 ganglioside. Although these strategies are in the very early stages of development, they represent concrete examples in animal models where endogenous trophic molecules potentially could be used to treat degenerative diseases such as AD.

ANTIOXIDANT THERAPY

Another potential strategy for treating degenerative diseases is currently being tested for Parkinson's disease. As described in Chapter 2, excessive oxidation of catecholamine in nigra striatal neurons has been implicated in the pathogenesis of Parkinson's disease. Antioxidant therapy, including vitamin E and monoamine oxidase inhibitor therapy, is being used in clinical trials to determine if the progress of Parkinson's disease can be reversed (see Chapter 2, reference 61). There is little concrete evidence to suggest a similar process in AD, though this type of antioxidant preventive therapy might also be used to slow the progress.

COGNITIVE DISORDERS IN YOUNG PEOPLE

Learning disabilities and mental retardation are disorders of the developing brain that result in fixed cognitive deficits in adults. While interest in degenerative cognitive diseases of adults has increased dramatically during the past decade, attention to the more static problems in children has plateaued during the same period, after a surge of research effort in the 1960s and 1970s.

Until recently, little direct neurobiologic or therapeutic connection has been drawn between these disorders and degenerative cognitive disorders in adults. New research, however, suggests the possibility that there may be common molecular links that could lead to therapeutic strategies. Such a connection has been drawn between mental retardation found in Down's syndrome and AD. Middle-aged Down's syndrome patients uniformly develop neuropathologic features of AD and become demented at a higher-than-expected rate. Also, brains from Down's syndrome patients accumulate pre-A4 amyloid protein at a much earlier age than in the normal aging population.[138] Since the gene for this protein found in excess in AD is on chromosome 21, its overexpression may be a result of extra chromosome 21 material. Neuropathologic and experimental studies indicate that brains of Down's syndrome and AD patients share a similar defect in cortical innervation by acetylcholine-con-

taining neurons. These observations suggest that in the future certain cognitive deficits in Down's syndrome might be altered by early pharmacologic intervention. The neurobiologic substrate for other types of mental retardation, which might be relevant to therapy, is not understood.

Dyslexia and Learning Disabilities

Learning disabilities produce relatively specific patterns of cognitive deficit and impede information acquisition, processing, and memory storage in children and adults. The neurobiologic basis of these abnormalities are not known, although defects in neuron migration to the cerebral cortex have been suggested. In clinical practice, many children with learning disabilities also have disorders of attention.

Dyslexia, in which processing of written language is disturbed, is a common component of many learning disabilities. Surprisingly, certain cognition-enhancing drugs such as piracetam have been reported to improve the reading ability of dyslexic children in several careful studies. Wilsher and associates[181] tested piracetam in 14 student volunteers and 16 male dyslexic boys, ages 17 to 24 years, in a double-blind, crossover technique. In a later study,[182] they found improvement in reading rate and in performance on a complex cognitive task. They also found that piracetam increased verbal learning by 15% in the dyslexic students and by 8.6% in the control group. Other researchers[78,79] reported that piracetam improved the performance of 30 boys, 8 to 13 years of age, on reading accuracy and also reported that short-term memory was improved. They also found improved immediate and delayed recall. Others[23,24] have investigated visual event-related potentials in a double-blind, placebo-controlled study and reported increased amplitude of the late positive component related to seeing a letter.

Tallal and colleagues[165] gave piracetam in a dose of 3300 mg/d to half of a group of 55 dyslexic boys, ages 8 to 13 years, in a 12-week, double-blind, placebo-control study. These subjects had normal intelligence and normal educational opportunities, no severe emotional problems or neurologic handicaps, and were in good general health and not taking other medication. They were, however, 1.5 years below their mental-age equivalent on an oral reading test. Compared with placebo, piracetam increased reading speed and the number of words written in a fixed time interval. This suggested that piracetam improves verbal fluency and increases rates of reading and writing accuracy. These studies are interesting because they provide the most well-documented evidence that this class of drugs does improve cognitive function in humans. However, their practical relevance is not established and this form of therapy is not yet approved by the Food and Drug Administration.

Attention Deficit Disorder

Attention deficit disorder is a relatively common problem in children who manifest developmentally inappropriate inattention, impulsivity, and hyperactivity. Therapy usually includes special help in the classroom and may also include stimulant medications that can help focus attention including methylphenidate (Ritalin), pemoline (Cylert), and dextroamphetamine (Dexedrine). These medications enhance the activity of catecholamine pathways in the cerebral cortex and the rest of the brain, enhancing learning and attention. Their action on catecholamine nerve terminals is to promote catecholamine release and inhibit reuptake into nerve terminals.

Whether the success of these medications for hyperactivity indicates that there is an underlying defect in catecholamine metabolism in children with hyperactivity remains uncertain. One study[146] reported a group of hyperactive boys who had low cerebrospinal fluid concentrations of the dopamine metab-

olite HVA. On the other hand, hyperactivity with attention deficit disorder may be found in children with Tourette's syndrome, who reportedly may have excessive activity in central dopamine pathways (see Chapter 2, p 72). Dextroamphetamine has also been shown to improve attention even in normal teenagers, suggesting that the effects of stimulants may be to enhance normal functioning rather than to replace a deficiency.[132]

Titration of the dose of stimulant medication is important for achieving a beneficial effect. Sprague and Sleator[156] examined the dose response to methylphenidate in hyperactive children for effects on learning and social behavior. They found that peak enhancement of learning occurred after a dose of 0.3 mg/kg body weight, while peak enhancement of social behavior occurred after a dose of 1 mg/kg. The results suggest that learning may actually be degraded at doses that produce the most decrease in hyperactivity.

Treatment with methylphenidate is generally started with 5 to 10 mg/d and gradually increased to a maximum dose of 60 mg/d. A once-daily dose may produce enough improvement in schoolwork and attention that further doses are unnecessary, although patients are often given twice-daily doses. A sustained-release preparation is available that lasts approximately 8 hours. Dextroamphetamine sulfate is given in doses approximately one half the dose of methylphenidate. Pemoline is longer-acting than either of the other stimulant medications and is generally given once daily. The recommended starting dose is 37.5 mg, and it is increased by increments of 18.75 mg until the desired response is achieved. Doses are generally limited to 112.5 mg.

All the stimulant medications share the adverse effects of anorexia, insomnia, risk of paradoxic hyperactivity, and delirium in some patients. Their use must be monitored carefully, with periodic physical examination, measurement of blood pressure, and assessment of learning and behavior. An uncommon side effect is precipitation of motor tics. This is especially likely to occur in children genetically predisposed to Tourette's syndrome. Withdrawal of the medication generally leads to reduction in the tics. However, many experts believe that tics are not a contraindication to continued use of stimulants.

SUMMARY

Therapy for cognitive disorders is an emerging field stimulated by the enlarging aged population and a more sophisticated understanding of the neurobiology of cognitive brain disorders. Current standard therapy is focused on managing attention and behavior disorders that accompany cognitive disabilities such as dementia, but active investigational efforts are directed at treating synaptic neurotransmitter abnormalities and underlying neurochemical abnormalities. The most prominent neurotransmitter "replacement" or augmentation strategy for AD has focused on the defect in acetylcholine neurotransmission. Although the improvements achieved have not been dramatic, modest effects continue to stimulate interest. Other neurotransmitter strategies are being explored. Another group of cognition-enhancing (nootropic) compounds show some promise for certain disorders such as dyslexia, and may be developed in the future. On the horizon are strategies to retard certain degenerative processes by using specific neuron growth factors or antioxidant compounds. This area of therapy will be an increasingly important one in the coming years.

REFERENCES

1. Anderson, LT, David, R, Bonnet, K, and Dancis, J: Passive avoidance learning in Lesch-Nyhan disease: Effect of 1-desamino-8-arginine-vasopressin. Life Sci 24:905–910, 1979.
2. Arnsten, AFT and Goldman-Rakic, PS: Noradrenergic mechanisms in age-related cognitive decline. J Neural Transm (Suppl 24) 24:317–324, 1987.
3. Barany, M, Chang, YC, Arus, C, Ruston, T, and Frey, WH: Increased glycerol-3-phosphorylcholine in post-mortem Alzheimer's brain. Lancet 1:517, 1985.
4. Bartus, RT, Dean, RL, Beer, B, and Lippa, AS: The cholinergic hypothesis of geriatric memory dysfunction. Science 217:408–417,1982.
5. Bartus, RT, Dean, RL, Sherman, KA, Friedman, E, and Beer, B: Profound effects of combining choline and piracetamin memory enhancement and cholinergic function in aging rats. Neurobiol Aging 2:105–111, 1981.
6. Beal, MF, MacGarvey, U, and Swartz, KJ: Galanin immunoreactivity is increased in the nucleus basalis of Meynert in Alzheimer's disease. Ann Neurol 28:157–161, 1990.
7. Beller, SA, Overall, JE, and Swann, AC: Efficacy of oral physostigmine in primary degenerative dementia. Psychopharmacology (Berlin) 87:147–151, 1985.
8. Blass, JP, and Weksler, ME: Toward an effective treatment of Alzheimer's disease. Ann Neurol 98:251–252, 1983.
9. Blessed, G, Tomlinson, BE, and Roth, M: The asociation between quantitative measures of dementia and of senile change in the cerebral gray matter of elderly subjects. Br J Psychiatry 114:797–801, 1968.
10. Blusztajn, JK, Liscovitch, M, Mauron, C, Richardson, UI, and Wurtman, RJ: Phosphatidylcholine as a precursor of choline for acetylcholine synthesis. J Neural Transm (Suppl 24) 24:247–259, 1987.
11. Blusztajn, JK and Wurtman, RJ: Choline and cholinergic neurons. Science 221:614–620, 1983.
12. Bowen, DM and Davison, AN: Biochemical studies of nerve cells and energy metabolism in Alzheimer's disease. Br Med J 42:75–80, 1986.
13. Bowen, DM, Smith, CB, White, P, and Davison, AN: Neurotransmitter related enzymes and indices of hypoxia in senile dementia and other abiotrophies. Brain 99:459–496, 1976.
14. Brinkman, SD, Pomara, M, Gordnick, PH, Barnett, N, and Domino, EF: A dose-

ranging study of lecithin in the treatment of primary degenerative dementia (Alzheimer disease). Journal of Clinical Psychopharmacology 2:281–285, 1982.

15. Brinkman, SD, Smith, RC, Meyer, JS, Vroulis, G, Shaw, T, Gordon, JR, and Allen, RH: Lecithin and memory training in suspected Alzheimer's disease. J Gerontol 37:4–9, 1982.

16. Brozoski, TJ, Brown, RM, Rosvold, HE, and Goldman, PS: Cognitive deficit caused by regional depletion of dopamine in prefrontal cortex of rhesus monkey. Science 205:929–931, 1979.

17. Bruno, G, Mohr, E, Gillespie, M, Fedio, P, and Chase, TN: Muscarinic agonist therapy of Alzheimer's disease: A clinical trial of RS-86. Arch Neurol 43:659–661, 1986.

18. Caine, ED: Cholinomimetic treatment fails to improve memory disorders. N Engl J Med 303:585–586, 1980.

19. Caltagirone, C, Goinotti, C, and Masullo, O: Oral administration of chronic physostigmine does not improve cognitive or amnestic performances in Alzheimer's presenile dementia. Int J Neurosci 18:248–249, 1982.

20. Christie, JE: Physostigmine and arecoline infusions in Alzheimer's disease. Aging 19:413–419, 1982.

21. Christie, JE, Blackburn, IM, Glen, AIM, Zeisel, S, Shering, A, and Yates, CM: Effects of choline and lecithin on CSF choline levels and on cognitive function in patients with presenile dementia of the Alzheimer type. Brain 5:377–387, 1979.

22. Cohen, BM, Zubenko, GS, and Babb, SM: Abnormal platelet membrane composition in Alzheimer's type dementia. Life Sci 40:2445–2451, 1987.

23. Conners, CK, Blouin, AG, Winglee, M, Lougee, L, O'Donnell, D, and Smith, A: Piracetam and event-related potentials in dyslexic children. Psychopharmacol Bull 20:667–673, 1984.

24. Conners, CK, Blouin, AG, Winglee, M, Lougee, L, O'Donnell, D, and Smith, A: Piracetam and event-related potentials in dyslexic males. International Journal of Psychophysiology 4:19–27, 1986.

25. Cook, P and James, I: Cerebral vasodilators, I. N Engl J Med 305:1508–1513, 1981.

26. Cook, P and James, I: Cerebral vasodilators, II. N Engl J Med 305:1560–1564, 1981.

27. Cost, JR: Double blind evaluation of naftidrofuryl in treating elderly, confused, hospitalized patients. Gerontology Clinic 17:160–167, 1975.

28. Coyle, JT, Price, DL, and DeLong, MR: Alzheimer's disease: A disorder of cortical cholinergic innervation. Science 219:1184–1190, 1983.

29. Davies, G, Hamilton, S, Hendritcoon, E, Levy, R, and Post, F: The effect of cyclandelate in depressed and demented patients: A controlled study in psychogeriatric patients. Age Ageing 6:156–162, 1978.

30. Davies, P: A critical review of the role of the cholinergic system in human memory and cognition. In Olton, DS, Gamzu, E, and Corkin, S (eds): Memory Dysfunctions: An Integration of Animal and Human Research from Preclinical and Clinical Perspectives. New York Academy of Sciences, New York, 1985, pp 212–217.

31. Davies, P, Katzman, R, and Terry, RD: Reduced somatostatin-like immunoreactivity in cerebral cortex of cases of Alzheimer disease. Nature 288:279–288, 1980.

32. Davis, GE, Blaker, SN, Engvall, E, Varon, S, Manthorpe, M, and Gage, FH: Human amnion membrane serves as a substratum for growing axons in vitro and in vivo. Science 236:1106–1109, 1987.

33. Davis, KL, and Mohs, RC: Enhancement of memory processes in Alzheimer's disease with multiple dose intravenous physostigmine. Am J Psychiatry 139:1421–1424, 1982.

34. Davis, KL, Mohs, RC, Rosen, WG, Greenwold, BS, Levy, MI, and Horvath, TB: Oral physostigmine in Alzheimer's disease. N Engl J Med 308:721, 1983.

35. Davis, KL, Mohs, RC, Tinklenberg, JE, Hollister, LE, Pefferbaum, A, and Kopell, BS: Cholinomimetics and memory: The effect of choline chloride. Arch Neurol 37:49–52, 1980.

36. Davis, KL, Mohs, RC, Tinklenberg, JR, Pfefferbaum, A, Hollister, LE, and Ko-

pell, BS: Physostigmine: Improvement of long-term memory processes in humans. Science 201:272–274, 1978.

37. Davous, P and Lamour, Y: Bethanecol decreases reaction time in senile dementia of the Alzheimer type. J Neurol Neurosurg Psychiatry 48:129709, 1985.

38. Decker, MW, Pelleymounter, MA, and Galagher, M: Effects of training on a spatial memory task on high affinity choline uptake in hippocampal and cortex in young adults and aged rats. J Neurosc 8:90–99, 1988.

39. Decker, MW: The effects of aging on hippocampal and cortical projections of the forebrain cholinergic system. Brain Research Reviews 12:423–438, 1987.

40. DeSouza, EB, Whitehouse, PJ, Kuhar, MJ, Price, DL, and Vale, WW: Reciprocal changes in corticotropin-releasing factor (CRF)-like immunoreactivity and CRF receptors in cerebral cortex of Alzheimer's disease. Nature 319:593–595, 1986.

41. deWied, D and van Ree, JM: Neuropeptides, mental performance and aging. Life Sci 31:709–719, 1982.

42. Deyo, RA, Straube, KT, and Disterhoft, JF: Nimodipine facilitates associative learning in aging rabbits. Science 243:809–812, 1989.

43. Dipken, MW, Foval, P, Harris, CM, Avertano, H, Bergen, D, Hoeppner, T, and Davis, JM: Lecithin administration in patients with primary degenerative dementia and in normal volunteers. Aging 19:385–392, 1982.

44. Drachman, DA and Leavitt, J: Human memory and the cholinergic system: A relationship to aging? Arch Neurol 30:113–121, 1974.

45. Ellison, DW, Beal, MF, and Martin, JB: Phosphoethanolamine and ethanolamine are decreased in Alzheimer's disease and Huntington's disease. Brain Res 417:389–392, 1987.

46. Emson, PC and Lindvall, O: Neuroanatomical aspects of neurotransmitters affected in Alzheimer's disease. Br Med Bull 42:57–62, 1986.

47. Etienne, P, Dastoor, D, Gautlier, S, Ludwich, R and Collier, B: Lecithin in the treatment of Alzheimer's disease.

Aging 19:369–372, 1982.

48. Etienne, P, Gauthier, S, Dastoor, D, Collier, B, and Ratner, J: Lecithin in Alzheimer's disease. Lancet 2:1206, 1978.

49. Ezzat, DH, Ibraheem, MM, and Makhawy, B: The effect of piracetam on ECT-induced memory disturbances. Br J Psychiatry 147:720–721, 1985.

50. Ferris, SH, Reisberg, B, Freedman, E, and Gershon, S: Combination of choline and piracetam treatment of senile dementia. Psychopharmacol Bull 18:96–98, 1982.

51. Ferris, SH, Sathananthon, G, Gershon, S, and Clark, C: Senile dementia: Treatment with deanol. J Am Geriatr Soc 25:241–244, 1977.

52. Ferris, SH, Sathananthon, G, Gershon, S, Clark, C, and Moshinsky, J: Cognitive effects of ACTH 4-10 in the elderly. Pharmacol Biochem Behav 5(Suppl):73–78, 1976.

53. Fischer, W, Wictorin, K, Bjorklund, A, Williams, LR, Varon, S, and Gage, FH: Amelioration of cholinergic neuron atrophy and spatial memory impairment in aged rats by nerve growth factor. Nature 329:65–68, 1987.

54. Fisman, M, Mersky, H, and Helmes, H: Double-blind trial of dimethylaminoethanol in Alzheimer's disease. Am J Psychiatry 138:970–972, 1981.

55. Fleishhacker, WW, Buchgeher, A, and Schubert, H: Memantine in the treatment of senile dementia of the Alzheimer type. Prog Neuropsychopharmacol Bio Psychiatry 10:87–93, 1986.

56. Florian, A, Casamenti, F, and Pipeu, G: Recovery of cortical acetylcholine output after ganglioside treatment in rats with lesion of the nucleus basalis. Neurosci Lett 75:313–316, 1987.

57. Folstein, MF, Folstein, SE, and McHugh, PR: "Mini-mental state": A practical method for grading the cognitive state of patients for the clinician. J Psychiatr Res 12:189–198, 1975.

58. Foster, NL, Aldrich, MS, Bluemlein, L, White, RF, and Bereut, S: Failure of cholinergic agonist RS-86 to improve cognition and movement in PSP despite effects on sleep. Neurology 39:257–261, 1989.

59. Francis, PT, Palmer, AM, Sims, NR,

Bowen, DM, Davidson, AN, Esiri, MM, Neary, D, Snowden, JS, and Wilcock, GK: Neurochemical studies of early-onset Alzheimer's disease. N Engl J Med 313:7–11, 1985.

60. Friedman, E, Sherman, KA, Ferris, SH, Reisberg, B, Bartos, RT, and Schneck MK: Clinical response to choline plus piracetam in senile dementia: Relation to red cell choline levels. N Engl J Med 304:1490–1491, 1981.

61. Gage, FH and Bjorklund, A: Cholinergic septal grafts into the hippocampal formation improve spatial learning and memory in aged rats by an atropine-sensitive mechanism. J Neurosci 6: 2837–2847, 1986.

62. Gamzu, E: Animal behavioral models in the discovery of compounds to treat memory dysfunction. In Olton, DS, Gamzu, E, and Corkin, S (eds): Memory Dysfunction: An Integration of Animal and Human Research from Preclinical and Clinical Perspectives. New York Academy of Sciences, New York, 1985, pp 370–393.

63. Gauthier, S, Bouchard, R, Lamontagne, A, et al: Tetrahydroaminoacridine-lecithin combination treatment in patients with intermediate stage Alzheimer's disease. N Engl J Med 322:272–276, 1990.

64. Gerin, J: Double-blind trial of naftidrofuryl in treating elderly, confused, hospitalized patients. Br J Clin Pract 28:177–178, 1974.

65. Gibson, GE, Peterson, C, and Sansone, J: Neurotransmitter and carbohydrate metabolism during aging and mild hypoxia. Neurobiol Aging 2:165–172, 1981.

66. Goldman, JE, and Yen, SH: Cytoskeletal protein abnormalities in neurodegenerative disease. Ann Neurol 19: 209–223, 1986.

67. Goodnick, P and Gershon, S: Chemotherapy of cognitive disorders in geriatric subjects. J Clin Psychiatry 45:196–209, 1984.

68. Greenamyre, JT, Penney, JB, Young, AB, D'Amato, CJ, Hicks, SP, and Shoulson, I: Alterations in L-glutamate binding in Alzheimer's and Huntington's disease. Science 227:1496–1499, 1985.

69. Greenamyre, JT, Penney, JB, D'Amato, CJ, and Young, AB: Dementia of the Alzheimer type: Changes in hippocampal L-3H-glutamate binding. J Neurochem 48:543–551, 1987.

69a. Greenblatt, DJ, Harmatz, JS, Shapiro, L, Engelhardt, N, Gouthro, TA, and Shader, RI: Sensitivity to triazolam in the elderly. N Engl J Med 324:1691–1698, 1991.

70. Growdon, JH, Corkin, S, Huff, FJ, and Rosen, TJ: Piracetam combined with lecithin in the treatment of Alzheimer's disease. Neurobiol Aging 7:269–276, 1986.

71. Growdon, JH, Corkin, S, and Huff, FJ: Clinical evaluation of compounds for the treatment of memory dysfunction. In Olton, DS, Gamzu, E, and Corkin, S (eds): Memory Dysfunction. An Integration of Animal and Human Research from Preclinical and Clinical Perspectives. New York Academy of Sciences, New York, 1985, pp 437–449.

72. Hachinski, V: Cerebral blood flow: Differentiation of Alzheimer's disease from multi-infarct dementia. In Katzman, RD and Bick, KP (eds): Alzheimer's Disease: Senile Dementia and Related Disorders. Raven Press, New York, 1978, p 97.

73. Hamot, HB, Patin, JR, and Singer, JM: Factor structure of Sandoz Clinical Assessment-Geriatric (SCAG) scale. Psychopharmacol Bull 20:142–150, 1984.

74. Harbaugh, RE: Intracerebroventricular cholinergic drug administration in Alzheimer's disease: Preliminary results of a double-blind study. J Neural Transm (Suppl 24) 24:271–277, 1987.

75. Hardy, J, Cowburn, R, Barton, A, Reynolds, G, Dodd, R, Wester, P, O'Carroll, AM, Lofdahl, E, and Winblad, B: A disorder of cortical GABAergic innervation in Alzheimer's disease. Neurosci Lett 73:192–196, 1987.

76. Hefti, F and Will, B: Nerve growth factor is a neurotrophic factor for forebrain cholinergic neurons: Implications for Alzheimer's disease. J Neural Transm (Suppl 24) 24:309–315, 1987.

77. Heiss, WD, Hebold, P, Klinkhammer, PK, Ziffling, P, Szelies, B, Pawlik, F, and

Herholz, K: Effect of piracetam on cerebral glucose metabolism in Alzheimer's disease as measured by positron emission tomography. Journal of Cerebral Blood Flow and Metabolism 8:613–617, 1988.

78. Helfgott, E, Rudel, RG, and Kairam, R: The effect of piracetam on short and long term verbal retrieval in dyslexic boys. International Journal of Psychophysiology 4:53–61, 1986.

79. Helfgott, E, Rudel, RG, and Krieger, J: Effect of piracetam in the single word and prose reading of dyslexic children. Psychopharmacol Bull 20:688–690, 1984.

80. Henderson, VW, Roberts, E, Wimer, C, Bardolph, MD, Chui, HC, Damasio, AR, Eslinger, PJ, Folstein, MF, Schneider, MD, Teng, EL, Tune, LE, Weiner, LP, and Whitehouse, PJ: Multicenter trial of naloxone in Alzheimer's disease. Ann Neurol 25:404–406, 1989.

81. Herrmann, WM, Kern, U, and Rohmel, J: Contribution to the search for vigilance indicative EEG variables: Results of a controlled double-blind study with pyitonol in elderly patients with symptoms of mental dysfunction. Pharmacopsychiatria 19:75–83, 1986.

82. Heyman, A, Schmechal, D, Wilkinson, W, Rogers, H, Krishnan, R, Holloway, D, Schultz, K, Gwyther, R, Peoples, R, Utley, C, and Haynes, C: Failure of long term high-dose lecithin to retard progression of early-onset Alzheimer's disease. J Neural Transm (Suppl 24) 24:279–286, 1987.

83. Hollander, E, Mohs, RC, and Davis, KL: Review: Antemortem markers of Alzheimer's disease. Neurobiol Aging 7:367–387, 1986.

84. Hollander, E, Mohs, RC, and Davis, KL: Cholinergic approaches to the treatment of Alzheimer's disease. Br Med J 42:97–100, 1986.

85. Hollister, LE and Yesavage, J: Ergoloid mesylates for senile dementias: Unanswered questions. Ann Intern Med 100:894–898, 1984.

86. Irle, E and Markowitsch, HJ: Basal forebrain-lesioned monkeys are severely impaired in tasks of association

and recognition memory. Ann Neurol 22:735–743, 1987.

87. Jenden, DJ: An overview of choline and acetylcholine metabolism in relation to the therapeutic uses of choline. Nutrition and the Brain 5:13–24, 1979.

88. Jenden, DJ, Russell, RW, Booth, RA, Lauretz, SD, Knusel, BJ, Roch, J, Rice, KM, Geoge, R, and Waite, JJ: A model hypocholinergic syndrome produced by a false choline analog, N-aminodeanol. J Neural Transm (Suppl 24) 24:325–329, 1987.

89. Jenden, DJ, Weiler, MH, and Gundersen, CB: Choline availability and acetylcholine synthesis. Aging 19:315–326, 1982.

90. Jenkins, JS, Mather, HM, Coughlen, AK, and Jenkins, DG: Desmopressin and desglycinamide vasopressin in post-traumatic amnesia. Lancet 1:39, 1981.

91. Johnson, K, Presley, AS, and Ballinger, BR: Levo-dopa in senile dementia. Br Med J 1:1625, 1978.

92. Johnston, MV, McKinney, M, and Coyle, JT: Evidence for a cholinergic projection to neocortex from neurons in the basal forebrain. Proc Natl Acad Sci USA 76:5392–5396, 1979.

93. Kanfer, JN, Hattori, H, and Oribel, D: Reduced phospholipase D activity in brain tissue samples from Alzheimer's disease patients. Ann Neurol 20:265–267, 1986.

94. Kanfer, JN and McCartney, DG: Phosphatase and phospholipase activity in Alzheimer brain disease. J Neural Transm (Suppl 24) 24:183–188, 1987.

95. Kaye, WH, Sitaram, N, Weingartner, H, Ebert, MH, Smallberg, S, and Billin, JC; Modest facilitation of memory in dementia with combined lecithin and anticholinesterase treatment. Biol Psychol 17:275–280, 1982.

96. Kopelman, MD and Lishman, WA: Pharmacological treatments of dementia. Brit Med Bull 42:101–105, 1986.

97. Kristensen, V, Olsen, M, and Theilgaard, A: Levo-dopa treatment of presenile dementia. Acta Psychiatr Scand 55:41–51, 1977.

98. Kromer, LF: Nerve growth factor treat-

ment after brain injury prevents neuronal death. Science 235:214–216, 1987.

99. Laczi, R, Ven Ree, JM, and Wagner, A: Effects of desglycinamide-arginine and vasopressin (DGAVPP) on memory processes in diabetes insipidus patients and non-diabetes subjects. Acta Endocrinol (Copenh) 102:206–212, 1983.

100. Lewis, C, Ballinger, BR, and Presly, A: Trial of levodopa in senile dementia. Br Med J 1:550–551, 1978.

101. Lipowski, ZJ: Delirium in the elderly patient. N Engl J Med 320:578–582, 1989.

102. Little, A, Levy, R, Charqui-Kidd, P, and Hnad, D: A double blind placebo controlled trial of high dose lecithin in Alzheimer's disease. J Neurol Neurosurg Psychiatry 48:736–742, 1985.

103. Marsh, GR and Linnorta, M: The effects of deanol on cognitive performance and electrophysiology in elderly humans. Psychopharmacology (Berlin) 66:99–104, 1979.

104. Martinez, HJ, Dreyfus, CF, Jonakait, GM, and Black, IB: Nerve growth factor selectively increases cholinergic markers but not neuropeptides in rat basal forebrain in culture. Brain Res 412:295–301, 1987.

105. McDonald, RJ: Hydergine: A review of 26 clinical studies. Pharmacopsychiatria 12:407–422, 1979.

106. McEntee, WJ and Mair, RG: Memory enhancement in Korsakoff's psychosis by clonidine: Further evidence of a noradrenergic defect. Ann Neurol 7:466–470, 1980.

107. McKhann, G, Drachman, D, Folstein, M, Katzman, R, Price, D, and Stadlam, EM: Clinical diagnosis of Alzheimer's disease: Report of the NINCDS-ADRDA work group. Neurology 34: 939–945, 1984.

108. Mesulam, MM, Geula, C, and Moran, MA: Anatomy of cholinesterase inhibition in Alzheimer's disease: Effect of physostigmine and tetrahydroaminoacridine on plaques and tangles. Ann Neurol 22:683–691, 1987.

109. Mesulam, MM, Mufsan, EJ, Levey, AI, and Wainer, BH: Cholinergic innervation of cortex by the basal forebrain: Cytochemistry and cortical connections. J Comp Neurol 214:170–179, 1983.

110. Miatto, O, Gonzalez, RG, Buonanno, F, and Growdon, SH: In vitro 31P NMR spectroscopy detects altered phospholipid metabolism in Alzheimer's disease. Can J Neurol Sci 13:535–539, 1986.

111. Mishkin, M: Memory in monkeys severely impaired by combined but not by separate removal of amygdala and hippocampus. Nature 273:297–299, 1978.

112. Mobley, WC, Rutkowski, JL, Tennekoon, GI, Gemski, J, Buchanan, K, and Johnston MV: Nerve growth factor increases choline acetyltransferase activity in developing basal forebrain neurons. Molecular Brain Research 1:53–62, 1986.

113. Moglia, A, Sinforiani, E, Zandrini, C, Gualtieri, G, Corsico, R, and Arriga, A: Activity of piracetam in patients with organic brain syndrome: A neuropsychological study. Clinical Neuropharmacol (Suppl 3) 9:573–578, 1986.

114. Mohs, E, Schlegel, J, Fabbrini, G, Williams, J, Mouradian, MM, Mann, UM, Claus, JJ, Fedio, P, and Chase, TN: Clonidine treatment of Alzheimer's disease. Arch Neurol 46:376–378, 1989.

115. Mohs, PC, Davis, BM, Johns, CA, Mathe, AA, Greenwald, BS, Horvath, TB, and Davis, KL: Oral physostigmine treatment of patients with Alzheimer's disease. Am J Psychiatry 142:28–33, 1985.

116. Mohs, PC, Rosen, WG, and Davis, KL: Defining treatment efficacy in patients with Alzheimer's disease. Aging 19: 351–356, 1982.

117. Muramato, O, Sugishita, M, Kazuya, H, et al: Cholinergic system and contructional apraxis: A further study of physostigmine in AD. J Neurol Neurosurg Psychiatry 47:485–491, 1984.

118. Oliverso, JC, Jandali, MK, and Timsit-Berthier, M: Vasopressin in amnesia. Lancet 1:42, 1978.

119. Olton, DS, Gamzu, E, and Corkin, S: Memory Dysfunctions: An Integration of Animal and Human Research from Preclinical and Clinical Perspectives.

New York Academy of Sciences, New York, 1985.

120. Passeri, M: Therapy of chronic consequences of brain ischemia. Comparison between two drugs acting on brain circulation and metabolism. Eur Neurol 17:150–158, 1978.

121. Peabody, CA, Davis, H, Berger, PA, and Tinklenberg, JR: Desamino-D-arginine-vasopressin (DDAVP) in Alzheimer's disease. Neurobiol Aging 7:301–303, 1986.

122. Pearson, RCA and Powell, TPS: Anterograde vs retrograde degeneration of the nucleus basalis medialis in Alzheimer's disease. J Neural Transm (Suppl 24) 24:139–146, 1987.

123. Penn, RD, Martin, EM, Wilson, RS, Fox, JH, and Savoy, SM: Intraventricular bethanechol infusion for Alzheimer's disease: Results of double-blind and escalating-dose trials. Neurology 38:219–222, 1988.

124. Perry, EK: The cholinergic hypothesis —Ten years on. Brit Med Bull 42:63–69, 1986.

125. Peters, BH and Levin, HS: Chronic oral physostigmine and lecithin administration in memory disorders of aging. Aging 19:421–426, 1982.

126. Peters, BH and Levin, HS: Memory enhancement after physostigmine treatment in the amnesic syndrome. Arch Neurol 34:215–219, 1977.

127. Pettegrew, JW, Kopp, SJ, Minshew, HJ, Glonek, T, Feliksik, JM, Tow, JP, and Cohen, MD: 31P nuclear magnetic resonance studies of phosphoglyceride metabolism in developing and degenerating brain: Preliminary observations. J Neuropathol Exp Neurol 46:419–430, 1987.

128. Pettegrew, JW, Withers, G, Panchalingam, K, and Post, JFM: 31P nuclear magnetic resonance (NMR) spectroscopy of brain in aging and Alzheimer's disease. J Neural Transm (Suppl 24) 24: 261–268, 1987.

129. Pfefferbaum, A, Davis, KL, Coulter, CL, Mohs, RC, Tinklenberg, JR, and Koppell, BS: EEG effects of physostigmine and choline chloride in humans. Psychopharmacology (Berlin) 62:225–233, 1979.

130. Phelps, CW, Gage, FH, Growdon, JH, Hefti, F, Harbaugh, R, Johnston, MV, Khachaturian, ZS, Mobley, WC, Price, DL, Rashkind, M, Simpkins, J, Thal, LJ, and Woodcoche, J: Potential use of nerve growth factor to treat Alzheimer's disease. Neurobiol Aging 10:247–249, 1989.

131. Poschel, BPH, Marriott, JG, and Gluckman, MI: Pharmacology underlying the cognition activating properties of piracetam (CI-879). Psychopharm Bull 19:720, 1983.

132. Rapoport, JL, Buschsbaum, MS, Zahn, TP, Weingartner, H, Ludlow, C, and Mikkelsen, EJ: Dextroamphetamine, cognitive and behavioral effects in normal prepubertal boys. Science 199:560–563, 1978.

133. Reinikainen, KJ, Reikkinen, PJ, Jolkkonen, J, Kosma, M, and Soininen, H: Decreased somatostatin-like immunoreactivity in cerebral cortex and cerebrospinal fluid in Alzheimer's disease. Brain Res 402:103–108, 1987.

134. Reisberg, B, Ferris, SH, Anand, R, Mir, P, Geibel, V, DeLeon, MJ, and Roberts E: Effects of naloxone in senile dementia: A double blind trial. N Engl J Med 308:621–722, 1983.

135. Reisberg, B, Ferris, SH, and Gershon, S: An overview of pharmacologic treatment of cognitive decline in the aged. Am J Psychiatry 138:593–599, 1981.

136. Roman, GC: Senile dementia of the Binswanger type: A vascular form of dementia in the elderly. JAMA 258:1782–1788, 1987.

137. Rosser, M and Iverson, LL: Non-cholinergic neurotransmitter abnormalities in Alzheimer's disease. Br Med J 42:70–74, 1986.

138. Rumble, B, Retallack, R, Hilbich, C, Simms, G, Multhaup, G, Martins, R, Hockey, A, Montgomery, P, Beyreuther, K, and Masters, MD: Amyloid A4 protein and its precursor in Down's syndrome and Alzheimer's disease. N Engl J Med 320:1446–1452, 1989.

139. Sara, SJ and Lefevre, D: Hypoxia-induced amnesia in one trial learning and pharmacological protection by piracetam. Psychopharmacologia 25:32–40, 1972.

140. Sara, SJ and David-Remacle, M: Recovery from electroconvulsive shock-induced amnesia by exposure to the training environment: Pharmacological enhancement by piracetam. Psychopharmacologia 36:59–66, 1974.

141. Sarter, M, Schneider, N, and Stephans, D: Treatment strategies for senile dementia: Antagonist B-carbolines. Trends in Neuroscience 11:13–17, 1988.

142. Schneck, MK, Reisberg, B, and Ferris, SH: Neurotransmitter treatment of senile dementia, Alzheimer type. International Drug Therapy Newsletter 16:5–8, 1981.

143. Schoenberg, BS, Kokmen, E, and Okazaki, H: Alzheimer's disease and other dementing illnesses in a defined United States population: Incidence rates and clinical features. Ann Neurol 22:724–729, 1987.

144. Schwartz, AS and Kohlstaedt, E: Physostigmine effects in Alzheimer's disease: Relationship to dementia severity. Life Sci 38:1021–1028, 1986.

145. Selkoe, D: Aging, amyloid and Alzheimer's disease. N Engl J Med 320:1484–1486, 1989.

146. Shaywitz, BA: CSF monoamine metabolites in children with minimal brain dysfunction. J Pediatr 90:67–71, 1977.

147. Sims, NR, Bowen, DM, Neary, D, and Davison, AN: Metabolic processes in Alzheimer's disease: Adenine content and production of $14CO_2$ from U-14C glucose in vitro in human neocortex. J Neurochem 41:1329–1334, 1983.

148. Sims, NR, Finegan, JM, Blass, JP, Bowen, DM, and Neary, D: Mitochondrial function in brain tissue in primary degenerative dementia. Brain Res 436:30–38, 1987.

149. Sims, NR, Finegan, IM, and Blass, JP: Altered metabolic properties of cultured skin fibroblasts in Alzheimer's disease. Ann Neurol 21:451–457, 1987.

150. Sitaram, N, Weingartner, H, and Gillin, JC: Human serial learning; enhancement with arecholine and choline and impairment with scopolamine. Science 201:274–276, 1978.

151. Smith, CM, Semple, SA, and Swash, M: Effects of physostigmine on responses in memory tests in patients with Alzheimer's disease. Aging 19:405–411, 1982.

152. Smith, CCT, Bowen, DM, Francis, PT, Snowden, JS, and Neary, D: Putative amino acid transmittors in lumbar CSF of patients with histologically verified Alzheimer's dementia. J Neurol Neurosurg Psychiatry 48:469–471, 1985.

153. Smith, CM and Swash, M: Physostigmine in Alzheimer's disease. Lancet 1:42, 1979.

154. Soininen, H, Koskinen, T, Helkala, EL, Pigache, R, and Riekkinen, PJ: Treatment of Alzheimer's disease with a synthetic ACTH 4-9 analog. Neurology 35:1348–1351, 1985.

155. Sofroniew, MV, Pearson, RCA, Cuello, AC, Tagari, PC, and Stephens, PH: Parenterally administered GM1 ganglioside prevents retrograde degeneration of cholinergic cells of the rat basal forebrain. Brain Res 398:393–396, 1986.

156. Sprague, RL and Sleator, EK: Methylphenidate in hyperkinetic children: Differences in dose effects on learning and social behavior. Science 198:1274–1276, 1977.

157. Squire, LR: Mechanisms of memory. Science 232:1612–1619, 1986.

158. Steiger, NA, Medelson, M, Jenkins, T, Smith, M and Goy, R: Effects of naloxone in treatment of senile dementia. J Am Geriatr Soc 33:155, 1985.

159. Stern, Y, Sano, M and Mayeux, R: Long-term administration of oral physostigmine in Alzheimer's disease. Neurology 38:1837–1841, 1988.

160. Stokes, CE and Hawthorne, JN: Reduced phosphoinositide concentrations in anterior temporal cortex of Alzheimer-disease brains. J Neurochem 48:1018–1021, 1987.

161. Summers, WK, Majovski, LV, Marsh, GM, Tachiki,K, and Kling, A: Oral tetrahydroaminoacridine in long-term treatment of senile dementia, Alzheimer type. N Engl J Med 315:1241–1245, 1986.

162. Summers, WK, Viesselman, JO, Marsh, GM, and Candelora, K: Use of THA in the treatment of Alzheimer-like dementia: Pilot study in twelve patients. Biol Psychiatry 16:145–153, 1981.

163. Sunderland, T, Tariot, PM, Weingartner, H, Murphy, DL, Newhouse, PA, Mueller, CA, and Cohen, RM: Pharmacologic modeling of Alzheimer disease. Prog Neuropsychopharmacol and Mol Psychiat 10:599–610, 1986.

164. Tacconi, MT and Wurtman, RJ: Piracetam: Physiological disposition and mechanism of action. Adv Neurol 43:675–685, 1986.

165. Tallal, P, Chase, C, Russell, G, and Schmitt, RL: Evaluation of the efficacy of piracetam in treating information processing, reading and writing disorders in dyslexic children. International Journal of Psychophysiology 4:41–52, 1986.

166. Tamminga, CA, Foster, NL, Fedio, P, Bird, ED, and Chase, TW: Alzheimer's disease: Low cerebral somatostatin levels correlated with impaired cognitive function and cortical metabolism. Neurology 37:161–165, 1987.

167. Tazaki, Y, Omae, T, Kuromaru, SH, Ohtomo, E, Hasegawa, K, Mori, A, Kurihara, M, Mutsusawa, M, and Otada, T: Clinical effects of encephabol (Pyritinol) in the treatment of cerebrovascular disorders. J International Journal of Medical Research 8:118–126, 1980.

168. Thal, LJ and Fuld, PA: Memory enhancement with oral physostigmine in Alzheimer's disease. N Engl J Med 308:720, 1983.

169. Thal, LJ, Fuld, PA, Masur, DM, and Sharpless, NS: Oral physostigmine and lecithin improve memory in Alzheimer's disease. Ann Neurol 13:491–496, 1983.

170. Thompson, TL, Filley, CM, Mitchell, WD, Culig, KM, LoVerde, M, and Byyny, RL: Lack of efficiency of Hydergine in patients with Alzheimer's disease. N Engl J Med 323:445–448, 1990.

171. Villardita, C, Parini, J, Grioli, S, Quattropani, M, Lomea, C, and Scapagnine, U: Clinical and neuropsychological study with piracetam versus placebo in patients with mild to moderate dementia. J Neural Transm (Suppl 24) 24:293–298, 1987.

172. Wade, IPH, Mirsin, TR, Hachinski, VC, Fisman, M, Lau, C, and Merskey, H: The clinical diagnosis of Alzheimer's disease. Arch Neurol 44:24–29, 1987.

173. Wecker, L: Influence of dietary choline availability and neuronal demand on acetylcholine synthesis by rat brain. J Neurochem 51:497–504, 1988.

174. Weingartner, H, Kaye, W, Gold, P, Smallberg, S, Peterson, R, Gillin, JC, and Ebert, M: Vasopressin treatment of cognition dysfunction in progressive dementia. Life Sci 29:2721–2726, 1981.

175. Weintraub, S and Mesulam, M-M: Mental state assessment of young and old adults in behavioral neurology. In Mesulam, M-M (ed): Principles of Behavioral Neurology. FA Davis, Philadelphia, 1986, pp 71–123.

176. Westreich, G, Alter, M, and Lundgren, S: Effect of cyclandelate on dementia. Stroke 6:535–538, 1975.

177. Wettstein, A: No effect from double-blind trial of physostigmine and lecithin in Alzheimer's disease. Ann Neurol 13:210–212, 1983.

178. Wettstein, A and Spiegel, R: Clinical trials with cholinergic drug RS-86 in Alzheimer's disease (AD) and senile dementia in Alzheimer type (SDAt). Psychopharmacology (Berlin) 84:571–573, 1984.

179. Whitehouse, PJ and Kellar, KJ: Nicotinic and muscarinic cholinergic receptors in Alzheimer's disease and related disorders. J Neural Transm (Suppl 24) 24:175–182, 1987.

180. Whitehouse, PJ, Price, DL, Struble, RG, Clark, AW, Coyle, JT, and DeLong MR: Alzheimer's disease and senile dementia: Loss of neurons in the basal forebain. Science 215:1237–1239, 1982.

181. Wilsher, C, Atkins, G, and Manfield, P: Piracetam as an aid to learning in dyslexia. Psychopharmacology (Berlin) 65:107–109, 1979.

182. Wilsher, CR: Effects of piracetam on developmental dyslexia. International Journal of Psychophysiology 4:29–39, 1986.

183. Wurtman, RJ: Precursor control of transmitter synthesis. In Barbeau, A, Growdon, JA and Wurtman, RJ (eds): Nutrition and the Brain 5:1–12, 1979.

184. Wurtman, RJ: Strategies in the development of drugs that might be useful in cognitive disorders. Clin Neuropharmacol (Suppl 3) 9:53–57, 1986.

185. Wurtman, RJ, Magil, SG, and Reinstein, DK: Piracetam diminishes hippocampal acetylcholine levels in rats. Life Sci 28:1091–1093, 1981.

186. Yesavage, JA, Tinklenberg, JR, Hollister, LE, and Berger, PA: Vasodilators in senile dementias. Arch Gen Psychiatry 36:220–223, 1979.

187. Young, AB: Cortical amino acidergic pathways in Alzheimer's disease. J Neural Transm (Suppl 24) 24:147–152, 1987.

Chapter 9

PAIN

Richard Payne, M.D., and
Gavril W. Pasternak, M.D.,
Ph.D.

The International Association for the Study of Pain classifies pain "an unpleasant sensory and emotional experience associated with actual or potential tissue damage, or described in terms of such damage."[78] However, the perception of pain for an individual remains very subjective and is related to nociceptive input in a very complex and poorly understood manner.[139] Nonetheless, advances in our understanding of the neuropharmacology and neurophysiology of pain and nociception have provided a more rational basis for therapy of acute and chronic pain in man,[23,39,67,97,123,141] as has the development of more sophisticated measurements of subjective responses.[15] This chapter will review current concepts of the mechanisms of pain and nociception and their therapeutic implications, emphasizing the pharmacologic management of pain. (See Chapter 5 for information on headache pain).

TYPES OF PAIN

Three basic types of pain in humans have been described. They often occur in combination, however, and patients may not be able to distinguish among them.

Somatic Pain

Somatic or "nociceptive" pain is a consequence of tissue injury, such as muscle, tendon, or ligament tears or strains; traumatic bone fractures; bone metastasis; or postoperative wound pain. Activation of specific sensory receptors termed *nociceptors* are responsible for this sensation.[139] Somatic pain is typically well localized and is usually familiar to the patient and easily described. It is frequently described as aching, sharp, and occasionally gnawing in quality.

Visceral Pain

This type of pain typically results from trauma, inflammation, infection, or tumor growth in thoracic or abdominal viscera. Nociceptors have been identified in visceral tissues and their activation by noxious stimuli probably accounts for the perception of visceral pain.[114,139] Common examples of visceral pain include cholecystitis, pancreatitis and pancreatic carcinoma, angina pectoris, and peptic ulcer pain. Unlike somatic pain, visceral pain is usually poorly localized and often referred to cutaneous sites, which may themselves be tender,[114] such as right shoulder pain accompanying diaphragmatic irritation in cholecystitis or the neck and left arm pain associated with myocardial ischemia. Clearly, ignorance of referral patterns for visceral pain may lead to diagnostic confusion. The neural mechanisms underlying referred pain may relate to convergence of visceral afferent input and cutaneous afferent input into common pools of somatosensory neurons in the dorsal horn of the spinal cord.[80,139]

Deafferentation Pain

Deafferentation pain, the third major category, is a consequence of neural injury.[123] This type of pain is usually exceedingly unpleasant, often has a very different quality than somatic or visceral pain, and is often unfamiliar to the patient.[4,123] Typically, deafferentation (neuropathic) pain is described as "squeezing" or "vise-like," "burning," or "shooting and electric-like." Typical examples include diabetic sensory neuropathies, acute zoster neuralgia and postherpetic neuralgia, idiopathic metastatic brachial or lumbosacral plexopathy, and "central" or "thalamic" pain complicating stroke.

The pathophysiology of pain complicating neural injury is complex and incompletely understood.[27,124] After injury to peripheral nerves, ectopic discharges have been noted at the level of peripheral nerve and within the dorsal horn and even the thalamus, which may be responsible for some components of deafferentation pain following peripheral nerve injury.[1,25,27,108,134] Deafferentation pain does not involve nociceptors, which may help explain its peculiar quality. Clinically, deafferentation pain is difficult to manage with conventional nonnarcotic and narcotic analgesic drugs and often is more easily treated with anticonvulsants such as carbamazepine, valproate, and phenytoin.[70,120] In specific cases, such as trigeminal neuralgia, anticonvulsants are clearly the agents of choice. Corticosteroids and antidepressants, which suppress ectopic discharges, also play a

major role in the management of deafferentation pain.[32]

The sympathetic nervous system may be involved in these pain syndromes, especially deafferentation pain. Causalgia complicating peripheral nerve injury represents a distinct, sympathetically mediated pain characterized by burning, dysesthetic pain associated with dystrophic changes in the skin, subcutaneous tissues, muscles, and joints.[84,98] Evidence implicating the sympathetic nervous system in pain include (1) the improvement of pain and dystrophic changes with sympathetic blockade in humans or sympatholytic drugs,[68] (2) the worsening of pain with sympathetic stimulation in patients with causalgia,[133] (3) the appearance of new alpha-adrenergic receptors on regenerating nerve sprouts following injury in animal studies,[27] (4) the demonstration of interactions between sympathetic efferent fibers and nonnociceptive afferent fibers and wide-dynamic range neurons in the dorsal horn following trauma,[111] and (5) microneurographic studies in humans that correlate the sensation of hyperpathia with the local application of norepinephrine and increased activity in C-fiber nociceptive units.[126]

ACUTE VERSUS CHRONIC PAIN

Clinically, it is important to distinguish acute from chronic pain. Acute pain usually has a well-defined onset and is often associated with a readily definable cause. Objective physical signs of autonomic nervous system (ANS) activity such as tachycardia, pupillary dilation, diaphoresis, and hypertension often occur concurrently. These signs serve to substantiate the patient's subjective report of pain. Acute pain is best managed by treating the underlying cause, thereby allowing the tissue to heal. Temporary relief may be obtained by administering analgesic drugs, both opiate and nonnarcotic.

The point at which acute pain becomes chronic is arbitrary, but is generally considered to be 6 months. Unlike the acute variety, chronic pain is often unassociated with ANS activity, and the temporal onset and etiology are often obscure. Chronic pain may be associated with symptoms and signs that mimic depression, and is often complicated by environmental and emotional factors that prolong pain in the absence of tissue damage. One cannot assume that the complaint of pain is due to depression, however. With few objective signs substantiating the report of chronic pain, the patient may not "look" as if he or she is experiencing any discomfort, leading the inexperienced physician to assume mistakenly that the patient is malingering. The treatment of chronic pain is based on identifying any potential causes of ongoing tissue damage, recognizing the significant affective and environmental factors that may contribute to the patient's pain experience, and then using psychologic, behavioral, and pharmacologic therapies to help the patient to maintain personally meaningful activities without risking further harm. Chronic cancer pain, unlike chronic pain of nonmalignant origin, often has a definable cause of ongoing tissue injury and is best treated like acute pain. For these reasons, it is best considered as persistent acute pain.

ANATOMY AND PHYSIOLOGY OF CENTRAL NOCICEPTIVE SYSTEMS

Nociceptors

Sensory receptors that respond to noxious or tissue-damaging stimuli can be found in skin and subcutaneous tissues, muscles, joints, and abdominal and thoracic viscera.[101,139] These nociceptors are defined by their morphologic characteristics and physiologic responses to noxious chemical, mechanical, or thermal stimuli. Although myelinated nociceptors respond almost exclusively to mechanical stimuli, the unmyelinated nociceptor is more typically polymodal, responding to noxious mechanical, thermal, and chemical stimuli with thresholds typically five-fold to 100-fold greater than for simple mechanoreceptors.[101] The morphology of nociceptors is still incompletely understood, but the unmyelinated or C-nociceptor may be simply a "free nerve ending." The cutaneous myelinated (A-delta) nociceptor, however, is apparently ensheathed in an axon–Schwann-cell–keratinocyte complex.[139] Although cutaneous nociceptors are not spontaneously active, animal studies indicate that thermal injury may sensitize them within minutes and the effect may last for hours.[79,101] This sensitization is characterized by (1) a decreased threshold for activation by mechanical stimuli, (2) an increased intensity of response to mechanical stimuli, and (3) spontaneous activity. The mechanism of nociceptor sensitization is unclear, but a number of chemical mediators have been proposed, including potassium, prostaglandins (especially PGE_1), bradykinin, and adenosine triphosphate.[79] Furthermore, sympathetic activity also may sensitize myelinated nociceptors,[111] an interesting observation in view of the relationship between the sympathetic system and causalgia.

Light myelinated ($6\,\mu$, A-delta; 35 m/s) or unmyelinated (1 to 2 μ, C fibers, 0.5 to 1 m/s) fibers conduct nociceptive afferent impulses and represent 10% of myelinated fibers and more than 90% of unmyelinated fibers.[130] Microneurography studies reveal that activation of a single myelinated nociceptor is sufficient to cause pain, often described as sharp and stinging in quality.[126] Stimulation of unmyelinated nociceptor afferents at frequencies greater than 1.5 per second is associated with dull, burning, or aching pain.[126] Microneurography has provided important insights into the transmission of nociceptive input and may prove valuable in future investigations of deafferentation pain states.[135]

Dorsal Horn and Spinothalamic Tracts

Nociceptive afferent fibers enter the spinal cord in the lateral segment of the dorsal root, although as many as 25% to 30% of unmyelinated ventral root fibers are afferent and may carry nociceptive information in humans.[20] The dorsal horn consists of six lamina[8], with lamina I, the marginal zone, being most dorsal (Fig. 9–1).[9] Nociceptive fibers, including those in the ventral root, synapse principally in laminae I, II, and V.[14,107] A-delta afferents synapse predominately in laminae I and V, while C-fiber afferents synapse directly in laminae II (the substantia gelatinosa) with polysynaptic relays into lamina V as well.[107] The substantia gelatinosa can be subdivided into outer (II_o) and inner (II_i) laminae, with lamina II_o receiving

some A-delta nociceptive input as well as nociceptive C-fiber input; lamina II_i receives no A-delta input and predominately nonnoxious C-fiber (mechanical and thermal) input.[107] Laminae III and IV receive largely nonnociceptive, large-fiber mechanoreceptor (A-beta) stimuli, and lamina VI receives no important nociceptive projections.

Neurons in laminae I and II are predominately "nociceptive-specific," and respond to a narrow range of noxious thermal, mechanical, or chemical stimuli, whereas neurons in lamina V, which receive major inputs from nonnoxious and noxious afferents, may respond to diverse sensory input and are termed *wide dynamic range* cells.[106] Both types of neurons are important in encoding for pain.[139] The substantia gelatinosa cells exert minor excitatory and major inhibitory effects at the local

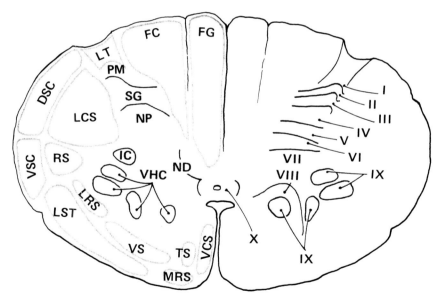

Figure 9–1. Cross section of the spinal cord at approximately the C-8/T-1 segmental level. Tracts and nuclei of the cord are illustrated on the left; Rexed's laminar organization of the gray matter is illustrated on the right. Abbreviations: DSC = dorsal spinocerebellar tract; FC = fasciculus cuneatus; FG = fasciculus gracilis; IC = intermediolateral cell column; LCS = lateral corticospinal tract; LRS = lateral reticulospinal tract; LST = lateral spinothalamic tract; LT = Lissauer's tract; MS = medial reticulospinal tract; ND = nucleus dorsalis; NP = nucleus proprius; PM = posteromarginal nucleus; RS = rubrospinal tract; SG = substantia gelatinosa; TS = tectospinal tract; VCS = ventral corticospinal tract; VHC = ventral horn cell columns; VS = vestibulospinal tract; VSC = ventral spinocerebellar tract. (From Gilman, S and Newman, SW: Manter and Gatz's Essentials of Clinical Neuroanatomy and Neurophysiology, ed 7. FA Davis, Philadelphia, 1987, p 16, with permission.)

segmental level; this is an important site in the modulation of nociceptive information. A small fraction of these cells contribute axons to the ascending spinothalamic tract.

Although axons from most cells in the dorsal horn contribute fibers to the ascending spinothalamic tracts, the predominant projections arise from cells in laminae I and V (Fig. 9–2).[139] The spinothalamic tract may be divided into two distinct physiological systems, the

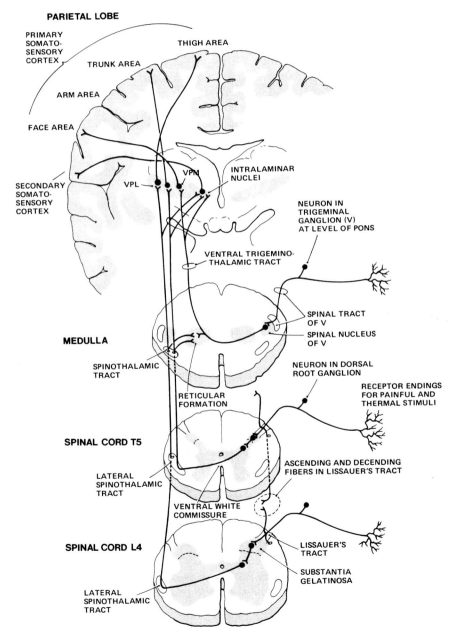

Figure 9–2. The central nervous system pathways that mediate the sensations of pain and temperature. (From Gilman, S and Newman, SW: Manter and Gatz's Essentials of Clinical Neuroanatomy and Neurophysiology, ed 7. FA Davis, Philadelphia, 1987, p 40, with permission.)

neospinothalamic tracts receive principally A-delta and C-fiber input respectively,[139] a subdivision thought to be responsible for the phenomenon of "first and second pain." For example, after cutaneous noxious stimulation by a pin, a well-localized prickling sensation is conveyed by A-delta neospinothalamic activity, followed by a less well-localized, more unpleasant "second pain" sensation thought to be conveyed by C-fiber paleospinothalamic afferent activity.

The neospinothalamic tract is a monosynaptic tract that projects to the ventroposterolateral nucleus of the thalamus and from there to the somatosensory cortex (Fig. 9–2).[71] It is topographically organized, overlaps with fibers conveying light touch sensation, and provides information concerning the quality, intensity, and location of noxious stimuli. In contrast, the paleospinothalamic tract, which is not topographically organized, is polysynaptic, with many projections into the brainstem reticular formation. It terminates in the medial and posterior thalamic nuclei.[71] Medial and intralaminar thalamic nuclei also receive efferents from the striatum, and it is speculated that this area of the thalamus may be involved in the reflex motor responses that often accompany painful stimulation.[139] Many of these thalamic cells receive convergent input from the skin, muscles, and viscera, perhaps explaining in part the phenomenon of referred pain.[139] After terminating in the thalamus, paleospinothalamic fibers project to diffuse limbic cortical and subcortical areas. This tract subserves the affective-motivational and "suffering" aspects of pain perception.

Mechanisms of Facial Sensation

The spinal trigeminal nucleus and adjacent reticular formation are directly continuous with the dorsal horn of the cervical spinal cord, and serve as the anatomic and physiologic equivalent of the dorsal horn.[29] Descending fibers in the spinal trigeminal tract convey nociceptive and nonnociceptive information for the ipsilateral face; forehead; and mucous membranes of the nose, mouth, and oral cavity. A subdivision of the spinal trigeminal nuclear complex, the subnucleus caudalis, is uniquely concerned with pain and thermal sensation and has a laminated structure analogous to the dorsal horn. Laminae I and V of this nucleus encode nociceptive information in a manner similar to the spinal dorsal horn.[29] Second-order neurons ascend to the contralateral ventroposteromedial thalamic nucleus as part of the medial lemniscus. Thus, the neural processing of facial and cranial nociceptive stimuli is entirely analogous to spinal mechanisms.

The Cortex and Pain

The role of the cerebral cortex in pain remains controversial. Although one can identify nociceptive-specific neurons in the primate cortex,[56] clinical effects of cortical lesions on pain perception remain enigmatic.[42,73,100] Marshall[73] reported that small lesions of the parietal cortex may be associated with the relatively selective loss of pain perception, whereas others have reported that large lesions of the cerebral hemispheres, including the somatosensory cortex, did not influence pain perception.[42] Although still unresolved, several clinical observations, in fact, suggest that the cortex does play a role in pain perception: (1) stimulation of the exposed cortex in humans sometimes produces pain,[100] (2) pain can be experienced during epileptic auras,[142] and (3) lesions of the parietal cortex rarely produce a syndrome mimicking "thalamic pain."[139]

ANTINOCICEPTIVE SYSTEMS IN THE CNS

The perception of nociceptive input in humans is highly dependent on the situation in which it occurs. Although the brain is continually bombarded with a variety of sensory stimuli, it retains the ability to focus on specific inputs without attending to others. Evidence from a variety of sources indicates that the central nervous system (CNS) has the ability to "filter" nociceptive input. When Beecher[9] compared the analgesic requirements of soldiers wounded during World War II to civilians undergoing surgery in the United States, he found that the soldiers required less medication despite their more extensive injuries. In recent years, endogenous pain-modulating systems capable of alleviating the perception of nociceptive input have been identified and extensively studied both physiologically and pharmacologically.[5,6,30,41]

Electrical stimulation of the periaqueductal gray (PAG), a region subsequently found to contain high levels of opioid peptides and receptors,[5,6,10,30,37] elicits a strong analgesia both in animals and in humans.[44,77] These actions are due, at least in part, to activation of descending systems of the nucleus raphe magnus, since lesions of this pathway abolish the analgesic response.[6] The microinjection of morphine into the PAG also produces analgesia,[10] whereas naloxone antagonizes both stimulation-produced analgesia and morphine analgesia from this region, implying that stimulation-produced analgesia results from the release of opioid peptides.

At the level of the spinal cord, both descending systems from the brainstem and local systems within the cord greatly influence nociceptive modulation. In the dorsal horn, small-diameter, primary afferent fibers terminating in lamina I and the outer substantia gelatinosa contain significant levels of substance P, a peptide thought to be important in pain transmission.[6,30] The complexity of spinal cord systems is illustrated by the large number of transmitters within the substantia gelatinosa, including enkephalins, bombesin, cholecystokinin, vasoactive intestinal polypeptide, neurotensin, and somatostatin; virtually all are able to modulate pain perception.[6,30,41] Additional transmitters involved with pain modulation within the CNS include acetylcholine, norepinephrine, dopamine, serotonin, gamma-aminobutyric acid, substance P, and adrenocorticotropic hormones. Although many of these drugs can influence pain perception, their actions are often limited and cannot compare to the potency of the opioid systems.

Endogenous Opioid Systems

We now know that the CNS contains sophisticated opioid systems important in a wide spectrum of CNS actions, of which pain perception is only one. The complexity of the endogenous opioid systems equals, or even exceeds, that of other classes of transmitters, such as the monoamines. In general, the localization of these peptides and their receptors correlates extremely well with those areas of the CNS described previously that have been implicated in pain perception. However, their presence in other brain regions emphasizes their wider importance in CNS function.

OPIOID PEPTIDES

The enkephalins are pentapeptides that share their first four amino acids and have either methionine or leucine as the fifth (Table 9–1). The additional opioid peptides, including the dynorphins and beta-endorphin, incorporate the sequence of either [leu^5]enkephalin or [met^5]enkephalin at their N-terminus. Despite the similarity in amino acid sequence, the enkephalins and the other endogenous opioid peptides are discrete gene products with distinct regional distributions and pharmacologies.[6,30]

In general, released neurotransmitters are inactivated within the brain either by reuptake and/or through enzymatic degradation (see Chapter 1). There is no convincing evidence for uptake of opioid peptides. Rather, the

Table 9–1 STRUCTURES OF SELECTED ENDOGENOUS AND SYNTHETIC OPIOID PEPTIDES

ENDOGENOUS OPIOID PEPTIDES

[Leu^5]enkephalin	H-**TYR-GLY-GLY-PHE**-Leu-OH
[Met^5]enkephalin	H-**TYR-GLY-GLY-PHE**-Met-OH
[Met^5]enkephalin-Arg^6-Phe^7 (heptapeptide)	H-**TYR-GLY-GLY-PHE**-Met-Arg-Phe-OH
β_h-endorphin	H-**TYR-GLY-GLY-PHE**-Met-Thr-Ser-Glu-Lys-Ser-Gln-Thr-Pro-Leu-Val-Thr- Leu-Phe-Lys-Asn-Ala-Ile-Ile-Lys-Asn-Ala-Tyr-Lys-Lys-Gly-Glu-OH
Dynorphin A	H-**TYR-GLY-GLY-PHE**-Leu-Arg-Arg-Ile-Arg-Pro-Lys-Leu-Lys-Trp-Asp-Asn-Gln-OH
Dynorphin A(1-8)	H-**TYR-GLY-GLY-PHE**-Leu-Arg-Arg-Ile-OH
Dynorphin A(1-9)	H-**TYR-GLY-GLY-PHE**-Leu-Arg-Arg-Ile-Arg-OH
Dynorphin B	H-**TYR-GLY-GLY-PHE**-Leu-Arg-Arg-Gln-Phe-Lys-Val-Val-Thr
α-neo-endorphin	H-**TYR-GLY-GLY-PHE**-Leu-Arg-Lys-Tyr-Pro-Lys-OH
β-neo-endorphin	H-**TYR-GLY-GLY-PHE**-Leu-Arg-Lys-Tyr-Pro-OH

EXOGENOUS OPIOID PEPTIDES

β-casomorphan	H-Tyr-Pro-Phe-Pro-Gly-Pro-Ile-OH
Dermorphin	H-Tyr-D-Ala-Phe-Gly-Tyr-Pro-Ser-NH$_2$
Kyotorphin	H-Tyr-Arg-OH

SYNTHETIC OPIOID PEPTIDES; ENKEPHALIN ANALOGUES

[D-Ala^2,Met^5]enkephalinamide (DAMEA)	H-Tyr-D-Ala-Gly-Phe-Met-CONH$_2$
[D-Ala^2,D-Leu^5]enkephalin (DADL)	H-Tyr-D-Ala-Gly-Phe-D-Leu-OH
FK-33824	H-Tyr-D-Ala-Gly-Phe(N-CH$_3$)-Met(O)ol
Morphiceptin	H-Tyr-Pro-Phe-Pro-CONH$_2$
Metkephamid	H-Tyr-D-Ala-Gly-Phe(N-CH$_3$)-Met-CONH$_2$
[D-Ala^2,MePhe^4,Gly(ol)^5]enkephalin (DAMPGO or DAGO)	H-Tyr-D-Ala-Gly-MePhe-Gly(ol)
[D-Ser^2,Leu^5]enkephalin-Thr^6 (DSLET or DSTLE)	H-Tyr-D-Ser-Gly-Phe-Leu-Thr-OH
[D-Pen^2,D-Pen^5]enkephalin (DPDPE)	H-Tyr-D-[Pen-Gly-Phe]-D-Pen

Amino acid sequences of selected endogenous and synthetic opioid peptides. Exact sequences of longer natural peptides will vary with different species. Bolded portions represent the four amino acids common to all opioid peptides occurring within the CNS.

opioid peptides are inactivated through the action of peptidases.[6,30] Substitution of the second amino acid, glycine, with D-amino acids, such as D-alanine, greatly stabilizes the peptides (see Table 9–1). Many of these compounds have now been examined both in animal studies and in humans and are potent analgesics. In recent years, a large number of peptides have been synthesized, including many with morphine-like, or mu, properties. Whereas the endogenous enkephalins act through both delta and mu$_1$ receptors, many of these analogues are highly selective for only mu or delta receptors, and others label a wide number of receptor classes. An alternative approach in analgesic development has been the development of inhibitors of these enkephalinases, which should increase the levels of enkephalins in vivo and induce analgesia. Although active in animal studies, clinical trials have not been promising.[30]

The opioid peptides are often present in neurons containing other neurotransmitters ("co-localization") (see Chapter 1). Although both transmitters are co-released, their ratios are not fixed and vary according to the conditions of release. Co-localization is interesting in view of the influence many neurotransmitter systems have on opioid analgesia.

OPIOID RECEPTORS

Early binding studies quickly established an excellent correlation between the affinity of opiates in binding assays and their pharmacologic potency in vivo.[91] Compounds with little analgesic activity had poor affinities at the receptor, including inactive opiate stereoisomers. Codeine was an exception, but it is demethylated to morphine, which is believed to be the active component. Binding sites were localized to neurons in general and to synaptasomal membranes in particular. Their regional distribution revealed a close association with areas known to be important in opiate analgesia, such as the PAG and medial thalamus within the brain and the substantia gelatinosa at the spinal cord level. High binding levels in other regions not associated with the modulation of pain, such as the striatum, suggested a more general role of opiate receptors beyond simply pain modulation. More recently, a number of distinct opioid receptor subtypes with unique binding profiles and pharmacologies have been reported (Table 9–2).[49,93]

Mu Receptors. The initial opiate receptors were identified by morphine and its analogues and were classified as mu.[75] Morphine produces is actions, including analgesia, constipation, and respiratory depression, through mu receptors. Evidence now suggests two subtypes of mu receptors: mu_1 and mu_2.[49,88,89,92,93,112,140] The mu_2 site is highly selective for morphine and binds the enkephalins poorly. The mu_1 site binds morphine with very high affinity, but it also binds a number of enkephalins, beta-endorphin and other opioids. However, the poor affinity of a number of highly selective delta and $kappa_1$ ligands for mu_1 receptors clearly demonstrates its unique binding selectivity profile.[18] The presence of two mu receptors through which morphine acts complicates the interpretation of actions mediated by morphine and the enkephalins. Actions elicited by morphine and not the enkephalins probably reflect mu_2 sites, whereas the reverse would

Table 9–2 TENTATIVE CLASSIFICATION OF OPIOID RECEPTOR SUBTYPES AND ACTIONS

Subtype	Active Drug Ligands	Proposed Actions
Mu		
Mu_1	Morphine and most opiates and opioid peptides	Supraspinal analgesia (including periaqueductal gray and locus ceruleus) Prolactin release Acetylcholine turnover
Mu_2	Morphine and most opiates	Respiratory depression Growth hormone release (?)* Dopamine turnover Gastrointestinal transit Guinea pig ileum bioassay Most cardiovascular actions
Delta	Enkephalins [D-Pen²,D-Pen⁵]enkephalin	Spinal analgesia Mouse vas deferens bioassay Modulation of epileptiform activity Growth hormone release (?)
Kappa		
$Kappa_1$	Dynorphin A U50,488H	Spinal analgesia Inhibition of ADH Sedation (?) Feeding
$Kappa_2$	No selective agents	Unknown
$Kappa_3$	Na1BzoH, nalorphine	Supraspinal analgesia
Epsilon	β-endorphin	Hormone (?) Rat vas deferens bioassay

*When questions remain about the assignment of receptors, a question mark is present.

correspond to delta receptors. Actions produced by both morphine and the enkephalins could be mediated independently through their selective sites or through the mu_1 receptor. The actions mediated by these receptors will be described subsequently.

Delta Receptors. Following the identification of the enkephalins, a receptor selective for the enkephalins, the delta receptor, was described.[69] Although both [met5]- and [leu5]enkephalin labeled both this delta receptor and the mu_1 receptor, a number of new derivatives have been synthesized that are highly selective for only the delta receptor, including [D-Pen2,D-Pen5] enkephalin (see Table 9–1). Delta receptors have a unique regional distribution[140] and pharmacology, as will be described later.

Kappa Receptors. Kappa receptors were initially proposed from in vivo studies based on a number of benzomorphan derivatives;[75] binding and pharmacologic evidence now has uncovered several kappa receptor subtypes.[18,35,38,105,143] $Kappa_1$ receptors are best defined by their selectivity for the agonist U50,488H and the antagonist nor-Binaltorphimine. Both $kappa_2$ and $kappa_3$ receptors are U50,488H-insensitive, but they differ significantly in the overall binding profile. The dynorphins are traditionally considered to be the endogenous ligand for kappa receptors. They have very high affinity for the $kappa_1$ receptor, but their association with the $kappa_2$ and $kappa_3$ receptors is not clear.

Other Classes of Opioid Receptors. A large number of different opioid peptides have been identified in the CNS, and it is reasonable to assume that they all have their own class of receptor subtype, raising the possibility for a number of additional opioid receptor subtypes. Several different receptor subtypes have been proposed,[49] including the epsilon receptor, which is presumably selective for beta-endorphin.[46,118] At this time, however, the pharmacologic and potential clinical importance of these additional receptor subtypes is not clear.

Opiate Actions

Understanding the pharmacologic actions of an opiate is dependent on knowing its receptor profile. Few drugs label a single site. Thus, the pharmacology of a drug is actually the summation of its interactions with all the receptors to which it binds. In addition, as the dose of drug is increased, it will interact with an increasing number of receptors, since almost all opioids will bind to any subpopulation of opioid receptor if the concentration of the ligand is sufficiently high. With these qualifications, some opiate actions are reviewed in Table 9–2.

OPIATE ANALGESIA

Opiates can elicit analgesia at several levels of the neuraxis. Indeed, epidural and intrathecal opiates have become increasingly popular during the past few years. Evidence from a number of animal studies, however, suggests that different subtypes of opioid receptors mediate analgesia in different regions of the CNS (Table 9–3). Supraspinal mechanisms predominate when drugs such as morphine are given systemically. Mu_1 and $kappa_3$ receptors have been implicated in supraspinal analgesia.[10,94] Following systemic administration, morphine produces analgesia through mu_1 receptors.[62,88–90]

At the spinal cord level, delta, mu_2 and $kappa_1$ receptors can modulate nociception.[43,62,94,95,121] These observations immediately raise important issues such as the choice of an epidural analgesic. Most physicians use morphine epidurally, but in patients already highly tolerant to morphine, its use epidurally may not be very effective. Drugs capable of activating delta and/or $kappa_1$ receptors might be more effective in this situation. An enkepha-

Table 9-3 SUBTYPES OF OPIOID RECEPTORS: REEGIONS OF THE CNS

Region	Receptor	Typical Ligands
Supraspinal	Mu_1	Morphindeltae
"		Most opiate analgesics
"	$Kappa_3$	Na1BzoH
		Nalorphine
		Levorphanol (in addition to mu)
Spinal	Mu_2	Morphine
"		Most opiate analgesics
"	Delta	[D-Ala^2,D-Leu^5] enkephalin and [D-Pen^2,D-Pen^5] enkephalin
"	$Kappa_1$	U50,488H

lin analogue active at delta receptors, [D-Ala^2,D-Leu^5]enkephalin, has been administered intrathecally in humans.[83] It was far more potent than morphine and was even effective in some patients highly tolerant to morphine. Although these findings are based on a small sample, they illustrate some of the potential advantages of understanding the receptor mechanisms of opiate action.

OPIATE TOLERANCE

With continuous use, opiates lose their effectiveness, a process termed "tolerance." Switching a patient from one opioid analgesic to another often restores effectiveness, raising the issue of incomplete cross-tolerance. Although differences in pharmacokinetics may play a role, the existence of multiple classes of opioid receptors capable of mediating analgesia independently of the others offers another possible explanation. Tolerance develops to each class of opioid receptor independently.[63] Exposure of an animal to a mu-selective drug produces tolerance to other mu drugs but not to agents acting through different classes of opioid receptors. This observation might explain incomplete cross-tolerance. For example, morphine and levorphanol are two widely used opioid analgesics. Whereas morphine interacts relatively selectively with mu receptors, levorphanol acts through a combination of mu and kappa receptors.[82] Animals tolerant to levorphanol demonstrated cross-tolerance to morphine, since the chronic levorphanol treatment produced tolerance to mu and kappa receptors. On the other hand, animals tolerant to morphine showed little cross-tolerance toward levorphanol, since the morphine-treated animals were tolerant only at mu receptors and levorphanol could produce analgesia through both mu and kappa receptors. This concept of unidirectional cross-tolerance (i.e., tolerance to morphine following levorphanol but little tolerance to levorphanol following morphine) may have important implications in the choice of opioids clinically.

RESPIRATORY DEPRESSION AND OTHER OPIATE ACTIONS

Many of the major recent advances in drug development have used the presence of subtypes of receptors to develop agents with very selective actions. Although respiratory depression is not a major issue in most patients, it can be troublesome in those with severe pulmonary difficulties or following general anesthesia. Animal studies indicate that respiratory depression produced by morphine is mediated through mu_2 receptors.[64,65] Thus, analgesics selective for mu_1, delta, or kappa receptors may not cause significant respiratory depression.

Morphine also inhibits gastrointestinal transit, resulting clinically in constipation. Like respiratory depression, this action also is mediated through mu² receptors.[43,96] Thus, drugs not acting through mu_2 receptors might have far less constipating actions in humans.

Finally, one of the major concerns regarding the prolonged use of opiates is the production of physical dependence. Discontinuing morphine after chronic use or challenging with an antagonist such as naloxone precipitates a well-described constellation of signs and symptoms collectively termed "opiate withdrawal." Although these signs and symptoms are due to actions mediated through more than one receptor, most, but not all, of the signs associated with precipitate withdrawal have been correlated to mu_2 receptors.[61] Thus, while morphine exerts its analgesic action primarily through mu_1 receptors, its concurrent activation of mu_2 receptors is responsible for the production of most aspects of physical dependence as well as a number of undesirable side effects. To further illustrate the difference between tolerance and withdrawal, animals tolerant to $kappa_3$ analgesia do not exhibit traditional withdrawal signs when challenged with an antagonist.[94]

PHARMACOLOGIC MANAGEMENT OF PAIN

Pain is a symptom, of course, and the most effective management of pain involves treatment of its cause. It is often necessary, however, to manage pain with analgesic drugs prior to the introduction of specific therapy. Indeed, inadequate pain control may preclude optimal diagnostic testing, thereby delaying definitive treatment. Further, acute pain may complicate medical or surgical therapy; treatment with analgesic drugs may be crucial to allow full recovery. Although a variety of non-pharmacologic approaches are available for the management of pain, drug therapy remains the mainstay of treatment of acute pain and chronic cancer-related pain. Drug therapy of pain has improved, but is often limited by mis-

conceptions and ignorance concerning the basic and clinical pharmacology of analgesic drugs, particularly opioids.[11,19,72]

Analgesic drugs can be divided into three major classes for the purposes of this overview: (1) aspirin and other nonsteroidal anti-inflammatory drugs (NSAIDs), which act on peripheral nerve endings at the site of injury and produce analgesia by altering the prostaglandin system; (2) narcotic analgesics (opioids), which act by binding to opioid receptors and activating endogenous pain suppression systems in the CNS; and (3) adjuvant analgesics, which act centrally to produce analgesia in certain pain states. The choice of the specific drug approach is based on an assessment of the pain syndrome, the severity of the pain, and an understanding of the clinical pharmacology of specific analgesics.

Clinical Use of NSAIDs

The NSAIDs are useful as "general purpose analgesics" in mild-to-moderate pain, especially if related to bone destruction and/or tissue inflammation.[55] These drugs include aspirin, fenoprofen, ibuprofen, diflunisal, and naproxen among others (Table 9–4). In addition to their actions as analgesics, they have antipyretic, antiplatelet, and anti-inflammatory effects.[55] There is a ceiling effect to analgesia, however. That is, increasing the dose of aspirin beyond 975 to 1300 mg/d will produce no increase in peak effect but may increase the duration of analgesia. An important mechanism of their action is the prevention of the conversion of arachidonic acid to prostaglandins, which can sensitize nociceptors on peripheral nerves to the nociceptive actions of bradykinin and other chemical mediators of inflammation. Thus, NSAIDs can influence pain at the level of the peripheral nervous sytem and may act synergistically with narcotic analgesics, which modulate pain in the CNS. Specific NSAIDs differ in their pharmacokinetics (i.e., plasma half-lives) and duration of analgesia.[132] Ibuprofen and fenoprofen have short half-lives and the same duration of action as aspirin. Diflunisal and naproxen have longer half-lives and longer durations of action and can be administered twice a day (see Table 9–4). Prolongation of the bleeding time may occur due to inhibition of platelet cyclo-oxygenase and reduced formation of thromboxane A_2. Gastric irritation also occurs commonly with this class of drugs.

Acetaminophen is also grouped in this class. It is roughly equipotent to aspirin in its analgesic and antipyretic potency, but has no anti-inflammatory or antiplatelet effects.[2] Side effects include hepatotoxicity at doses greater than 10 to 15 g/d. Choline magnesium trisalicylate (Trilisate) is also an effective analgesic, lacks antiplatelet effects, and has fewer gastrointestinal side effects than aspirin.

Nonsteroidal anti-inflammatory analgesics (especially indomethacin) may have a unique role in the management of bone pain secondary to tumor metastasis.[31] With the exception of acetaminophen and perhaps choline magnesium trisalicylate, however, the use of NSAIDs in oncology is limited by their effects on platelet function, which may increase the risk of hemorrhage in patients with thrombocytopenia and coagulation defects.

Clinical Use of Opioid Analgesics

Opioid analgesics (Tables 9–4 and 9–5) are indicated to manage moderate to severe acute pain and occasionally severe chronic pain, especially cancer-related pain and pain related to chronic medical illness.[33,102] Misconceptions by both patients and caregivers regarding intolerance, physical dependence, and psychologic dependence ("addiction") have limited their use. When used properly, however, opioids can be effective in the vast majority of patients.

OPIATE TOLERANCE, PHYSICAL DEPENDENCE, AND ADDICTION

Fears of making patients addicts is evident throughout all levels of health-care professionals, despite studies indicating that this is a very rare event in medical patients.[104] The terms "tolerance" "physical dependence," and "addiction" each describe a different effect that can be distinguished both clinically and pharmacologically.[11,31,33,50,54,61]

Any patient chronically taking opiates will develop both tolerance and physical dependence. The degree of both is related to both the dose and duration of treatment,[33,129] often beginning within the first several weeks of therapy. Although tolerance occurs in association with physical dependence, it does not imply psychologic dependence, or addiction.[50] Both tolerance and physical dependence are normal physiologic responses that should not interfere greatly in patient management.

The first sign of tolerance is a decease in the duration of effective analgesia,[45] but increasing analgesic requirements in cancer patients may also be associated with progression of disease. To minimize tolerance, many clinicians will combine opiates with nonopiates, such as the NSAIDs or acetaminophen, which do not develop tolerance, and use oral dosing, since some anecdotal evidence suggests that tolerance develops more rapidly with a parenteral administration.[103] Once tolerance develops, switching patients to an alternative opiate may be helpful since they often demonstrate incomplete cross-tolerance. To do this, start with one half of the predicted equianalgesic dose from Tables 9–4 and 9–5 and gradually increase the dose as needed.

Tolerance develops to all opiate actions, including respiratory depression. Thus, the fear of respiratory depression, which often leads physicians to underdose patients,[72] is greatly overstated, except in the presence of signifi-

Table 9-4 ANALGESICS COMMONLY USED ORALLY FOR MILD-TO-MODERATE PAIN

Name	*Equianalgesic Dose (mg)	Oral Dose Range (mg)	Duration of Analgesia (h)	Plasma Half-life (h)	Pediatric Dose (mg/kg per dose)	Comments
NONNARCOTICS						
Aspirin	650	650 qid	4–6	3–5	10	Standard of comparison for nonopioids; often used in combination with opioid-type analgesics; papillary necrosis and interstitial nephritis with chronic use; avoid during pregnancy, in hemostatic disorders, and in combination with steroids
Acetaminophen	650	650 qid	4–6	1–4	10	Like aspirin (but no anti-inflammatory or antiplatelet effects)
Ibuprofen (Motrin)	—	200–400 qid	4–6	2		Higher analgesic potential than aspirin
Fenoprofen (Nalfon)	—	200–400 qid	4–6	3		Like ibuprofen
Diflunisal (Dolobid)	—	500–1000 bid	8–12	8–12		Longer duration of action than ibuprofen; higher analgesic potential than aspirin
Naproxen (Naprosyn)	—	250–500 bid	8–12	14		Like diflunisal
Choline magnesium trisalicylate (Trilisate)	—	500–750 bid, tid	8–12	9–17		Anti-inflammatory potency similar to aspirin; few antiplatelet or gastrointestinal effects
Piroxicam (Feldene)	—	20–40 bid	8–12	45		Steady-state concentrations not reached for 7–10 d; maximal therapeutic effect in 2 wk
Indomethacin (Indocin)	—	25–50 tid	4–6	4.5		Gastrointestinal ulcers and bleeding possible
NARCOTICS						
Codeine	32–65	32–65 q4h	4–6	3	0.5–1	"Weak" morphine; often used in combination with nonopioid analgesics; biotransformed, in part, to morphine; nausea and sedation common with dose escalation
Oxycodone	5	5–10 q3h	3–5	—	0.08	Short acting; also formulated in combination with nonopioid analgesics (Percodan, Percocet) which limits dose escalation
Meperidine	50	50–100 q3h	3–5	3–4	0.75	Short acting; biotransformed to normeperidine, a toxic metabolite; normeperidine ($t_{1/2} = 12–16$ h) accumulates with repetitive dosing, causing CNS excitation; not for patients with impaired renal function receiving monoamine oxidase inhibitors

(continued)

281

Table 9–4—*Continued*

Name	*Equianalgesic Dose (mg)	Oral Dose Range (mg)	Duration of Analgesia (h)	Plasma Half-life (h)	Pediatric Dose (mg/kg per dose)	Comments
Propoxyphene HCl (Darvon) Propoxyphene napsylate (Darvon-N)	65–130	65–130 q4h	4–6	12	—	"Weak" narcotic; often used in combination with non-narcotic analgesics; long half-life biotransformed to potentially toxic metabolite (norpropoxyphene); propoxyphene and metabolites accumulate with repetitive dosing; overdose complicated by convulsions
Pentazocine (Talwin)	50	50–100 q4h	4–6	2–3	0.75	In combination with nonopioids; in combination with naloxone to discourage parenteral abuse; may cause psychotomimetic effects; mixed agonist-antagonist and therefore, may precipitate withdrawal in opioid-dependent patients

*These doses are recommended starting doses from which the optimal dose for each patient is determined by titration and maximal dose limited by adverse effects. For nonopioid analgesics, relative potency was compared to aspirin. For opioid analgesics, relative potency was compared to 10 mg IM morphine.

Source: Adapted from Payne, R: Pain. In Wittes, RE (ed): Manual of Oncological Therapeutics. JB Lippincott, Philadelphia, 1987.

Table 9–5 OPIOID ANALGESICS COMMONLY USED FOR SEVERE PAIN

Name	*Equianalgesic IM Dose (mg)	IM/PO Potency Ratio	Starting Oral Dose Range (mg)	Pediatric Dose Ranges IM PO (mg/kg per dose)	Plasma Half-life (h)	Comments
MORPHINE-LIKE AGONISTS						
Morphine	10	6	30–60	0.1–0.2 0.5–1.2	2–3	Standard of comparison for opioid analgesics; lower doses for aged patients with impaired ventilation; bronchial asthma; increased intracranial pressure; liver failure
Hydromorphone (Dilaudid)	1.5	5	4–8	0.015–0.3 0.04–0.08	2–3	Slightly shorter acting than morphine; high potency IM dosage form for tolerant patients
Methadone (Dolophine)	10	2	5–20	0.1–0.2 0.2–0.4	24–36	Good oral potency; long plasma half-life; may accumulate with repetitive dosing causing excessive sedation (on days 2–5)
Levorphanol (Levo-Dromoran)	2	2	2–4		12–16	Like methadone, may accumulate on days 2–3; delirium and hallucinations may occur
Oxymorphone (Numorphan)	1	—	—		—	Not available orally; like IM morphine
Heroin	5	6–10	—		0.5	Slightly shorter acting than morphine; biotransformed to active metabolites (e.g., morphine); not available in the United States
Meperidine (Demerol)	75	4	—		3–4	Slightly shorter acting than morphine; used orally for less severe pain (see Table 9–4); toxic metabolite, normeperidine, accumulates with repetitive dosing, causing CNS excitation; not for patients with impaired renal function or receiving monoamine oxidase inhibitors
MIXED AGONIST-ANTAGONISTS						
Pentazocine (Talwin)	60	3	50–100		2–3	Used orally for less severe pain; ?less abuse liability than morphine; included in Schedule IV of Controlled Substances Act; may cause psychotomimetic effects; may precipitate withdrawal in opioid-dependent patients; not for myocardial infarction

(continued)

Table 9–5—*Continued*

Name	*Equianalgesic IM Dose (mg)	IM/PO Potency Ratio	Starting Oral Dose Range (mg)	Pediatric Dose Ranges IM PO (mg/kg per dose)	Plasma Half-life (h)	Comments
Nalbuphine (Nubain)	10	—	—		5	Not available orally; like I.M. pentazocine but not scheduled; incidence of psychotomimetic effects lower than with pentazocine
Butorphanol (Stadol)	2	—	—		2–4	Not available orally; like nalbuphine
PARTIAL AGONISTS						
Buprenorphine (Temgesic)	0.4	—	—		—	Not available orally; sublingual preparation not yet in U.S.; less abuse liability than morphine; does not produce psychotomimetic effects; may precipitate withdrawal in opioid-dependent patients

*These doses are recommended starting IM doses from which the optimal dose for each patient is determined by titration and the maximal dose limited by adverse effects. Equianalgesic doses are based on single-dose studies in which an intramuscular dose of each drug listed was compared with morphine to establish relative potency.

For these equianalgesic IM doses, the time to peak analgesia in nontolerant patients ranges from 1/2 to 1 hour and the duration from 4 to 6 hours. The peak analgesic effect is delayed and the duration prolonged after oral administration.

Source: Adapted from Payne, R: Pain. In Wittes, RE (ed): Manual of Oncologic Therapeutics. JB Lippincott, Philadelphia, 1987.

cant pulmonary disease or in conjunction with general anesthetics or other respiratory depressants.[45,47,103] In the event of an overdose with an opioid with a short half-life, physical stimulation may be enough to prevent significant hypoventilation. No patient has succumbed to respiratory depression while awake. If an opioid antagonist is required, it should be used cautiously.[33] The dose of naloxone (0.4 mg) should be diluted to at least 10 mL and administered slowly. Patients tolerant to opiates can be extraordinarily sensitive to antagonists, and the naloxone dose should be titrated to avoid precipitation of profound withdrawal, seizures, and severe pain. Naloxone has a short half-life and may have to be given repeatedly, especially when reversing a long-acting opiate such as methadone. Comatose patients should be intubated prior to naloxone administration to prevent pulmonary aspiration. Patients receiving meperidine chronically are particularly likely to develop seizures when reversed by naloxone.

Physical dependence represents a syndrome of specific signs and symptoms associated with either the abrupt discontinuation of an opioid or the administration of an opioid antagonist. Clinically, it should not be a problem provided that the patient is not withdrawn from medication too rapidly. It is characterized by anxiety, nervousness, irritability, chills alternating with hot flashes, salivation, lacrimation, rhinorrhea, diaphoresis, piloerection, nausea, vomiting, abdominal cramps, insomnia, and, rarely, multifocal myoclonus.[74] The time course of this abstinence syndrome is a function of the specific opioid and its elimination half-life.[74,75] Symptoms may appear within 6 to 12 hours and peak at 24 to 72 hours for drugs with short half-lives, such as morphine or hydromorphone, but are usually delayed for several days and are typically less florid with drugs possessing longer half-lives, such as methadone and levorphanol. The abstinence syndrome can be avoided by slowly lowering the dose by 50% to 75% every sev-

eral days until low doses are reached, after which the medication can be discontinued.[57]

Psychologic dependence (addiction) is defined as a pattern of compulsive drug use characterized by a continued craving for the drug and the need to use an opioid for effects other than pain relief.[50] The addict exhibits drug-seeking behavior, leading to overwhelming involvement with the use and procurement of the drug. Although most patients with psychologic dependence are also physically dependent, the reverse is rarely the case in patients using opioids for management of pain.[54,104] The risk of addiction should not be a primary concern to the physician prescribing opioids for the management of pain, particularly cancer pain. Drug use alone is not the major factor in the development of psychologic dependence; other medical, social, and economic factors appear to play a more important role.[85]

GENERAL GUIDELINES IN THE USE OF OPIOID ANALGESICS

A number of general issues should be considered when administering opiates in the management of severe pain (Table 9–6).[31,33,47,50] Pain is a subjective sensation and the only way of assessing its severity is to ask the patient. While the presence of many of the autonomic signs seen in acute pain can be helpful, their absence, particularly in chronic pain patients, does not indicate the absence of pain. The autonomic signs attenuate over time despite the presence of severe pain. Furthermore, the sensitivity of patients to analgesics can vary widely. Similar observations have been made in animals, where the sensitivity of different strains of mice to morphine can vary by 20-fold. Thus, each patient must be titrated individually, slowly increasing the dose until pain relief is obtained and adjusting the dosing interval. The half-life does not always correspond well with the duration of analgesia, which rarely exceeds 6 to 8 hours regardless of analgesic.

Table 9–6 GENERAL GUIDELINES IN THE USE OF OPIOID ANALGESICS IN ACUTE AND CHRONIC PAIN

1. Respect individual differences among patients in:
   a. Starting doses (see Tables 9–4, 9–5)
   b. Duration of pain relief
2. Dose titration is the rule and not the exception:
   a. Slowly increase the dose until pain relief or limiting side effects occur.
   b. Administer opioids "around-the-clock," not "prn," after optimal dose is established by dose titration.
   c. Remember "equieffective" doses when switching drugs or routes of administration (see Tables 9–4, 9–5).
3. Anticipate and treat side effects:
   a. Constipation — daily bowel regimen
   b. Sedation — decrease dose and increase frequency
   c. Nausea and vomiting — use antiemetics and/or switch drugs
4. Anticipate tolerance and treat the tolerant patient with analgesics:
   a. Increase dose appropriately.
   b. Switch drugs.
   c. Use adjuvant analgesics.
   d. Use other therapeutic modalities (i.e., anesthetic, surgical, psychologic approaches).

It is often best to administer analgesics regularly, not prn.[122] However, administration of opioids around-the-clock should be done only after establishing the optimal dose by titration. Particular care should be exercised when using long-half-life agents since blood levels require approximately five half-lives to stabilize after changing doses. For example, it may take up to 5 days to stabilize at a new methadone dose. Once the dose requirements for a 24-hour period have been established, then analgesics can be administered on an around-the-clock basis with fewer side effects. Lower doses of medicine are needed to maintain pain relief than to "take" it away. For the patient's comfort, try to use oral administration, remembering that higher doses relative to parenteral administration are needed due to the "first-pass" effect, which greatly diminishes the potency of the drug. It is tempting to use parenteral agents because of their rapid onset of action, but this route is also associated with more side effects and perhaps faster development of tolerance. Unconventional routes of administration are discussed later.

Opiates have a number of side effects that should be anticipated and treated symptomatically if they occur, including sedation, constipation, nausea, vomiting, and respiratory depression.[31,33] Laxatives with stool softeners (e.g., sodium sulfosuccinate [Colace]) are particularly important since virtually all patients become constipated. Sedation is best treated by reducing the dose and increasing the frequency of administration, which avoids high peak concentrations of drug. In select patients in whom sedation is the only problem, dextroamphetamine (2.5 to 7.5 mg PO bid) may be added to increase alertness. Nausea and vomiting may be treated symptomatically by administering antiemetics (hydroxyzine or a phenothiazine) or by switching to another opiate. The appropriate management of respiratory depression has been discussed previously.

Choosing an opioid analgesic can be confusing. It is best to choose several drugs and learn them well. Morphine is the standard against which all opiates are compared; all physicians should be familiar with its use. In general, all narcotics provide similar qualities of analgesia, and as a class, they have similar qualities and frequency of side effects as well.[33,47] Thus, choosing a drug is often empirical. Mild-to-moderate pain is best treated by oral medications, and most physicians initiate treatment with either codeine, oxycodone, or propoxyphene. All three can be effective agents, particularly in conjunction with aspirin, acetaminophen, or another NSAID. If more potent agents are needed, drugs such as methadone, dihydromorphone, morphine, and levorphanol are available.

Certain drugs should be used cautiously. Meperidine is demethylated to normeperidine, a toxic metabolite that can accumulate and produce tremors, seizures, and myoclonus (see Chapter

10).[51] Patients with renal failure are particularly vulnerable since normeperidine is eliminated by the kidney. Mixed agonist/antagonists, such as pentazocine, can induce withdrawal in highly tolerant patients, since these patients are highly sensitive to the antagonists. Addicts often report that they are "allergic" to these medicines.

The half-lives of opioids can vary from minutes to days (see Tables 9-4 and 9-5). The very short-acting compounds are used almost exclusively during anesthesia. Of the more commonly used analgesics, methadone and levorphanol have much longer elimination half-lives (18 to 24 and 24 to 36 hours, respectively) than morphine (2 to 3 hours), and may provide a slightly longer duration of analgesia than morphine, especially in the opioid-naive patient. Despite these long half-lives, methadone and/or levorphanol should be given every 4 to 6 hours to obtain constant pain relief. The discrepancy between the duration of analgesic action and the plasma half-life of the drug remains unclear.

When facing limiting side effects, try switching opiates. Often patients are more sensitive to the side effects of one drug than another. In addition, opiates often demonstrate incomplete cross-tolerance, which may reflect differences in pharmacokinetics between the drugs or might be due to unidirectional cross-tolerance at the receptor level, as discussed previously.

HEROIN AND CANCER PAIN

Although oral or parenteral diacetylmorphine (heroin) provides pain relief in cancer patients,[53,127] it offers no unique pharmacokinetic or pharmacodynamic advantage over morphine or other more easily available opiates for the management of pain.[48,53] Heroin is deacetylated to 6-acetylmorphine very rapidly after administration and is then deacetylated again to morphine. Its analgesic actions are thought to result from the 6-acetylmorphine and morphine, rather than from heroin itself.

Although more soluble in water than morphine and thus easier to formulate in concentrated solutions, this advantage is no longer important with the availability of high-potency hydromorphone preparations (Dilaudid-HP, 10 mg/mL) which are even more potent than heroin.[48]

NOVEL ROUTES OF OPIOID ADMINISTRATION

Administration of opioids by routes other than oral ingestion or intermittent subcutaneous or intravenous injection may be necessary when these routes are impractical or the physician wishes to minimize side effects, provide a more rapid onset and longer duration of action, or to facilitate nursing care to provide smoother pain control (Table 9-7).[97] Clinically important differences in drug effects may occur as a result of changes in dosing regimens.[36,116] Guidelines have been published recently for the use of subcutaneous and intravenous infusions of opioids,[81,81a,103,131] and there is nearly a 10-year experience with spinal opioid administration.[23,97,141] Although the safety of these routes of administration has been demonstrated, their use requires sound knowledge of the clinical pharmacology of opioid analgesics and should only be undertaken if patients can be monitored carefully, particularly when used outside of the hospital. In addition, careful clinical studies documenting the efficacy of these routes in the management of specific pain syndromes have been sparse. Thus, these unconventional routes of administration should not be used as first-line treatments.

Sublingual and Buccal Administration. Sublingual and buccal administration of opioids may be desirable in patients with bowel obstruction who cannot absorb oral drugs. An additional advantage is that these routes avoid the first-pass metabolism effect when drugs are absorbed through the bowel wall (see Chapter 1). Currently, only bu-

Table 9–7 NOVEL ROUTES OF OPIOID ADMINISTRATION

Route	Indications	Comment
Sublingual	Bowel obstruction	Easy to administer
	Avoid constipating effects of oral analgesics	Swallowing will reduce potency
	Prolonged administration of opioids	No FDA-approved formulations in the United States
Buccal	Same as sublingual	May be associated with less salivation and swallowing than sublingual route
Continuous infusion		
Intravenous	Rapid pain relief desired	Use limited by need for IV access
	Prominent "bolus effects" on intermittent parenteral dosing	Rapid dose escalation in some patients
	Frequent injections required	
Subcutaneous	Prolonged parenteral administration (especially outside of hospital)	Avoids need for IV access
		Readily managed by patients and families at home
		Fewer side effects as compared to IM or PO
Transdermal	Prolonged parenteral administration; stable pain baseline	Recently available. Very convenient form of administration.
Patient-controlled analgesia	Postoperative pain	Smoother pain control
	Incident pain	Fewer side effects as compared to conventional repetitive dosing
Spinal	Postoperative pain	Long duration of pain relief possible
	Obstetric analgesia	Rapid tolerance may develop
	Cancer pain	Spinal (urinary retention) and supraspinal (nausea, sedation, respiratory depression, pruritus) side effects may occur
		Can be given by intermittent injection and continuous infusion
Intraventricular	Diffuse cancer pain	Long duration of pain relief with small dose
	Head and neck cancer pain	Ommaya reservoir placement is necessary

prenorphine is marketed in a sublingual formulation, and it is not yet available in the United States. In single-dose, cross-over analgesic studies, buprenorphine is 25 times as potent as morphine in terms of total analgesic effect (see Table 9–5).[136] Further controlled clinical studies investigating the bioavailability and potencies of opioids by sublingual or buccal routes are needed.

Intravenous Infusion. Continuous intravenous infusion of opioids is indicated when (1) patients require parenteral injections more frequently than every 3 hours, (2) patients experience prominent "bolus effects" such as sedation and rapid return of pain corresponding to peak and trough drug levels, or (3) rapid titration of drug doses is required to produce rapid pain relief. This mode of drug administration has become increasingly common in the management of postoperative and cancer pain.[103,116] In the management of postoperative pain, morphine requirements during a 72-hour period in patients receiving intramuscular doses prn were nearly fourfold greater (mean dose 140 mg) than a comparable group receiving continuous infusion (mean dose 36 mg). Portenoy[103] has reviewed continuous infusion in patients with cancer pain and proposed guidelines in its use. Pain relief was "acceptable" in 70% of patients, and side effects were similar to those seen with opiates given through alternative routes. Of note, respiratory depression occurred in only one patient and was easily reversed with naloxone. The most common cause for rapid dose escalation was progression of disease and impending death. The problems of chronic intravenous access and the availability of continuous subcutaneous infusion as an alternative have limited this mode of administration primarily to hospitalized patients.

Subcutaneous Infusion. Subcutaneous infusion obviates the need for intravenous access and allows long-term parenteral administration of opioids outside the hospital.[13,24,131] In hospitalized patients, continuous subcutaneous infusion frees patients from delays in obtaining medication from the nursing staff, and patients can be discharged without compromising pain management. In addition, continuous subcutaneous infusion has been associated with fewer adverse side effects, particularly constipation, in comparison to intramuscular dosing.[131]

Any opioid may be infused subcutaneously, although it is perhaps best to use short half-life drugs such as morphine or hydromorphone to avoid drug accumulation over time. Meperidine should be avoided due to the toxicity of its metabolite normeperidine, as noted earlier.[51] In Great Britain, heroin has been used.[115] Although its greater solubility permits the use of smaller volumes than morphine, pharmacologically it offers no advantage over morphine. Hydromorphone, which also is quite soluble, may provide a satisfactory substitute in countries where heroin is not available.

In summary, the safety, efficacy, and ease of use of continuous subcutaneous infusions, even in the home, make this route of administration an attractive alternative for many patients in whom prolonged parenteral narcotic administration is required.

Patient-Controlled Analgesia. In patient-controlled analgesia (PCA), the patient controls the frequency of intermittent drug boluses through a drug delivery device in which the physician programs the amount and frequency of the drug.[12,38,122] PCA has been studied most extensively in postoperative pain using intravenous drugs. This approach has a number of significant advantages and is preferred by most patients. The patient has a sense of "control" and is less dependent on busy nursing staff. The knowledge that he or she can easily obtain medication when needed eliminates a lot of anxiety, and studies indicate that patients using PCA actually require far less medication then when they use traditional dosing regimens. Incident pain, in which the pain is associated with movement, is often quite difficult to treat and, in theory, PCA may be advantageous in its management, since patients can anticipate movement and "premedicate" themselves.

Spinal Epidural and Intrathecal Administration. Spinal epidural or intrathecal (subarachnoid) opioids have the advantage of providing prolonged durations of pain relief with fewer side effects.[76,97] Drugs can be administered by intermittent injection through reservoir devices or by continuous infusion through implantable and external pumps.[21,76,97] The indications for spinal opioid administration are still not well defined, but this route is commonly used for management of obstetric analgesia, postoperative pain, and in cancer patients with bilateral or midline opioid-responsive pain below the level of the umbilicus, in whom adequate pain relief cannot be obtained with systemic opioids because of dose-limiting side effects.[3,23] Cross-tolerance develops between spinally and systemically administered opioids, however, and chronic spinal opioid administration may be associated with the need for rapid dose escalation.[39,82,87]

Epidural or intrathecal administration produces cerebrospinal fluid morphine concentrations 10 to 100 times greater than those obtained with systemic administration[86] and also is associated with significant levels of drug in plasma,[16] explaining the occurrence of unwanted supraspinal effects such as nausea and vomiting, pruritus, sedation, and respiratory depression. Factors that predispose to respiratory depression in postoperative pain management with spinal opioids include old age, use of large doses of hydrophilic opioids (e.g., morphine), lack of systemic opioid tolerance, and rapid changes in intrathoracic pressures such as might occur with positive end-expiratory ventilation.[23,97] Urinary retention is also seen in up to 30% of patients, but this may be related to a spinal effect of morphine.

Spinally administered opioids clearly have a role in pain management but further clinical studies are needed to optimize the use of this route of administration. Recent studies in animals and humans indicate that the opioid receptor subtypes active at the spinal level differ from those active supraspinally (see p 277 and Table 9–3). As already mentioned, for example, the enkephalin derivative [D-Ala^2,D-Leu^5]enkephalin, a delta-receptor agonist, is more potent in humans at the spinal level than morphine and was effective in some patients who were markedly tolerant to morphine.[83] Understanding the mechanisms involved with spinal analgesia will undoubtedly help in the development of new analgesic agents. Further studies in the optimal use of the drugs currently available are also needed.

Intracerebroventricular Administration. In humans, intracerebroventricular (ICV) administration of single doses of morphine ranging from 0.25 to 7 mg produces analgesia starting within 15 to 50 minutes and lasting for more than 24 hours in some patients.[59,60,66] Most patients obtained "good" to "excellent" pain relief even if pain arose from distal body segments. Side effects were not serious, the most common being confusion, sedation, pruritus, nausea, and respiratory depression. Respiratory depression may be delayed for up to 9 hours after ICV administration, but in all instances responded to intravenous naloxone.[66] There appears to be some cross-tolerance between ICV and systemically administered opioids, and tolerance develops with continued ICV administration. The drugs are directly injected into the cerebral ventricles through an indwelling ventricular catheter that is attached to a subcutaneous reservoir. Reservoir malfunction and infection were not major problems. Although potent total-body analgesia with rapid onset and long duration may be achieved with smaller doses of morphine than would be required with systemic administration, the advantage of ICV morphine over more conventional routes is still unclear and awaits further studies.

Adjuvant Analgesics

A number of other drugs are useful in the management of pain, either alone or in conjunction with opioid or nonopioid analgesics.[32] In some neuropathic pain syndromes, they are the drug of choice (Table 9–8).[32,120]

ANTICONVULSANTS

This category of drugs can be particularly useful for the management of pain in chronic neuralgias such as trigeminal neuralgia, postherpetic neuralgia, glossopharyngeal neuralgia, and post-traumatic neuralgias.[120] Carbamazepine (400 to 800 mg/d or higher) is the drug of choice for management of any painful peripheral neuropathy, including trigeminal neuralgia, that produces a paroxysmal, "shooting," "electric shock"-like pain.[32] It is generally less useful in managing the burning and aching sensations associated with neuropathic pain.

PHENOTHIAZINES

Methotrimeprazine (Levoprome) is a potent analgesic that can produce analgesia equivalent to moderate doses of morphine.[8] It does not interact with

Table 9–8 ADJUVANT ANALGESIC DRUGS

Drug	Usual Dose and Route of Administration	Indications for Use	Comment
Amitriptyline (Elavil, others)	10–125 mg PO/d *2–5 mg/kg per day	Deafferentation pain	Start treatment at 10 mg hs for elderly (25 mg hs for others) and slowly escalate to 125 mg as tolerated over 1–2 wk *Side effects:* sedation, dry mouth, urinary retention (especially in elderly men)
Fluphenazine (Prolixin, others)	1–3 mg PO/d *0.02–0.05 mg/kg per dose to 1 mg/8 h	Deafferentation pain	Usually used in combination with amitriptyline (50–100 mg) or imipramine (50–100 mg) *Side effects:* sedation, orthostatic hypotension, extrapyramidal effects, including tardive dyskinesia
Methotrimeprazine (Levoprome)	10–15 mg IM; then 10–20 mg IM q6–8h	Opioid-tolerant patients; to avoid severe opioid-induced constipation or respiratory depression	Not available orally; should give 10–15 mg IM test dose; analgesic effects are independent of opioid effects; 15 mg IM equipotent to 15 mg IM morphine *Side effects:* orthostatic hypotension, sedation, extrapyramidal effects, including tardive dyskinesia
Haloperidol (Haldol)	0.5–1.0 mg PO, bid, or tid *0.05–0.075 mg/kg per day	Co-analgesic (with opioids) in acutely agitated or psychotic patients	May potentiate morphine analgesia and allow reduction in dose; antipsychotic dose is higher (10 mg bid or tid) *Side effects:* sedation, hypotension, extrapyramidal effects, including tardive dyskinesia
Dextroamphetamine (Dexedrine)	5–10 mg PO, bid *2–10 mg/d	Reduce sedative effects of opioids; potentiate opioid analgesia in postoperative pain	Avoid giving last dose in evening to minimize insomnia; may be co-analgesic with morphine in postoperative pain management. *Side effects:* tachycardia, agitation, insomnia
Dexamethasone (Decadron)	4–8 mg PO qid	Refractory bone and deafferentation pain; epidural spinal cord compression (ESCC)	May have specific oncolytic effects; dose and route of administration vary depending on clinical situation (may give up to 100 mg IV bolus for acute ESCC); usually give over 1–2-wk period; may give equivalent in prednisone *Side effects* (with acute use): weight gain, gastrointestinal hemorrhaging, myopathy, psychosis (rare); avoid concomitant NSAID use. Should check blood counts at regular intervals.
Carbamazepine (Tegretol)	200 mg/d (start) 800–1200 mg/d	Deafferentation pain (especially with lancinating or shooting qualities)	*Side effects:* nausea, dizziness, ataxia
Hydroxyzine (Vistaril, others)	25–50 mg PO/IM q6h *0.2–0.5 mg/kg per day	Co-analgesic in anxious, nauseated patient	Synergistic analgesic effect with opioids *Side effect:* drowsiness

Source: Adapted from Payne, R: Pain. In Wittes, RE (ed): Manual of Oncologic Therapeutics. JB Lippincott, Philadelphia, 1987, and from Davis et al.[26]
*Recommended pediatric doses.

opioid receptors and its analgesia is insensitive to reversal by naloxone, indicating a nonopioid mechanism of action. It can be useful in the treatment of opioid-tolerant patients and helps to avoid the constipating and respiratory depressant effects of those drugs, but sedation and orthostatic hypotension are limiting side effects. Fluphenazine (Prolixin) has been used as an adjuvant analgesic, particularly in combination with tricyclic antidepressants, in the management of painful neuropathies such as diabetic sensory neuropathy[26] and postherpetic neuralgia.[125] Its use remains controversial, however, and additional studies are needed to evaluate its actions. A number of other phenothiazines are also useful in the treatment of opiate-induced emesis, but they may exacerbate sedative effects. Their chronic use should be limited because of the possibility of tardive dyskinesias.

TRICYCLIC ANTIDEPRESSANTS

These agents possess direct analgesic effects in animal models[119] and are the drugs of choice for a number of chronic pain syndromes, neuropathic pains, and migraine.[22,32,137] Their mechanisms of action are still not clear, but may be related to their blockade of serotonin and norepinephrine uptake. Amitriptyline has the best-documented analgesic actions,[137] but its anticholinergic actions, such as dry mouth, orthostatic hypotension, and, rarely, urinary retention or delirium, can interfere with its use. It is generally administered once a day and at doses far lower (10 to 125 mg/d) than those used to treat depression. Should side effects interfere with therapy, switching to an alternative antidepressant can be helpful. The choice of agent is empirical. They are often used in conjunction with opiates, where they enhance the analgesia.

DEXTROAMPHETAMINE

Amphetamines also enhance opioid analgesia when combined with opiates in the postoperative period,[34] but are rarely used. Dextroamphetamine is more commonly employed to reduce the sedative effects of opioids, though even this use is uncommon.

STEROIDS

Prednisone, hydrocortisone, and dexamethasone have specific and nonspecific effects in pain management. They are the drugs of choice for temporal arteritis[28] and may prove useful in intractable migraine or cluster headaches (see Chapter 5). They may be oncolytic for some tumors (e.g., lymphoma) and may ameliorate painful nerve or spinal cord compression or bone metastases by reducing edema in tumor and nervous tissue. Their use is standard practice in the treatment of suspected malignant spinal cord compression and they often markedly relieve the pain. Their use is usually based on the underlying disease, however, and they are not often prescribed specifically for pain. They retain their typical side effects, some of which may prove helpful, such as an increase in appetite and euphoria. Others, including the propensity to cause gastrointestinal bleeding, proximal myopathy, and (rarely) psychosis, may prove troublesome. Rapid withdrawal of steroids may exacerbate pain independent of the progression of systemic cancer ("pseudorheumatoid syndrome").[113]

ANTIHISTAMINES

Hydroxyzine has analgesic and antiemetic activity in addition to its antihistamine effects. It may produce additive analgesia when combined with opioids, with only slightly more sedation, so that it is a useful adjuvant for the anxious, nauseated patient.[7]

Agents to Be Avoided in the Pharmacologic Management of Pain

Benzodiazepines are effective for treatment of acute anxiety attacks and muscle spasm, but do not have analgesic properties. Their routine use is not recommended for the treatment of chronic pain. Although acute pain is often associated with typical signs of anxiety, treatment should focus on the cause of pain and the use of specific analgesic agents.

Barbiturates and other sedative-hypnotic drugs also lack intrinsic analgesic properties and should generally be avoided in the management of pain. Many commonly used analgesics are formulated in combination with barbiturates (Belladenal, Fiorinal, Axotal) and must be prescribed with caution.

Although delta-9-tetrahydrocannabinol has some analgesic properties in controlled clinical studies,[40] it is associated with high incidence of dysphoria, drowsiness, hypotension, and bradycardia. Its routine use cannot be recommended for management of pain in cancer, although it does have some efficacy as an antiemetic for chemotherapy-induced nausea and vomiting.

Finally, cocaine has local anesthetic properties, but controlled trials have demonstrated no efficacy as an analgesic alone or in combination with opiates.[128]

Placebo Response

The placebo response is common.[138] Thus, testing patients with saline to see if their pain is "real" provides no useful information. In fact, many patients with a documented organic basis for their pain will obtain a temporary response when given a placebo. The deceptive use of placebos to distinguish "psychogenic" from "real" pain should be avoided.

Pain in Children

Children may have acute or chronic pain, but inadequate verbal skills and/or their misconceptions about the etiology or consequence of pain may alter the symptoms and signs. Children should receive opioid analgesics when confronted with surgical procedures

and/or painful complications of disease, such as that accompanying cancer.[117] Assessing pain in young children can be difficult. As in adults, autonomic signs may not be present in chronic pain. Young children may refuse to take oral medication or intermittent injections and in this situation the intravenous route is used.

Children 12 years of age and older generally require adult doses of medications. Between the ages of 7 and 12, children generally require 50% of adult doses and this drops to approximately 20% to 25% in children 2 to 6 years of age. For infants younger than 2 years of age, the starting morphine dose is generally 0.1 to 0.2 mg/kg per dose IV or 0.5 to 1.2 mg/kg/per dose PO.[117] These are starting doses and, as in the adult patient, dose titration up or down is often necessary to maintain analgesia with a minimum of side effects. There is no evidence to suggest that preadolescent or adolescent children are at a higher risk for addiction than the general population when opiates are administered for pain. Like adults, they will develop tolerance with chronic therapy and may require larger doses to adequately control their pain, particularly with advanced cancer.

Analgesics in the Elderly

Analgesics may be given safely to geriatric patients, although adjustments of doses are usually required.[52,99] The elderly are usually more sensitive to opiates such as morphine and starting doses are generally smaller. In addition, elderly (as well as younger patients) with CNS disease may be more sensitive to opiates. Elderly patients are also more sensitive to the actions of the tricyclic antidepressants; therapy is usually initiated at very low doses and increased gradually. The tricyclics must be used cautiously in older men with prostatic hypertrophy due to their predisposition toward urinary retention, as well as in patients with cardiac conduction problems.

SUMMARY

Advances in understanding the neuropharmacology and neurophysiology of pain have provided a more rational basis for its treatment. Pain can be classified according to its source into somatic, visceral, and deafferentation types. The three types of pain are mediated by distinct networks of neuron receptors and neuroanatomic pathways. Deafferentation pain from nerve damage typically has a very unpleasant, burning quality that distinguishes it from somatic or visceral pain. Analgesics that control other pain are often ineffective for deafferentation pain, and "adjuvant" drugs such as anticonvulsants may be more helpful. It is also useful to classify pain as either acute (less than 6 months duration) or chronic.

For mild-to-moderate pain, the "general purpose" NSAIDs such as aspirin, fenoprofen, and naproxen are commonly useful. Acetaminophen is also in this class but does not have an anti-inflammatory effect. These drugs act in a similar fashion to block chemical mediators that activate pain in peripheral nerve endings. They may also act synergistically with opioid analgesics in the CNS.

Opioid analgesics such as morphine, meperidine, hydromorphone, and codeine are the most effective class of drugs for treatment of moderate or severe visceral and somatic pain. Addiction to opiates rarely develops during the treatment of acute pain, although clinicians tend to undertreat patients because they fear this effect. Opioids work by activating the brain's own opioid antinociceptive system composed of neurotransmitters (enkephalins, dynorphins, and endorphins) and specific opioid receptors. The drugs act at one or more subtypes of opioid receptors (mu, delta, kappa, and numerous others) that are distributed at different levels of the nervous sytem and mediate distinct actions. The first opiate receptor to be discovered, the mu receptor, mediates actions of morphine. It has been divided into distinct subtypes that mediate analgesia and respiratory depression independently. This kind of information on receptor pharmacology has been used to design new drugs that act on a variety of opioid receptors. Switching from one opioid to another that has a different spectrum of receptor action may renew an analgesic effect to which a patient has become tolerant or reduce unwanted side effects. Differences in route of administration or duration of action may also be important determinants of which drug to prescribe. New methods of opioid administration such as buccal administration, continuous subcutaneous infusion, PCA, and ICV administration have been developed to provide adequate analgesia for severe pain in special situations.

Adjuvant drugs, not usually thought of as analgesics, may relieve pain in conjunction with other drugs or alone. This group includes anticonvulsants (e.g., carbamazepine), phenothiazines, tricyclic antidepressants, steroids, and antihistamines. These drugs act by diverse mechanisms, some of which are related to the roles of nonopioid neurotransmitter systems (e.g., serotonin) in the control of pain perception.

REFERENCES

1. Albe-Fessard, D, Condes-Lara, M, Sanderson, P, et al: Tentative explanation of the special role played by the areas of paleospinothalamic projection in patients with deafferentation pain syndromes. In Krueger, L and Liebskind, JC (eds): Advances in Pain Research and Therapy, Vol. 6. Raven Press, New York, 1984, pp 167–182.
2. Ameer, B and Greenblatt, DJ: Acetaminophen. Ann Intern Med 87:202–209, 1977.
3. Arner, S, and Arner, B: Differential effects of epidural morphine in the treatment of cancer-related pain. Acta Anesthesiol Scand 29:32–36, 1985.
4. Asbury, AK and Fields, HL: Pain due to peripheral nerve damage: An hypothesis. Neurology 34:1587–1590, 1984.

5. Atweh SF, and Kuhar MJ: Distribution and physiological significance of opioid receptors in the brain. Br Med Bull 39:47–52, 1983.

6. Basbaum, AI: Anatomical substrates of pain and pain modulation and their relationship to analgesic drug action. In Kuhar, MJ and Pasternak, GW (eds): Analgesics: Neurochemical, Behavioral and Clinical Perspectives. Raven Press, New York, 1984, pp 97–124.

7. Beaver, WT and Feise, G: Comparison of the analgesic effects of morphine, hydroxyzine and their combination in patients with post-operative pain. In Bonica, JJ and Albe-Fessard, D (eds): Advances in Pain Research and Therapy. Raven Press, New York, 1976, pp 553–557.

8. Beaver, WT, Wallenstein, SL, Houde, RW, and Rogers, A: A comparison of the analgesic effect of methotrimeprazine and morphine in patients with cancer. Clin Pharmacol Ther 7:436–446, 1966.

9. Beecher HK: Pain in men wounded in battle. Ann Surg 123:96–105, 1946.

10. Bodnar, RJ, Williams, CL, Lee, SJ, and Pasternak, GW: Role of mu_1 opiate receptors in supraspinal opiates analgesia. Brain Res 447;25–37, 1988.

11. Bonica, JJ: The treatment of cancer pain: Current status and future needs. In Fields, HL, et al (eds): Advances in Pain Research and Therapy, Vol. 9. Raven Press, New York, 1985, pp 589–616.

12. Bullingham, RES, Jacobs, OLR, McQuay, HJ, and Moore RA: The Oxford system of patient-controlled analgesia. In Foley, KM and Inturrisi, CE (eds): Advances in Pain Research and Therapy, Vol. 8. Raven Press, New York, 1986, pp 319–324.

13. Campbell, CF, Matson, JB and Weiler, JM: Continuous subcutaneous infusion of morphine for the pain of terminal malignancy. Ann Intern Med 98:51–52, 1983.

14. Cervero, F and Iggo, A: The substantia gelatinosa of the spinal cord. A critical review. Brain 103:717–772, 1980.

15. Chapman, CR, Casey, KL, Dubner, R, Foley, KM, Graceley, RH, and Reading, AE: Pain measurement: An overview. Pain 22:1–31, 1985.

16. Chauvin, M, Samii, K, Schermann, JM, Sandouk, P, Bourdon, R, and Viars, P: Plasma pharmacokinetics of morphine after i.m., extradural and intrathecal administration. Br J Anesth 54:843–848, 1982.

17. Clark, JA, Houghten, R, and Pasternak, GW: Opiate binding in calf thalamic membranes: A selective mu_1 binding assay. Mol Pharmacol 34:308–317, 1988.

18. Clark, JA, Liu, L, Price, M, Hersh, B, Edelson, M, and Pasternak, GW: κ opiate receptor multiplicity: Evidence for two U50,488-sensitive κ_1 subtypes and a novel κ_3 subtype. J Pharmacol Exp Ther 251:461–468, 1989.

19. Cleeland, CS, Cleeland, LM, Dar, R, and Rinehart, LL: Factors in influencing physician management of cancer pain. Cancer 1986, 58:796–800.

20. Coggeshall, RE, Applebaum, ML, Fabn, M, et al: Unmyelinated axons in human ventral roots, a possible explanation for the failure of dorsal rhyzotomy to relieve pain. Brain 98:157–166, 1975.

21. Coombs, DW, Saunders, RL, Gaylor, MS, Block, AR, Colton, T, Harbaugh, R, Pageaa, MG, and Mroz, W: Relief of continuous chronic pain by intraspinal narcotics infusion via an implanted reservoir. JAMA 250:2336–2339, 1983.

22. Couch, JR, Ziergler, DK, and Hassanein R: Amitriptyline on the prophylaxis of migraine. Neurology 26:121–127, 1976.

23. Cousins, MJ and Mather, LE: Intrathecal and epidural administration of opioids. Anesthesiology 61:276–310, 1984.

24. Coyle, N, Mauskop, A, Maggard, and J, Foley, KM: Continuous subcutaneous infusion of opiates in cancer patients with pain. Oncology Nursing Forum 13:53–57, 1986.

25. Culp, WJ and Ochoa, J: Abnormal Nerves and Muscles as Impulse Generators. Oxford University Press, New York, 1982.

26. Davis, JL, Lewis, SB, Gerich, JE, Kaplan, RA, Schultz, TA, and Wallin, JD:

Peripheral diabetic neuropathy treated with amitriptyline and fluphenazine. JAMA 238:2291–2292, 1977.

27. Devor, M: The pathophysiology and anatomy of damaged nerve. In Wall, PD and Melzack, R (eds): Textbook of Pain. Churchill Livingstone, Edinburgh, 1984, pp 49–64.

28. Diamond, S and Dallessio, DJ: Traction and inflammatory headache and cranial neuralgias. In Diamond, S and Dallessio, DJ (eds): The Practicing Physician's Approach to Headache, ed 4. Williams & Wilkins, Baltimore, 1986, pp 84–98.

29. Dubner, R and Bennett, GJ: Spinal and trigeminal mechanisms of nociception. Ann Neurol 6:381–418, 1983.

30. Evans, CJ, Hammond, DL, and Frederickson, RCA: The opioid peptides. In Pasternak, GW (ed): The Opiate Receptors. Humana Press, Clifton Park, NJ, pp 23–74, 1988.

31. Foley, KM: The treatment of cancer pain. N Engl J Med 313:84–95, 1985.

32. Foley, KM: Adjuvant analgesic drugs in cancer pain management. In Aronoff, GM (ed): Evaluation and Treatment of Chronic Pain. Urban and Schwarzenberg, Baltimore-Munich, pp 425–434, 1985.

33. Foley, KM: The practical use of narcotic analgesics. Med Clin North Am 66:1091–1104, 1982.

34. Forrest, WH, Brown, BW, Brown, CR, et al: Dextroamphetamine with morphine for the treatment of postoperative pain. N Engl J Med 296:712–715, 1977.

35. Gistrak, MA, Paul, D, Hahn, EF, and Pasternak, GW: Pharmacological actions of a novel mixed opiate agonist/antagonist: Naloxone benzoylhydrazone. J Pharmacol Exp Ther 251:469–476, 1989.

36. Goldman, P: Rate-controlled drug delivery. N Engl J Med 307:286–290, 1982.

37. Goodman, RR, and Pasternak, GW: Visualization of mu_1 opiate receptors in rat brain using a computerized autoradiographic subtraction technique. Proc Natl Acad Sci USA 82:6667–6671, 1985.

38. Graves, D, Foster, TS, Batenhorst, RL, Bennett, RL, and Baumann, TF: Patient-controlled analgesia. Ann Intern Med 99:360–366, 1983.

39. Greenberg, HS, Taren, J, Ensminger, W, et al: Benefit from and tolerance to continuous intrathecal infusion of morphine for intractable cancer pain. J Neurosurg 57:360–364, 1982.

40. Harris, LS: Cannabinoids as analgesics. In Beers, RF and Bassett, EG (eds): Mechanism of Pain and Analgesic Compounds. Raven Press, New York, 1979.

41. Haubrich, R, Baizman, ER, Morgan, BA, and Saelens, JK: The role of endogenous nonendorphin substances in nociception. In Kuhar, MJ, and Pasternak, GW (eds): Analgesics: Neurochemical, Behavioral and Clinical Perspectives. Raven Press, New York, 1984, pp 195–234.

42. Head, H and Holmes, G: Sensory disturbances from cerebral lesions. Brain 34:102–254, 1911.

43. Heyman, JS, Williams, CL, Burks, TF, Mosberg, HI and Porreca, F: Dissociation of opioid antinociception and central gastrointestinal propulsion in the mouse: Studies with naloxonazine. J Pharmacol Exp Ther 245:238–243, 1988.

44. Hosobuchi, Y: The majority of unmyelinated afferent axons in human ventral roots probably conduct pain. Pain 8:167–180, 1980.

45. Houde, RW: The use and misuse of narcotics in the treatment of chronic pain. Adv Neurol 4:527–536, 1974.

46. Houghton, RA, Johnson, N, and Pasternak, GW: ^{3}H-Endorphin binding in rat brain. J Neurosci 4:2460–2465, 1984.

47. Inturrisi, CE and Foley, KM: Narcotic analgesics in the management of pain. In Kuhar, MJ and Pasternak, GW (eds): Analgesics: Neurochemical, Behavioral and Clinical Perspectives. Raven Press, New York, 1984, pp 257–288.

48. Inturrisi, CE, Max, MB, Foley, KM, Schultz, M, Shin, S-C, and Houde, RW: The pharmacokinetics of heroin in patients with chronic pain. N Engl J Med 210:1213–1217, 1984.

49. Itzhak, Y: Multiple opioid binding

sites. In Pasternak, GW (ed): The Opiate Receptors. Humana Press, Clifton, NJ, 1988, pp 95–142.

50. Jaffe, JH: Drug addiction and drug abuse. In Gilman, AG, Gooodman, LS, Rall, TW, and Murad, F (eds): The Pharmaceutical Basis of Therapeutics, ed 7. Macmillan, New York, 1985, pp 532–581.

51. Kaiko, RF, Foley, KM, Grabinski, PY, Heidrich, G, Rogers, AG, Inturrisi, CE, and Reidenberg, MM: Central nervous system excitatory effects of meperidine in cancer patients. Ann Neurol 13:180–185, 1983.

52. Kaiko, RF, Wallenstein, SL, Rogers, AG, Grabinski, PV, and Houde, RW: Narcotics in the elderly. Med Clin North Am 66:1079–1089, 1983.

53. Kaiko, RF, Wallenstein, SL, Rogers, AG, Grabinski, PV, and Houde, RW: Analgesic and mood effects of heroin and morphine in cancer patients with postoperative pain. N Engl J Med 304:1501–1505, 1981.

54. Kanner, RM and Foley, KM: Patterns of narcotic drug use in a cancer pain clinic. Ann NY Acad Sci 362:161–172, 1981.

55. Kantor, TG: The control of pain by nonsteroidal anti-inflammatory drugs. Med Clin North Am 66:1053–1059, 1982.

56. Kenshalo, DR and Isensee, O: Responses of primate SI cortical neurons to noxious stimuli. J Neurophysiol 50:1479–96, 1983.

57. Kolb, L and Himmelsbach, CK: Clinical studies of drug addiction. III. A critical review of withdrawal treatments with methods of evaluating abstinence syndromes. Am J Psychiatry 94:759–797, 1938.

58. Kosterlitz, HW, Paterson, SJ, and Robson, LE: Characterization of the kappa-subtype of the opiate receptor in the guinea pig brain. Br J Pharmacol 73:939–949, 1981.

59. Leavens, ME, Hill, CS, Cech, DA, Weyland, JB, and Weston, JS: Intrathecal and intraventricular morphine for pain in cancer patients: Initial study. J Neurosurg 56:241–242, 1982.

60. Lenzi, A, Galli, G, Gandolfini, M, and Marini, G: Intraventricular morphine in paraneoplastic painful syndrome of the cervicofacial region: Experience in thirty-eight cases. Neurosurgery 17:6–11, 1985.

61. Ling, GSF, Macleod, JM, Lee, S, Lockhart, S, and Pasternak, GW: Separation of morphine analgesia from physical dependence. Science 226:462–464, 1984.

62. Ling, GSF and Pasternak, GW: Spinal and supraspinal analgesia in the mouse: The role of subpopulations of opioid binding sites. Brain Res 271:152–156, 1983.

63. Ling, GSF, Paul, D, Simantov, R, and Pasternak, GW: Differential development of acute tolerance to analgesia, respiratory depression, gastrointestinal transit and hormone release in a morphine infusion model. Life Sci 45:1627–1636, 1989.

64. Ling, GSF, Spiegel K, Lockhart SH, and Pasternak GW: Separation of opioid analgesia from respiratory depression: Evidence for different receptor mechanisms. J Pharmacol Exp Ther 232:149–155, 1985.

65. Ling, GSF, Spiegel K, Nishimura S, and Pasternak GW: Dissociation of morphine's analgesic and respiratory depressant actions. Eur J Pharmacol 86;487–488, 1983.

66. Lobato, RD, Madrid, JL, Fatela, LV, Rivas, JJ, Reig, E, and Lamas, E: Analgesia elicited by low-dose intraventricular morphine in terminal cancer patients. In Fields, HL, Dubner, R, and Cerveno, F (eds): Advances in Pain Research and Therapy, Vol 9, Raven Press, New York, 1985, pp 673–681.

67. Lobato, RD, Madrid, JL, Fatela, LV, Rivas, JJ, Reig, E, and Lamas, E: Intraventricular morphine for control of pain in terminal cancer patients. J Neurosurg 59:6627–6633, 1983.

68. Loh, L and Nathan, PW: Painful peripheral states and sympathetic blocks. J Neurol Neurosurg Psychiatry 41:664–671, 1978.

69. Lord, JH, Waterfield, AA, Hughes, J, and Kosterlitz, HW: Endogenous opioid peptides: Multiple agonists and receptors. Nature 267:495–499, 1977.

70. Maciewicz, R, Bouckoms, A, and Martin, JB: Drug therapy for neuropathic pain. The Clinical Journal of Pain 1:39–49, 1985.

71. Maciewicz, R and Sandrew, BB: Physiology of pain. In Aronoff, GM (ed): Evaluation and Treatment fo Chronic Pain. Urban and Schwarzenberg, Baltimore-Munich, 1985, pp 17–39.

72. Marks, RM and Sachar, EG: Undertreatment of medical inpatients with narcotic analgesics. Ann Intern Med 78:173–181, 1973.

73. Marshall, J: Sensory disturbances in cortical wounds with special reference to pain. J Neurol Neurosurg Psychiatry 14:187–204, 1951.

74. Martin, WR: Opioid antagonists. Pharmacol Rev 19:463–521, 1967.

75. Martin, WR, Eades, CG, Thompson, JA, Huppler, RE, and Gilbert, PE: The effects of morphine- and nalorphine-like drugs in the nondependent and morphine-dependent chronic spinal dog. J Pharmacol Exp Ther 197:517–532, 1976.

76. Max, MB, Inturrisi, CE, Kaiko, RF, Som, J, Grabinski, PY, Li, CH, and Foley, KM: Epidural and intrathecal opiates: Cerebrospinal fluid and plasma profiles in patients with chronic cancer pain. Clin Pharmacol Ther 38:631–641, 1985.

77. Mayer, DJ, and Liebeskind, JC: Pain reduction by focal electrical stimulation of the brain: An anatomical approach. Brain Res 68:73–93, 1974.

78. Mersky, H (ed): Classification of chronic pain: Description of chronic pain syndromes and definitions of pain terms. Pain (Suppl)3:S217, 1986.

79. Meyer, RA and Campbell, JN: Myelinated nociceptive afferents account for the hyperalgesia that follows a burn to the hand. Science 213:1527–1529, 1981.

80. Milne, RJ, Foreman, RD, Giesler, GJ, and Willis, WD: Convergence of cutaneous and pelvic visceral nociceptive inputs onto primate spinothalamic neurons. Pain 11:163–181, 1981.

81. Miser, AW, Davis, DM, Hughes, CS, Mulne, AF, and Miser, JS: Continuous subcutaneous infusions of morphine in children with cancer. Am J Dis Child 137:383–385, 1983.

81a. Miser, AW, Miser, JS, and Clark, BS: Continuous intravenous infusion of morphine sulfate for control of severe pain in children with terminal malignancy. J Pediatr 5:930–932, 1980.

82. Moulin, DE and Pasternak, GW: Unidirectional analgesic cross tolerance between morphine and levorphanol in the rat. Pain 33:233–239, 1988.

83. Moulin DE, Max M, Kaiko RF, Inturrisi, CE, and Foley, KM: The analgesic efficacy of intrathecal (IT) [D-Ala, D-Leu]enkephalin in cancer patients with chronic pain. Pain 23:213–221, 1985.

84. Nathan, PW: Pain and the sympathetic nervous system. J Auton Nerv Sys 7:363–370, 1983.

85. Newman, RG: The need to redefine "addiction". N Engl J Med 308:1096–1098, 1983.

86. Nordberg, G: Pharmacokinetic aspects of spinal morphine analgesia. Acta Anesth Scand 28(Suppl)79:6–38, 1984.

87. Onofrio, BM, Yaksh, TL, and Arnold, PG: Continuous low-dose intrathecal morphine administration in the treatment of chronic pain of malignant origin. Mayo Clin Proc 56;516–520, 1981.

88. Pasternak, GW: Opiate, enkephalin and endorphin analgesia: Relations to a single subpopulation of opiate receptors. Neurology 31:1311–1315, 1981.

89. Pasternak, GW, Childers SR, and Snyder SH: Opiate analgesia: Evidence for mediation by a subpopulation of opiate receptors. Science 208:514–516, 1980.

90. Pasternak, GW, Childers SR, and Snyder SH: Naloxazone, a long-acting opiate antagonist: Effects on analgesia in intact animals and on opiate receptor binding in vitro. Pharmacol Exp Ther 214;455–462, 1980.

91. Pasternak, GW: Early studies of opiate binding. In Pasternak, GW (ed): The Opiate Receptors. Humana Press, Clifton, NJ, 1988, pp 75–94.

92. Pasternak, GW and Snyder SH: Identification of novel high affinity opiate re-

ceptor binding in rat brain. Nature 253:563–565, 1975.

93. Pasternak, GW and Wood, PL: Multiple mu opiate receptors. Life Sci 38:1889–1898, 1986.

94. Paul, D, Levison, JA, Howard, DH, Pick, CG, Hahn, EF, and Pasternak, GW: Naloxone benzoylhydrazone (NalBzoH) analgesia. J Pharmacol Exp Ther 255:769–799, 1990.

95. Paul, D, Bodnar, RJ, Gistrak, MA, and Pasternak, GW: Different mu receptor subtypes mediate spinal and supraspinal analgesia in mice. Eur J Pharmacol 168:307–314, 1989.

96. Paul, D and Pasternak, GW: Differential blockade by naloxonazine of two μ opiate actions: Analgesia and inhibition of gastrointestinal transit. Eur J Pharmacol 149:403–404, 1988.

97. Payne, R: The role of epidural and intrathecal narcotics and peptides in the management of cancer pain. Med Clin North Am 71:313–327, 1987.

98. Payne, R: Neuropathic pain syndromes, with special reference to causalgia and reflex sympathetic dystrophy. The Clinical Journal of Pain 2:59–73, 1986.

99. Payne, R and Pasternak GW: Pain and pain management in the elderly. In Cassel, CK, Sorensen, L, Riesenberg, D, and Walsh, JR, (eds): Geriatric Medicine, ed 2. Springer-Verlag, New York, 1990, pp 585–606.

100. Penfield, W and Boldrey, E: Somatic motor and sensory representation in the cerebral cortex of man as studied by electrical stimulation. Brain 60:389–443, 1937.

101. Perl, ER: Characterization of nociceptors and their activation of neurons in the superficial dorsal horn: First steps for the sensation of pain. In Kruger, L and Liebeskind, JC (eds): Advances in Pain Research and Therapy, Vol 6. Raven Press, New York, 1984, pp 23–52.

102. Portenoy, RK and Foley, KM: Chronic use of opioid analgesics in non-malignant pain: Report of 38 cases. Pain 25:171–186, 1986.

103. Portenoy, RK, Moulin, DE, Rogers, A,

Inturrisi, CE, and Foley, KM: I.V. infusion of opioids for cancer pain: Clinical review and guidelines for use. Cancer Treat Rep 70:575–581, 1986.

104. Porter, J and Jick, H: Addiction rare in patients treated with narcotics. N Engl J Med 302:133, 1980.

105. Price, M, Gistrak, MA, Itzhak, Y, Hahn, EF, and Pasternak, GW: Receptor binding of ^{3}H-naloxone benzoylhydrazone: A reversible κ and slowly dissociable mu opiate. Mol Pharmacol 35:67–74, 1989.

106. Price, DD and Dubner, R: Neurons that subserve the sensory-discriminative aspects of pain. Pain 3:307–338, 1977.

107. Ralston, HJ: The fine structure of laminae IV, V and VI of the macaque spinal cord. J Comp Neurol 212:425–434, 1982.

108. Rasminsky, M: Ectopic impulse generation in pathological nerve fibers. Trends in Neuroscience 1983, pp 388–390.

109. Rexed, B: The cytoarchitectonic organization of the spinal cord in the cat. J Comp Neurol 96:415–494, 1952.

110. Reynolds, DV: Surgery in the rat during electrical analgesia induced by focal brain stimulation. Science 164:444–445, 1969.

111. Roberts, WJ and Elardo, SM: Sympathetic activation of A-delta nociceptors. Somatosensory Research 3:33–44, 1985.

112. Rothman, RB, Jacobson, AE, Rice, KC, and Herkenham, M: Autoradiographic evidence for two classes of mu opioid binding sites in rat brain using [^{125}I]FK33824. Peptides 8:1015–1021, 1987.

113. Rotstein, J and Good, RA: Steroid pseudorheumatism. Arch Intern Med 99:545–555, 1957.

114. Ruch, TC: Visceral sensation and referred pain. In Fulton, J (ed): Howell's Textbook of Physiology, ed 15. WB Saunders, Philadelphia, 1946, pp 385–401.

115. Russell, PSB: Heroin for the relief of pain [letter]. N Engl J Med 311:1633–1634, 1984.

116. Rutter, PC, Murphy, F, and Dudley, AF: Morphine: Controlled trial of different methods of administration for postoperative pain relief. Br Med J 12–13, 1980.

117. Schlechter, NE: Pain and pain control in children. Cur Prob Pediatr 15:1–67, 1985.

118. Schulz, R, Wuster, M, and Herz, A: Pharmacological characterization of the epsilon opiate receptor. J Pharmacol Exp Ther 216:604–606, 1981.

119. Spiegel, K, Kalb, R, and Pasternak, GW: Analgesic activity of tricyclic antidepressants. Ann Neurol 13:462–465, 1983.

120. Swerdlow, M: Anticonvulsant drugs and chronic pain. Clin Neuropharmacol 7:51–82, 1984.

121. Takemori, AE, Ho, YH, Naeseth, JS, and Portoghese, PS: Nor-Binaltorphimine, a highly selctive κ-opioid antagonist in analgesic and receptor binding assays. J Pharmacol Exp Ther 246:255–258, 1988.

122. Tameson, A, Sjoestroem, S, and Hartvig, P: The Uppsala experience of patient-controlled analgesia. In Foley, KM and Inturrisi, CE (eds): Advances in Pain Research and Therapy, Vol 8. Raven Press, New York, 1986, pp 325–335.

123. Tasker, RR: Deafferentation. In Wall, PD and Melzack, R (eds): Textbooks of Pain. Churchill Livingstone, New York, 1984, pp 119–132.

124. Tasker R, Organ, LW, and Hawrylyshyn, P: Deafferentation and causalgia. In Bonica, JJ (ed): Pain: Association for Research in Nervous and Mental Disease. Vol 58. Raven Press, New York, 1980, pp 305–330.

125. Taub, A and Collins, WF: Observations on the treatment of denervation dysesthesia with psychotropic drugs: Postherpetic neuralgia, anesthesia dolorosa, peripheral neuropathy. In Bonica, JJ (ed): Advances in Neurology, Vol 4. Raven Press, New York, 1974, pp 309–315.

126. Torebjork, HE and Hallin, RG: Microneurographic studies of peripheral pain mechanisms in man. In Bonica, JJ (ed): Advances in Pain Research and Therapy, Vol. 3. Raven Press, New York, 1979, pp 121–131.

127. Twycross, RG: Choice of strong analgesic in terminal cancer: Diamorphine or morphine? Pain 3:93–104, 1977.

128. Twycross, RG, and Lack, SA: Value of cocaine in opiate-containing elixirs. Br Med J 2:1348, 1977.

129. Twycross, RG and Lack SA: Symptom Control in Far Advanced Cancer: Pain Relief. Pitman Publishing, London, 1983.

130. Vallbo, AB, Hagbarth, K-E, Torebjork, HE, and Wallin, BG: Somatosensory, proprioceptive, and sympathetic activity in human peripheral nerves. Physiol Rev 59:919–957, 1979.

131. Ventafridda, V, Spoldi, E, Caraceni, A, et al: The importance of continuous subcutaneous morphine administration for cancer pain. The Pain Clinic 1:47–55, 1986.

132. Verbeeck RK, Blackburn, JL, and Loewen GR: Clinical pharmacokinetics of non-steroidal anti-inflammatory drugs. Clin Pharmacokinet 8:297–331, 1983.

133. Walker, AE and Nulson, F: Electrical stimulation of the upper thoracic portion of the sympathetic chain in man. Archives of Neurology and Psychiatry 5:559–560, 1948.

134. Wall, PD and Gutnick, M: Ongoing activity in peripheral nerves: The physiology and pharmacology of impulses originating from a neuron. Exp Neurol 43:580–593, 1974.

135. Wall, PD, and McMahon, SB: Microneuronography and its relation to perceived sensation. A critical review. Pain 21:209–229, 1985.

136. Wallenstein, SL, Kaiko, RF, Rogers, AG, and Houde, RW: Clinical analgesic assay of sublingual buprenorphine and intramuscular morphine. In Cooper, JR, Altman, F, Brown, BS, and Czechowicz, D (eds): NIDA Research Monograph, Vol. 41: Problems of Drug Dependence. Rockville, MD, US Department of Health and Human Services, 1981, pp 288–293.

137. Watson, CP, Evans, RJ, Reid, K, et al:

Amitriptyline vs. placebo in postherpetic neuralgia. Neurology 32:671–673, 1982.

138. White, L, Tursky, B, and Schwartz, GE: Placebo: Theory, Research and Mechanisms. Guilford Press, New York, 1985.

139. Willis, WD: The Pain System: The Neural Basis of Nociceptive Transmission in the Mammalian Nervous System. S. Karger, Basel, Switzerland, 1985.

140. Wolozin BL and Pasernak GW: Classification of multiple morphine and enkephalin binding sites in the central nervous system. Proc Natl Acad Sci USA 78:6181–6185, 1981.

141. Yaksh, TL and Rudy, TA: Studies on the direct spinal action of narcotics in the production of analgesia in the rat. J Pharmacol Exp Ther 202:411–428, 1977.

142. Young, GB and Blume, WT: Painful epileptic seizure. Brain 106:537–554, 1983.

143. Zukin, RS, Eghbali, M, Olive, D, Unterwald, EM, and Tempel, A: Characterization and visualization of rat and guinea pig brain κ opioid receptors: Evidence for κ_1 and κ_2 opioid receptors. Proc Natl Acad Sci USA 85:4061–4065, 1988.

Chapter 10

ACUTE DRUG INTOXICATION

*Daniel H. Lowenstein, M.D.,
and Roger P. Simon, M.D.*

ALTERATIONS IN CONSCIOUSNESS CAUSED BY DRUGS AND TOXINS SEIZURES CAUSED BY DRUG INTOXICATION

Previous chapters in this book discussed the therapeutic use of drugs and their unwanted side effects. The practitioner is also confronted with disorders caused by accidental or willful intoxication with neuroactive drugs. The variety of serious neurologic and psychiatric disorders caused by abuse of drugs seems to expand steadily as new drugs and methods for administering them are invented. The neurologic manifestations of acute intoxication, specifically drug-induced alterations in consciousness, coma, and seizures, are discussed in this chapter with emphasis on mechanisms of action and their various clinical presentations. Treatment is discussed if it is specific to a particular toxin. The general approach to supportive management of intoxicated patients is discussed in numerous monographs and papers.[61] We have focused our discussion on substances of abuse, including sedative-hypnotics, alcohol, psychotropics, stimulants, hallucinogens, and inhalants.

Most intoxicated patients will respond to appropriate intervention. The critical determinant of outcome for the majority of patients should be the interval between intoxication and arrival at the emergency room. This assumes an ability of the physician to (1) differentiate other forms of disease from the alterations in central nervous system (CNS) function due to exogenous agents, (2) recognize the patterns of dysfunction caused by various drugs, and (3) promptly initiate appropriate therapy.

ALTERATIONS IN CONSCIOUSNESS CAUSED BY DRUGS AND TOXINS

As described in Chapter 8, a number of drugs can disrupt cognitive function and produce confusion, delirium, and coma (Table 10–1). In addition, certain drugs are particularly prone to cause behavior disinhibition, agitation, panic, or acute signs of organic psychosis. In some cases, observations of the toxic actions of drugs have provided insights into brain function, as when anticholinergic drugs produce amnesia and delirium. The same may be said for drugs that are abused, such as the opiates, cocaine, and amphetamine derivatives. The distinctive effects of these compounds are related to their interaction with specific neuron circuits.

Mechanisms of Alterations in Consciousness

A rich network of neuron pathways connecting the brainstem and diencephalon with the cerebral cortex is responsible for normal arousal and consciousness.[130] Ascending pathways originating in the brainstem and thalamus sustain normal arousal of the cerebral cortex. This ascending reticular activating system (ARAS) is a major target for drug intoxications that produce coma. The center of this system is a group of medium-sized neurons located within the core of the brainstem, extending from the medulla to the midbrain. The ARAS, however, is really a dispersed physiologic network rather than a precise anatomic structure. It makes a wide range of connections with the cerebral cortex, thalamus, hypothalamus, and every major sensory pathway.

The ARAS controls cortical activity through three principal circuits. One pathway projects to the thalamic reticular nucleus. Stimulation of the thalamic reticular nucleus predominately inhibits the cerebral cortex, and the ARAS modulates cortical activity through this mechanism. A second major pathway ascends to the hypothalamus to stimulate neuron structures within the limbic system and basal forebrain. The cholinergic neurons that project from the basal fore-brain to the cerebral cortex anatomically resemble neurons in the brainstem ARAS and probably should be grouped with them. The third principal group of pathways are the diffuse serotonergic and catecholamine projections to the cerebral cortex from the midbrain and pons. These pathways and their influence on the cerebral cortex are also discussed in Chapter 8. In addition to those mentioned, excitatory amino acid (EAA) neurotransmitter mechanisms may play a major role in arousal and consciousness. For example, dissociative anesthetics such as ketamine appear to exert their primary influence by blocking the N-methyl-D-aspartate (NMDA)-type glutamate receptor channel complex. Differing effects of drugs on these pathways may be responsible for the varied clinical presentations of drug intoxication (see Chapter 1).

Drugs that impair consciousness do so by several general mechanisms. These include a generalized increase in the activity of inhibitory neurotransmitter function, blockade of excitatory neurotransmitter pathways, and nonspecific toxic effects on neuron membranes and neuron metabolism. These molecular mechanisms responsible for impaired consciousness are discussed in greater detail in Chapters 1 and 3. Sedative-hypnotic drugs, benzodiazepines, and anticonvulsants impair consciousness by increasing inhibition within the nervous system, but very high doses also may produce nonspecific toxic effects. Anticholinergic drugs, heterocyclic antidepressants, cocaine, and amphetamine derivatives are examples of drugs that impair consciousness by disrupting the synaptic function of neurotransmitter-specific ascending pathways originating in the brainstem. Organic toxins that are inhaled probably cause impairment of consciousness through nonspecific toxic effects on many components of the brain. Although knowledge of the precise mechanisms responsible for disruption of consciousness by drugs is incomplete, the following sections attempt to delineate clinical syndromes of intoxication and relate them to potential mechanisms.

Distinguishing Intoxication from Other Causes of Coma

The major effects of acute intoxication on the CNS include alteration in level of consciousness, disturbances in central respiratory control, and seizures. There may also be dysfunction of ocular motility, the pyramidal and extrapyramidal systems, and autonomic control. A wide variety of different exogenous agents may cause similar effects. Fortunately, certain patterns of symptoms and signs suggest particular classes of agents.

INITIAL EVALUATION
AND MANAGEMENT

The depressive effects of exogenous toxins on consciousness range from mild confusion to deep coma. Regardless of the level of consciousness, the first task in the evaluation of the patient is to ensure adequate cardiorespiratory function and to institute prompt resuscitative measures if necessary. It is routine to draw venous blood samples and an arterial blood gas, and concurrently to administer intravenous dextrose (50 mL of a 50% dextrose solution), naloxone (0.8 to 2.0 mg), and thiamine (100 mg) to the comatose patient prior to any further evaluation.

The first diagnostic endeavor is to distinguish between structural and metabolic disease. Coma is generally a consequence of either bihemispheric or brainstem dysfunction. Structural disease, such as stroke or tumor mass, may affect both hemispheres by direct involvement of one side and subsequent compression of the other side, or by superimposing a new process on old disease of the contralateral hemisphere. Structural lesions may also impinge directly or secondarily on the brainstem (ARAS). Metabolic processes presumably have a diffuse effect on both hemi-

spheres, the brainstem, or both, yet certain pathways, such as those subserving the pupillary light reflex, are relatively resistant. Based on these concepts, the following principles have proved extremely useful:

1. Focal neurologic signs, in the absence of a history of prior focal CNS disease, suggest a structural cause of coma.

2. Preserved pupillary light reflexes and a nonfocal examination suggest a metabolic cause of coma.

There are exceptions to these rules, however. For example, asymmetric abnormalities of eye movement may be seen with certain toxins (e.g., phenothiazines), and the pupillary light reflex is lost in severe anticholinergic and barbiturate poisoning when ventilation is supported. Thus it is essential to search for other clues in the history or examination to confirm the diagnosis.

Another important distinguishing characteristic between coma of metabolic and structural origin is the evolution of signs over time. A fluctuating level of consciousness is exceedingly common in metabolic encephalopathy; it may be more common with endogenous than exogenous causes. Alternatively, patients with structural processes tend to have either fixed deficits or a progression of signs that may, in the case of supratentorial lesions, follow a "rostral-caudal" pattern.[130]

CLUES TO ETIOLOGY FROM
THE PHYSICAL EXAMINATION

Tables 10–2, 10–3, and 10–4 list a number of signs that may help in distinguishing different toxic causes of coma. For a detailed description of the examination of the comatose patient, the reader is referred to the Plum and Posner[130] and Fisher[41] monographs.

Hypothermia. In a review of 148 patients admitted to the San Francisco General Hospital from 1970 to 1979 with a temperature of 35°C (95°F) or less, 51 (34%) were intoxicated with alcohol and 15 (10%) with sedatives.[40] Hy-

Table 10-2 SYSTEMIC SIGNS IN DRUG INTOXICATION

Substance	Hypo-thermia	Hyper-thermia	Low Blood Pressure	High Blood Pressure	Arrhythmia	Skin Vesicles	Pulmonary Edema
Barbiturates	+		+		+	+	
Glutethimide (Doriden)	+	+	+			+	
Methaqualone (Quaalude)	+		+			+	+
Ethchlorvynol (Placidyl)	+		+		+		+
Benzodiazepines (Valium)	+		+				
Opioids	+		+			+	+
Ethanol	+		+				
Heterocyclic antidepressants		+	+		+	+	
Neuroleptics	+	+			+		
Amphetamines		+		+			
Cocaine		+		+	+		
Phencyclidine		+		+			

+ = positive for given sign.

pothermia has also been associated with coma due to overdose with glutethimide.[122] butyrophenones,[87] and certain phenothiazines such as chlorpromazine. Some patients become hypothermic because they lose the ability to recognize and take precautions in a cold environment.[137] In others, however, there appears to be a direct effect of the toxin on the thermoregulatory system.[137] Alcoholics are especially prone to accidental hypothermia,[2,39,186] and this has been attributed to the direct impairment of vasoconstriction by the alcohol itself, abnormalities in glucose metabolism,[46,177] and abnormalities of central control mechanisms.[68,84,99] Barbiturates also may influence central mechanisms.[33,98]

The hypothermic state, in itself, may cause profound abnormalities in neurologic function. Thus, a number of the patients mentioned earlier[40] who had severe hypothermia (20°C to 27°C) and no identifiable CNS structural lesions, were comatose and had sluggish or nonreactive pupils, increased muscle tone, and extensor plantar responses. A thorough reexamination is therefore necessary following rewarming procedures.

Hyperthermia. Fever in a comatose patient suggests an infectious process. Of course, this needs to be carefully pursued through the physical examination and appropriate laboratory investigations, including cerebrospinal fluid analysis. Hyperthermia is the hallmark of the patient with heat stroke.[27,144] It may also occur in patients following seizures.[4] Beyond these causes, however, unexplained hyperthermia with coma should prompt a search for an exogenous toxic etiology.[126,144]

Anticholinergic agents (including alkaloids, H_1 antihistamines, heterocyclic antidepressants, and certain phenothiazines) may cause fever, which has been attributed to suppression of sweating and possibly to central actions. Toxins with sympathomimetic properties, such as amphetamine, cocaine, and phencyclidine (PCP), will cause fever as well.[11,82,192] In these cases, the mechanism probably involves the hypothalamus[25,97] and is exacerbated by muscular hyperactivity.[192] Rosenberg and colleagues[142] described the clinical course of 12 patients with hyperthermia and drug intoxication (including anticholinergics, salicylates, diphenhydramine, a stimulant, and hallucinogens). Of the 12 patients, 11 were comatose, 4 were not sweating despite rectal temperatures greater than 40.5°C, 9 had increased muscle activity, and 5 were in status epilepticus. Other untoward effects included hypotension, arrhythmias, rhabdomyolysis, coagulopathies, and electrolyte disorders. Despite attempts at cooling, and the use of neuromuscular blockade or dantrolene in some cases, 5 patients died and 3 suffered from severe neurologic sequelae. The authors emphasized the need for early recognition of patients at risk and prompt, aggressive treatment.

The cardinal features of neuroleptic malignant syndrome include hyperpyrexia, altered level of consciousness, increased muscle tone with parkinsonian features, and autonomic instability.[32] Some patients initially present in coma. Most cases have been associated with haloperidol or fluphenazine, but various other neuroleptics have been implicated as well. Its pathogenesis and management are discussed in Chapter 7.

Skin Lesions. The comatose patient intoxicated with a sedative-hypnotic is prone to the development of pressure-associated skin lesions,[17,108,113,157] referred to as "barbiturate burns." We encountered a patient presenting with coma due to glutethimide overdose who had linear and angular bullous lesions in the pectoral, axillary, and shoulder region on one side. It was later discovered that these lesions corresponded exactly to the seams of the patient's polo shirt (including the shirt pocket and sleeve). More commonly, the lesions appear on the skin overlying the sacrum, the scapulae, and medial aspects of the knees and ankles, that is, regions subjected to sustained pressure due to the position of the patient. They usually begin as dusky, erythematous patches that eventually evolve into bullae or vesicles. Skin biopsies demonstrate necrosis of the sweat gland epithelium.[95,108] The exact pathogenesis of

these lesions remains unknown. Some have argued that the blisters are a very nonspecific consequence of prolonged local skin pressure. In the acute setting, however, their presence should lend supportive evidence to coma from either sedative-hypnotics or carbon monoxide poisoning.[17,157]

A related phenomenon is dermographism, that is, the appearance of erythema, flare, and wheal after stroking the skin firmly with a blunt implement. A study of 73 patients comatose from drug overdose found dermographism, or erythema and flare alone, in 28 (38%) of the patients.[29] None of the 30 control patients with coma from other causes demonstrated the response. Most of the patients with a positive response had ingested barbiturates. The histopathology appears similar to the pressure-related lesions described previously. Thus, this simple clinical test may further suggest drug intoxication.

Pupil Size and Responsiveness. Careful examination of pupil size and reactivity is a critical part of the examination of the comatose patient (see Table 10–3).[130] Bilateral alterations in pupil characteristics may be observed

Table 10–3 PUPILLARY SIGNS IN DRUG INTOXICATION

SMALL PUPILS
Opioids
Ethanol
Barbiturates
Chlorpromazine

LARGE PUPILS
Atropine
H_1-histamine antagonists
Heterocyclic antidepressants
Amphetamines
Cocaine
Thiopental
Glutethimide
Methaqualone

FIXED PUPILS*
Barbiturates
Heterocyclic antidepressants
Glutethimide

*Seen only with profound intoxication; patients are apneic and require assisted ventilation.

in *both* structural and metabolic disease; it is the presence or absence of associated focal signs that may help to exclude one or the other etiology. Furthermore, as emphasized earlier, a preserved pupillary light response in the setting of otherwise absent brainstem function is highly suggestive of a metabolic process.

A large number of exogenous agents may affect pupillary size, but relatively few are also associated with coma. Mydriatic pupils are seen following ingestion of antimuscarinic agents, sympathomimetic agents, and some sedative-hypnotics (see Table 10–3).

Opiates are the most common drugs that cause coma and miotic pupils; the changes in pupil size are probably due in part to a direct effect on the parasympathetic neurons within the oculomotor nucleus. Ethanol, barbiturates, and certain phenothiazines, most notably chlorpromazine, may cause miosis as well. Mitchell and associates[116] investigated drug-induced comas in children. The frequency of miosis was 88% for narcotics, 72% for phenothiazines, 35% for ethanol, and 31% for barbiturates, and was found to correlate with the level of obtundation. Although in most cases the size of both pupils remains the same in toxic coma, there are occasional reports of anisocoria.[18]

The pupillary light response may be significantly impaired. This certainly occurs when the coma is caused by a drug with antimuscarinic properties; in such cases there is direct blockade of the cholinergic neurons mediating the efferent arc of the reflex. Fixed midposition pupils are also seen with severe barbiturate or heterocyclic overdose.[12] Any degree of intoxication that causes loss of the light reflex will also impair respiratory function, however, so if the patient has fixed pupils and is breathing, one should suspect a structural lesion affecting the mesencephalon.

Abnormalities of Ocular Motility. Observations of eye position, movements, and response to oculocephalic and oculovestibular testing is essential (see Table 10–4). Once again, asym-

Table 10–4 EYE MOVEMENT ABNORMALITIES IN DRUG INTOXICATION

OPHTHALMOPLEGIA
Barbiturates, other anticonvulsants
Benzodiazepines
Heterocyclic antidepressants
Neuroleptics (may be asymmetric with phenothiazines)
Opioids
Ethanol

FORCED DOWNWARD EYE MOVEMENTS
Barbiturates
Glutethimide
Methaqualone
Ethchlorvynol
Benzodiazepines
Ethanol
Neuroleptics

NYSTAGMUS
Phencyclidine

OPSOCLONUS
Phencyclidine
Amitriptyline
Haloperidol plus lithium

metry of function favors the diagnosis of a structural rather than a metabolic process.[130] Nonetheless, a variety of abnormalities, some of them asymmetric, may be seen with toxic coma.

Impairment or complete loss of the oculocephalic and oculovestibular response is much more common in exogenous than endogenous metabolic coma. Ophthalmoplegia is the rule in barbiturate[41] and anticonvulsant overdose, and has been described in tricyclic overdose as well.[132,153,159] Internuclear ophthalmoplegia (INO) was seen in 7 of 70 cases of toxic coma.[8] In most instances, a barbiturate and/or benzodiazepine was involved. In 6 of the 70 cases, the INO was bilateral. Another group[28] reported two patients with phenothiazine overdose and unilateral INOs.

A finding with oculovestibular testing that appears to be rather common in sedative-induced coma is "forced downward ocular deviation."[152] In 24 of 32 patients with coma due to sedative-hypnotic overdose, caloric-induced lateral eye movements were followed by forced downward deviation of one or both eyes after a delay of 5 to 15 seconds, whereas none of the 15 patients with coma not due to toxins showed this response.[152] The pathophysiologic basis of these observations is not clear, but it may relate to a selective effect of sedative drugs on mechanisms for upgaze, coupled to activation of the oculovestibular pathways for downgaze through caloric stimulation of the posterior semicircular canal. Forced downward deviation may occur, but is uncommon, in structural and non–drug-induced metabolic comas. Its presence is therefore very suggestive of sedative-hypnotic drug overdose.

Horizontal, vertical, and rotatory nystagmus is a common accompaniment of PCP poisoning. In a review of 55 cases of PCP-induced coma,[112] approximately two thirds of patients had nystagmus, but its direction and amplitude did not correlate with the severity of intoxication.[111] Opsoclonus has also been reported as a manifestation of overdoses of PCP, amitriptyline, and haloperidol combined with lithium. Alternating skew deviation was described in one patient with coma due to methaqualone and diphenhydramine intoxication.[127]

Motor Abnormalities. In most cases, examination of the motor system offers few clues for distinguishing the various types of metabolic coma. Most depressant drugs, in sufficient quantities, cause generalized flaccidity and depressed or absent stretch reflexes. An identical picture is produced by a variety of metabolic processes of endogenous origin. The observation of flexor and extensor postural responses may have some discriminating value, however. Greenberg and Simon[55] described 10 patients with sedative drug overdose who had decorticate or decerebrate postures in response to noxious stimuli. None had evidence of structural CNS pathology or endogenous metabolic abnormalities. The posturing was bilateral, and was associated with hyperreflexia in 6 of the 10 patients. None had extensor plantar responses. These postural reflexes were transient; they disappeared within hours after first examination of the patient. Importantly, the oculocephalic and oculovestibular responses were abnormal in all patients tested, while the pupillary light response was spared. Although posturing may be observed in endogenous metabolic coma, oculovestibular responses are usually preserved. Thus, the triad of flexor and/or extensor postures, absent eye movements to oculovestibular stimulation, and preserved light response should suggest sedative overdose.

Spontaneous motor activity, such as tremor, myoclonus, or seizures, may be seen in both endogenous and exogenous metabolic coma. One review of PCP-induced coma[112] described tremor or twitching in 7 of 55 patients (13%). Tremor is part of a characteristic abstinence syndrome that occurs in the chronic barbiturate abuser[69] and is frequently seen in comatose patients recovering from barbiturate overdose.[2] Severe, diffuse tremor may occur in comatose patients recovering from long-term barbiturate anesthesia for refractory status epilepticus.[103] Athetosis and generalized muscular rigidity also have been described in barbiturate overdose.[113]

LABORATORY INVESTIGATIONS

A number of laboratory tests are routine in the emergency room evaluation of the comatose patient, and will readily identify important endogenous causes of metabolic coma. These include serum glucose concentration (preferably drawn before the intravenous administration of dextrose), electrolytes, creatinine, and blood urea nitrogen (BUN). Liver function tests, including prothrombin time and partial thromboplastin time, as well as a stool guaiac may provide evidence for hepatic encephalopathy.

Arterial blood gas analysis is essential as a test for adequate respiratory function, and may be used to discriminate exogenous from endogenous causes of coma when combined with other tests that can help to exclude or suggest other diseases.[130] That is, a metabolic acidosis occurs with certain drugs (e.g., salicylates, isoniazid, ethylene glycol, methanol, paraldehyde), but is also associated with a variety of endogenous metabolic abnormalities such as diabetic ketoacidoses, uremia, and lactic acidosis. Similarly, a respiratory alkalosis occurs during the early phase of salicylate poisoning, but also in hepatic encephalopathy, sepsis, and pulmonary disease. Sedative-hypnotics, as well as brainstem disease, may cause centrally induced hypoventilation and consequent respiratory acidosis; these must be distinguished from peripheral causes such as neuromuscular disease, acute pulmonary disease, and chest-wall injury.

The computed tomography (CT) or magnetic resonance imaging (MRI) scan is valuable in the evaluation of any patient with coma of unknown etiology because a structural lesion is not reliably excluded by clinical examination. The studies may reveal a chronic lesion that explains focal findings complicating the presentation of metabolic coma. Beyond this, however, they are of limited use because they fail to differentiate among most causes of metabolic coma. Diffuse edema following respiratory or circulatory arrest may appear on CT scan as generalized mass effect, blurring of the gray-white–matter border, or lack of contrast enhancement in hypodense regions. MRI scans show a prominent increased signal on T_2-weighted images. Certain CNS infections, such as herpes simplex encephalitis, are associated with characteristic CT or MRI appearances, although noninfectious processes can have similar findings.

A comparison of measured and calculated serum osmolality is a rapid and reliable screen for the presence of several important toxins.[49] Normal serum osmolality is principally determined by the serum concentration of sodium, glucose, and urea. With these values, serum osmolality can be calculated using the following formula:

$$mOsm/kg\ H_2O = (2\times sodium) + (glucose/18) + (BUN/2.8)$$

Empirically this has been shown to provide a valid estimate of actual measurements of osmolality in normal conditions.[36] A difference between the calculated and measured osmolality (the osmolar gap) arises from one of two situations. The most common is the presence of an additional osmotically active substance, such as ethanol, methanol, ethylene glycol, paraldehyde, or other toxins with a molecular weight of less than 150d.[51,101] The other situation is a decrease in serum water concentration, due to either hyperlipidemia or hyperproteinemia, but this is much less likely to be causally associated with coma.

A raised osmolar gap usually represents an ingestion. In the case of ethanol, a frequently suspected intoxicant, calculation of the osmolar gap can provide a rapid estimation of the serum ethanol level by use of the formula:

$$ETOH\ (mg/100\ mL) = osmolar\ gap \times 4.5$$

(This formula is based on the molecular weight of ethanol and the conversion of mmol/L to mg/100 mL). This estimate is of great assistance in correlating the degree of intoxication with the amount of ethanol ingested. It will also help exclude the presence of ethanol in cases of suspected alcohol-withdrawal seizures.

An even more sophisticated analysis combines the serum osmolality with the anion gap. Toxic agents such as methanol and ethylene glycol, by virtue of their metabolism to acids, will raise the anion gap, whereas other toxins will not.[75]

Electroencephalogram. Although electroencephalography will never, in itself, identify the etiology of metabolic coma, certain patterns on the electroencephalogram (EEG) may suggest one cause or another. The EEG may also be helpful in excluding certain nonmetabolic causes of coma, such as focal brain lesions and nonconvulsive status epilepticus. The EEG provides more accurate information about the depth of coma than clinical examination alone,[23] and is thus useful in serial assessment for some cases. Brainstem auditory evoked responses are usually normal in metabolic coma, and therefore may have diagnostic value as well.

Severity of acute intoxication with barbiturate or benzodiazepines correlates with a sequence of specific EEG changes.[93] In the earliest stage, there is fast activity (>14/s), primarily in frontal and central regions, admixed with theta and occasional delta activity. With deeper coma, theta and then delta activity come to predominate, with the latter having a frontal emphasis. This evolves into short bursts of slow waves followed by faster elements, separated by silent periods. Finally, in extreme degrees of intoxication, the EEG shows periods of electrocerebral silence, lasting from minutes to hours. At this point, the clinical examination usually shows complete neurologic unresponsiveness, including the lack of brainstem reflexes. Prolonged electrocerebral silence in overdose due to CNS depressants does not signify a poor outcome.[12,103] Thus, as long as there are measurable plasma levels of barbiturate, one cannot rely on the EEG as a guide to prognosis.

The EEG in patients comatose from phenothiazine or butyrophenone intoxication shows diffuse low-voltage activity in the theta and delta range, which may be interrupted by higher-voltage slow waves and sharp transients. Heterocyclic antidepressants may cause widespread and irregular activity in the alpha range, interposed theta and overt epileptiform discharges. Benzodiazepines produce an anterior predominant, unreactive 16/s rhythm mixed with diffuse theta.

Electroencephalogram findings in PCP-induced coma may be highly characteristic.[166] In deeper stages, there is a generalized, regular, sinusoidal theta activity interrupted by periodic slow-wave discharges and no reactivity to external stimuli. As coma lightens, the periodic activity is lost. A similar EEG pattern is seen with the anesthetic ketamine, a derivative of PCP.

Alpha-pattern coma may occur in drug intoxication. The term refers to coma in which the EEG shows diffuse, unreactive, alpha-frequency activity. Early reports of this pattern emphasized an association with either brainstem lesions or postanoxic encephalopathy, as well as the fact that it is a dismal prognostic sign. In the past decade, however, a number of reports describing alpha coma in acute drug intoxication have appeared. Although the EEG characteristics were indistinguishable from those seen in the previously mentioned settings, all reported drug cases survived without residual deficit.[92]

Toxicology Analysis. Without a precise history or clear physical signs, identification of a drug via toxicologic analysis of serum, urine, or gastric contents may be the only method of establishing a definitive diagnosis in the comatose patient. On the other hand, a negative toxicologic analysis may shift the focus of investigation back toward endogenous causes. When a particular agent is found, quantitative analysis sometimes provides important information with regard to degree of intoxication and treatment requirements. Judicious use of the toxicology laboratory requires several considerations: (1) ranking of clinical suspicion for various classes of agents; (2) availability and sensitivity of qualitative (screening) and quantitative tests; (3) optimal timing for specimen collection; and (4) selecting the preferred specimens for the various tests.

It is prudent to collect samples for toxicology during the initial evaluation of the patient (5 mL serum, 50 mL urine, 50 mL gastric emesis or lavage, if available). Later serum and urine samples may have a higher yield (e.g., acetaminophen, salicylates) depending on the time of ingestion. One then assesses the need for qualitative or quantitative analysis. Most toxicology laboratories run a "coma panel" that detects the presence of the more common drugs causing coma. A falsely negative screen may arise for a number of reasons including assay insensitivity for the unchanged drug or its metabolites, the causative agent not being included in the screen, and decreased renal clearance or variations in urine pH.

Few reports have clearly documented the value of toxicologic analysis in the evaluation of coma. One review[62] of 208 patients with coma of unknown origin found that toxicologic analysis disclosed the cause of coma in 106 (51%) of the cases; one half of these involved more than one drug. For 8 patients, the test results led to specific therapies (in addition to supportive care). In contrast, after a review of the use of toxicology for patients with suspected overdose (not all of whom were comatose), another group[187] concluded that emergency toxicology results rarely affected patient management. These studies are representative of the disagreement among toxicologists as to the true value of these tests.[64,114,179] We believe, however, that toxicologic analysis is an important resource in the evaluation of coma of unknown origin, if the physician bases his or her request on a careful clinical assessment and understands the test capabilities and limitations.

Specific Agents that Produce Alterations in Consciousness

SEDATIVE-HYPNOTICS

Barbiturates. Barbiturates produce coma through their direct suppression of neuron transmission (see Chapters 1 and 3). Barbiturates have been shown experimentally to decrease the amplitude of the action potential,[161] augment the presynaptic and postsynaptic inhibition mediated by gamma-aminobutyric acid, (GABA), modify transmitter release,[133] reduce excitatory postsynaptic potentials,[139] and prolong inhibitory postsynaptic potentials. Whether the observed decrement in cellular metabolism is a consequence of these changes in neuron function or is a separate mechanism is not clear.

All barbiturates are derivatives of barbituric acid; variations in side-chain length on the parent molecule determines the potency and duration of action. This correlates in part with the ionization constant (pK) and relative lipid solubility of the drug (see Chapter 1). Derivatives with increased lipid solubility are generally more potent and have a shorter onset and duration of action. Depending on the pK, alterations in blood pH will also determine the degree of passage into the CNS. Thus, phenobarbital, with a dissociation constant of 7.2, exists primarily in the ionized form at physiologic pH (7.4). A decrease in pH will favor changes to the un-ionized state, and hence, more drug will pass through membranes, such as those comprising the blood-brain barrier. For example, during bicuculline-induced status epilepticus in freely convulsing rats, blood pH fell to below 7.0 within 1 minute of status onset, and brain-to-blood phenobarbital ratios were twice those of nonconvulsing control animals by 2 minutes of status.[154] Besides differences in penetration into the CNS, there is also variation in activity of different barbiturates at the level of the neuron. For example, the anesthetic barbiturate pentobarbital has been shown to suppress spontaneous neuron activity directly, whereas phenobarbital, an anticonvulsant, does not (see Chapter 3).

The mechanism for elimination of barbiturates (i.e., whether renal or hepatic) also depends upon the relative lipid solubility. Because lipophilic compounds tend to bind to albumin, less drug is cleared by the kidney, and metabolism therefore depends on hepatic enzymatic systems. The reverse holds true for drugs that are less lipophilic. Duration of action of different compounds correlates with the mode of elimination; those cleared primarily by the kidneys are long acting and those by the liver, short acting.

Toxic doses of barbiturates cause a rapidly progressive decline in level of consciousness to coma, especially when the amount ingested is more than ten times the normal hypnotic dose. A correlation between degree of obtundation and serum levels has been demonstrated in short-acting barbiturate overdose,[58,113] but consideration must be made for patients with hepatic or renal disease,[60] and for the chronic abuser.[86] The use of other drugs concurrently, most notably alcohol, is relatively common and can significantly depress the CNS even further. The progression of barbiturate-induced coma is described in a classification scheme introduced by Reed and colleagues[135] in 1952.

Grade 0: asleep but arousable
Grade 1: withdrawal from painful stimuli, deep tendon reflexes intact
Grade 2: no response to painful stimuli, deep tendon reflexes intact, vital signs stable
Grade 3: deep tendon reflexes absent or markedly reduced, vital signs stable
Grade 4: respiratory depression and/ or circulatory instability

This scheme may misrepresent the variability in deep tendon reflexes seen at various stages. As mentioned previously, patients in more advanced grades may have Babinski's sign, flexor and extensor postural reflexes, and forced downward ocular deviation with testing of the oculovestibular response.[152] The oculocephalic response is usually absent. The pupils may be either miotic or mydriatic and may become sluggishly reactive to light.

In severe intoxication, respiration slows and changes to a Cheyne-Stokes pattern or ceases altogether. The skin may be cold and cyanotic, and may have bullous lesions in pressure-related areas. Cardiovascular instability results from a direct suppressant effect on myocardial contractility, as well as from arteriolar and venous dilation. The pupillary light response is lost. Life-threatening complications include pneumonia, pulmonary edema, adult respiratory distress syndrome, cardiac arrhythmias, and renal failure.[113]

Barbiturate overdose exemplifies the importance of monitoring respiratory function in the initial evaluation and treatment of the comatose patient. Any suspicion of sedative-hypnotic intoxication requires that an arterial blood gas be the first diagnostic test, given the unreliability of the history and the nonspecific nature of the physical examination. Mild hypoventilation demands vigilant observation; if there is any question as to the level or trend of respiratory function, the patient should be intubated and placed on a respirator. Hypotension and hypothermia should be aggressively treated. Gastric lavage and use of activated charcoal is suggested if the ingestion occurred less than 24 hours before presentation, although its value beyond 4 hours postingestion is questionable.[47] CNS stimulants, a therapy promoted in the 1950s, have been shown to increase morbidity as compared with supportive management and are contraindicated. Attempts to enhance drug elimination, such as alkaline diuresis for phenobarbital, hemodialysis,[6] or hemoperfusion,[141,188] are reserved for those cases with uncontrollable cardiovascular instability or renal failure. The technique used depends on the pharmacokinetics of the particular barbiturate.

Thus the therapy for barbiturate overdose is supportive, as in many intoxications. The outcome correlates primarily to the duration and degree of intoxication at initial presentation.[130]

Glutethimide. Glutethimide is a sedative-hypnotic, similar in structure and pharmacologic actions to the barbiturates. Although recognition of its abuse potential has caused a decline in its therapeutic use, it remains an important cause of fatal overdose.[10]

With a few minor variations, the coma of glutethimide overdose mimics that of barbiturates. Glutethimide has anticholinergic activity and may cause tachycardia, hyperpyrexia, ileus, urinary retention, and mydriasis. Hypotension is common and can be refractory to treatment.[189] Occasionally patients present with dilated, fixed pupils yet retain spontaneous respirations.[189] Unilateral fixed and dilated pupils and other focal abnormalities have been described as well.[18,122] Glutethimide may cause a waxing and waning level of consciousness,[122,130] which has been ascribed to variable absorption from the gastrointestinal tract, release from adipose tissue, or formation of other active metabolites.

Treatment is supportive, although some have advocated hemoperfusion in severe cases.[141,188] In one study, older age was the most important predictor of a poor outcome.[56]

Methaqualone. The mechanism(s) underlying the CNS-depressant effects of methaqualone are not known, but may involve inhibition of the formation of intermediate substances in the respiratory chain.[19] Patients abusing methaqualone usually present to the emergency room lethargic but arousable, but overdoses may cause coma and death, especially when the drug is used with other sedative-hypnotics, opiates, or alcohol.[7,189] The coma from methaqualone is usually nonspecific. Retinal hemorrhage, muscle hypertonicity, hyperreflexia, myoclonus, and seizures have been described and may offer a clinical clue to the diagnosis.[19]

Ethchlorvynol. Ethchlorvynol is a fast-acting sedative-hypnotic that can produce respiratory depression, hypothermia, hypotension, bradycardia, and prolonged coma. When ethchlorvynol is used intravenously, patients are at risk of developing pulmonary edema; presumably this is a consequence of a direct toxic effect on the alveolar-capillary membrane.[52,145] Peak serum levels are seen within 90 minutes of ingestion. Thus, a level obtained after a delay of 12 or more hours may represent a serious overdose despite the fact that it falls within the nontoxic range.[184] Charcoal and resin hemoperfusion have been advocated for severe overdose.

Benzodiazepines. Despite having a high margin of safety and a relatively low rate of abuse, benzodiazepines are still an important cause of toxic coma.[57,62] Their CNS-depressant effects arise, at least in part, from binding to specific receptors and consequent potentiation of GABA-mediated inhibitory systems (see Chapter 3). There are no distinguishing characteristics of the coma, although respiratory depression and hypotension are seen less often than with other sedative-hypnotics.[57,130] Toxic ingestions of benzodiazepines commonly involve other drugs, especially alcohol.[26] Combined actions of alcohol and benzodiazepines on GABAergic transmission probably explain the particular toxicity of this combination.[167] The recent development of benzodiazepine antagonists may prove valuable in reversing the coma induced by these agents.[148]

OPIOID ANALGESICS

Opioid analgesics, along with their endogenous counterparts (enkephalins, endorphins, and dynorphins) act on the CNS via specific receptors (see Chapter 9). Experimental work has demonstrated several distinct opioid receptor subtypes. Morphine exerts its effects, including respiratory depression, through mu_2 receptors. Drugs selective for mu_1, kappa, or delta opioid receptors do not induce respiratory depression. How receptor binding is translated into altered cellular function is not entirely clear, but changes in calcium or cyclic adenosine monophosphate homeostasis are likely mechanisms. Respiratory depression is partly caused by reduced brainstem responsiveness to increases in carbon dioxide tension (PCO_2). Miosis probably arises from a direct excitatory effect on the parasympathetic subnucleus within the oculomotor complex.

Heroin and methadone, both primarily mu-receptor agonists, are the most commonly abused opiates, and account for most overdoses.[54] Both the chronic addict and occasional recreational user may overdose by miscalculating the amount or quality of the drug to be taken, or as a suicide attempt. Overdoses occur after intravenous, nasal, and oral administration. Concurrent use of cocaine, alcohol, and other substances is common.[54]

The patient typically presents comatose and flaccid, occasionally with suggestive needle tracks or skin abscesses. The respiratory rate is often very slow and irregular. Noncardiogenic pulmonary edema, possibly due to a direct toxic effect of the drug, is a frequent complication and compromises respiratory function even further.[43,164] A metabolic acidosis due to hypoxia, added to the respiratory acidosis from hypoventilation, may cause myocardial depression, loss of vasomotor control, and eventual shock. If seen soon after the overdose, the patient may be hypothermic. However, a normal or elevated temperature is not unusual and may signify infection.

The character of the pupils is the key finding (see Table 10–3). They are pinpoint (i.e., less than 1 mm in diameter), responsive to light, and enlarge with administration of an opioid antagonist (see below). The oculocephalic response may be paralyzed. The casual observer may erroneously describe the pupillary light response as absent; more often than not this is due to the use of a relatively dim light source, or failure to use a magnifying glass to adequately visualize the pupils. The only structural process that mimics the pupillary findings of opiate overdose is a lesion of the pons. The absence of miotic pupils does not rule out opioid overdose, however. If anoxia and hypotension go untreated, the pupils may dilate and become unresponsive, consistent with the changes seen in hypoxic encephalopathy. In addition, meperidine, which has some anticholinergic activity, may cause the pupils to be of normal or even enlarged diameter.

Specific antagonists completely reverse the depressant effects of opioid overdose. A variety of mixed opioid antagonists and agonist-antagonists exist, each with specific activity on the different receptor subtypes. Naloxone hydrochloride is unique in being a competitive antagonist at all receptor subtypes, with the highest affinity for the mu receptor.[24] In overdose with the commonly abused opioids (i.e., mu-receptor agonists), appropriate doses of intravenous or intramuscular naloxone reverse the respiratory depression, hypotension, sedation, and miosis within minutes. Failure to observe a change in level of consciousness or pupillary size should suggest a different or additional diagnosis, including the effects of additional toxins.

One milligram of intravenous naloxone counters the effect of 25 mg of heroin (approximately equivalent to 80 mg of morphine). Since there is so much variability in the toxic dose of opioids, however, it is impossible to predict the optimal dose of naloxone for any given patient. For example, 30 mg of intravenous morphine will produce serious toxicity in a normal nontolerant adult, whereas the usual dose for a chronic addict may be 250 mg or more, and the toxic dose may exceed 2 g. The suggested initial dose of naloxone for treating opioid-induced coma in the adult is 2 mg intravenously (in children 0.01 mg/kg initially, then 0.1 mg/kg),[120] but higher doses may be necessary depending on the clinical circumstances.[54,76] The drug can also be given by the intramuscular, sublingual, or endotracheal route. The duration of action is approximately 30 to 45 minutes. The initial administration of naloxone is a diagnostic rather than a therapeutic maneuver. A careful comparison of the patient's level of consciousness, respiratory rate, and pupil size must be made before and 2 to 3 minutes following the bolus of naloxone. If there is any clinical improvement, the 2-mg dose should be repeated. If a further response is seen, naloxone can be mixed with maintenance intravenous solutions and given at a rate of 2.5 μg/kg per hour in adult patients.[15]

A few points deserve further comment. First, due to its lower affinity at the sigma receptor, significantly higher doses of naloxone (i.e., 15 mg or more) may be required to counteract the effects of drugs such as pentazocine (a sigma-receptor agonist), and higher doses may be needed for large intoxications with any of the opioids.[120] Second, there are few adverse reactions with naloxone used in the previously mentioned doses.[38] It can, however, provoke a potentially harmful abstinence syndrome in the dependent user. If signs of withdrawal occur, the dose of naloxone should be decreased to maintain the patient in a slightly narcotized state. Third, a partial but incomplete response to naloxone therapy suggests a concurrent process, such as other toxins, hypoxic encephalopathy due to a pulmonary edema, or a prolonged postictal state following a seizure. Finally, there are reports in the literature of naloxone reversing some of the effects of overdose with barbiturates, benzodiazepines, glutethimide,[76] chlorpromazine, and alcohol.[35,59,76,107,158]

ETHANOL

Although it is difficult to assign a precise incidence, ethanol abuse can be a cause of toxic coma,[180] and often plays a role in overdose with other substances. In a recent prospective study of the prevalence of ethanol intoxication in patients brought to the emergency room of a large urban hospital,[65] 15 of 20 comatose patients tested positive for ethanol, and in 13 of these the blood ethanol level was greater than 0.08% (80 mg/100 mL), the legal limit for intoxication. Another study[62] found that 10% of 208 patients with coma of unknown etiology had ingested ethanol, and in 5% this was the sole cause for coma.

Ethanol has a depressant effect on the CNS that is mediated, in part, by apparently nonspecific interactions with neuron membranes.[78] There is also evidence to suggest that these nonspecific effects, or a more direct action, alters the function of membrane-bound receptors. For example, ethanol has been shown to affect GABAergic transmission in a number of in vitro experiments,[67,91] and recent work has shown that certain GABA-benzodiazepine-

receptor antagonists block the effects of ethanol. Furthermore, alcohol has recently been shown to block excitatory (glutamate) neurotransmission at the NMDA receptor.[102]

Alcoholic coma is the extreme manifestation of the progressive deterioration in the level of consciousness observed in intoxicated patients. The amount of ethanol that will induce coma depends on (1) the amount ingested, (2) the rate of rise of serum ethanol concentration, and (3) individual tolerance. Ethanol concentrations greater than 0.4% (400 mg/100 mL) are associated with coma and death; the LD_{50} has been estimated to be 0.5% (500 mg/100 mL), which corresponds to a dose of 3 g/kg body weight. However, some chronic alcoholics appear only mildly intoxicated with blood ethanol levels greater than 0.4%. One report[79] described a patient with a level of 1.51% (1510 mg/100 mL) who was "agitated and slightly confused but alert."

The patient in alcoholic coma is unresponsive when left alone but may show some motor response with vigorous stimulation. The breathing is slow and noisy, and the pupils may become dilated and sluggishly reactive. Eye movements may be unresponsive to passive head movements. Hypothermia is relatively common in this form of intoxication and may depress CNS function even further. The characteristic odor associated with inebriation (due to impurities in the liquor and not the ethanol itself) is not helpful in assessing the level of coma. Furthermore, ethanol is often abused concurrently with other substances, and is so often associated with trauma and metabolic disorders that one cannot assume that "alcohol" on the breath explains the entire clinical picture. Laboratory investigations, including toxicology screen and CT scanning, are especially important in this setting. As mentioned previously, rapid determination of the osmolar gap can provide a quick assessment of how the patient's clinical state correlates with a calculated ethanol level.

Ethanol, benzodiazepines, and barbiturates have common neuropharmaco-logic actions and all interact with the GABA-receptor chloride channel complex. Like pentobarbital, ethanol enhances Cl uptake by brain synaptoneurosomes at concentrations that produce mild intoxication in vivo.[67,91] The imidazobenzodiazepine Ro15-4513 antagonizes ethanol's enhancement of GABA-mediated Cl-flux in vitro and blocks some of ethanol's intoxicating effects in vivo.[167] In rodents, Ro15-4513 decreases ethanol-induced sedation, ataxia, and impaired righting reflex, but does not appear to reverse coma or prevent lethal intoxication.[167] The role of Ro15-4513 and related compounds in the treatment of acute ethanol intoxication in humans will be determined by studies on their safety and efficacy.

Management of alcoholic coma is analogous to that of sedative-hypnotic overdose. Hemodialysis is effective in clearing ethanol, but is probably best reserved for patients with extremely high ethanol levels or for those with hemodynamic compromise.[61,65]

PSYCHOTHERAPEUTIC DRUGS

Heterocyclic Antidepressants. Heterocyclic antidepressants include the tricyclic compounds and newer agents such as amoxapine, maprotiline, and trazodone (see Chapter 7). In terms of abuse, these drugs are notable for their relatively low margin of safety and easy availability to substance abusers and patients with a high suicide risk, therefore acting as an important cause of lethal intoxication. The acute toxic effects of heterocyclic antidepressants are probably related to blockade of reuptake of one or more biogenic amines, including norepinephrine, 5-hydroxytryptamine (5-HT), acetylcholine, and dopamine (depending on the particular drug; see Chapter 7). The initial change in level of consciousness may be hyperalertness and restlessness, accompanied by seizures, myoclonus, or dystonia.[124] Obtundation follows, and is complicated by hypoven-tilation, hypotension, and hypothermia. Anticholinergic effects are characteristic (except with trazodone), and include tachycardia; flushed, dry skin; urinary retention; and dilated pupils.[66] The oculovestibular response may be lost, as in sedative overdose.[159] Pyramidal signs, including hyperreflexia and extensor plantar responses, are common.[124]

The patient comatose from heterocyclic antidepressant overdose usually survives with proper management. This is understood by the fact that 70% to 80% of patients who die do so before reaching the hospital,[20] whereas the in-hospital mortality rate is approximately 2% to 3%,[20,66,165,173,183] and most in-hospital deaths occur within a few hours of admission.[20] Vigilant monitoring of the cardiovascular system is important, because most lethal complications are cardiac arrhythmias and myocardial depression, and these may appear suddenly.[20] A limb-lead QRS interval greater than 100 milliseconds on electrocardiogram correlates with severe intoxication, and is probably a better predictor of cardiac toxicity than plasma levels.[14] Such patients require admission to the intensive care unit and aggressive management of cardiac disturbances.[16] Physostigmine has been advocated for certain cases with prominent anticholinergic features,[16] but exact indications for this therapy remain unclear due to the risk of complications from the physostigmine itself.[88]

Coma is not a major impediment to recovery per se, at least when unaccompanied by seizures.[90,100] Most patients regain consciousness in less than 24 hours[66,163] without specific therapy; the duration may be longer with some of the newer tetracyclic agents.[88] Respiratory depression due to heterocyclic antidepressants alone is relatively uncommon and of short duration.[163] When coma persists, other complications, including co-ingestion of other drugs, should be suspected.

Antipsychotic Agents. Other than as part of the neuroleptic malignant syndrome, isolated phenothiazine or butyrophenone overdose rarely causes coma.

STIMULANTS

Amphetamines. Amphetamines such as dextroamphetamine, methamphetamine, and methylphenidate are sympathomimetic CNS stimulants. A pure form of methamphetamine hydrochloride, referred to as "ice," can be inhaled and is becoming a very popular drug of abuse, especially in Hawaii and the West Coast of the United States.[26] Amphetamines act by stimulating release of catecholamines and serotonin from nerve endings and powerfully block reuptake of these neurotransmitters into nerve endings. They also inhibit neurotransmitter degradation by blocking monoamine oxidase activity (see Chapters 1 and 7; Table 10-5). Amphetamines produce a spectrum of altered consciousness, from agitation and psychotic-like behavior to coma in severe overdoses (Tables 10-6 and 10-7). Mild amphetamine toxicity causes restlessness, insomnia, tremor, hyperreflexia, sweating, dilated pupils, and flushing. Coma in amphetamine overdose is usually related in part to a combination of seizures, hyperthermia, extremes of blood pressure or cerebral ischemia, and hypoxia secondary to cardiorespiratory collapse (see Table 10-2).[185, 155]

Treatment of acute amphetamine overdose includes control of hyperthermia with cooling blankets, alpha-adrenergic blockade for extreme hypertension, and acidification of the urine in patients with intact renal function. If the drug has been taken orally and the patient is awake, ipecac syrup together with activated charcoal and a cathartic such as magnesium citrate have been recommended. Patients should be placed in a quiet environment. Chlorpromazine, haloperidol, droperidol, and diazepam may be effective for reducing overstimulation. Caution should be used if the diagnosis of amphetamine intoxication is uncertain, because neuroleptics are generally contraindicated in patients in whom PCP and other hallucinogens have been administered. Amphetamine psychosis, which generally follows severe, chronic amphetamine use, may cause repeated compulsive behaviors, vivid hallucinations, and a picture resembling paranoid schizophrenia. This syndrome usually fades a few days after the drug is discontinued.

Amphetamine-Like Compounds. A number of derivatives of amphetamines have proven to have powerful psychotropic effects and are widely abused.[147] These compounds include STP (2,5-dimethoxy-4-methylamphetamine), MDMA (3,4 methylene-dioxymethane-betamine), and Bromo-DMA. Some of these drugs have been called "designer drugs" because they have been custom synthesized by chemists who distribute them for use before they have been recognized and classified as drugs of abuse by the Food and Drug Ad-

Table 10-5 EFFECTS OF STIMULANT MEDICATIONS ON BRAIN NEUROTRANSMITTER SYSTEMS

Drug	Blocks Catecholamine Reuptake	Stimulates Dopamine Release	Enhances Release of Serotonin	Inhibits MAO	Acts as Local Anesthetic
Amphetamine	+++	++	++	+	+
Methylphenidate	+++	++	?	?	?
Cocaine	+++	++	++	?	+++

Key: MAO = monoamine oxidase; + = mild activity; ++ = moderate activity; +++ = high activity; ? = activity unknown

Source: Modified from Gawin and Ellinwood[48] p 1178.

Table 10-6 SIGNS OF AMPHETAMINE INTOXICATION

Mental status change: agitation, fighting, hypervigilance, coma
Tachycardia
Pupillary dilation
Elevated blood pressure
Perspiration
Chills
Nausea and vomiting
Convulsions

ministration. MDMA, a derivative of amphetamine, has activity resembling both the hallucinogen drug mescaline and the parent amphetamine. MDMA has been referred to popularly as "ecstasy" and is also referred to as "XTC," "ADAM," or "MDM."[119] The drug has been administered by a few psychiatrists to improve insight in psychotherapy. Until 1984, the drug was not a controlled substance, but in 1986 it was classified as a schedule I substance.

Severe overdoses of MDMA may produce prominent signs similar to those for amphetamine overdose. Death appears to be uncommon except in those patients with underlying cardiac disease. More troubling is the observation in monkeys that administration of MDMA in doses two to three times the typical self-administered human dose produces a profound decrease in immunoreactive serotonin fibers in the brain.[138] The mechanism by which MDMA and related drugs produce their toxic actions is not well understood. Some evidence in animals suggests that the drug may share toxic mechanisms with other serotonin neurotoxins by being taken up into the nerve terminal and causing acute release of serotonin.[119] Prevention of uptake of the neurotoxin into serotonin nerve terminals by a drug such as fluoxetine, which blocks the 5-HT carrier, may reduce neurotoxicity. It remains to be seen whether serotonin neurotoxicity observed in animals is a serious long-term problem for persons who have abused this and similar drugs. As the number of "designer drug" variations on this chemical theme increases, it seems likely that a variety of new toxic manifestations will present to clinicians.

Table 10-7 ORGANIC MENTAL SYNDROMES ASSOCIATED WITH PSYCHOACTIVE SUBSTANCES

Psychoactive Substance	Intoxication	Withdrawal	Delirium	Withdrawal Delirium	Delusional Disorder	Mood Disorder
Alcohol	X	X		X		
Amphetamine and related substances	X	X	X		X	
Caffeine	X					
Cannabis	X				X	
Cocaine	X	X	X		X	
Hallucinogen	X (hallucinosis)				X	X
Inhalant	X					
Nicotine		X				
Opioid	X	X				
Phencyclidine and related substances	X		X		X	X
Sedative, hypnotic, or anxiolytic	X	X		X		

Source: Adapted from American Psychiatric Association: Diagnostic and Statistical Manual of Mental Disorders, ed 3, Revised. Washington, DC, American Psychiatric Association, 1987, p 124.

Cocaine. This drug can produce a spectrum of altered consciousness and organic mental disorders (see Table 10–7). It is discussed on page 325, in the context of seizures.

HALLUCINOGENS

Hallucinogens such as D-lysergic acid diethylamide (LSD), PCP, mescaline, and psilocybin seldom cause coma, but they may produce prolonged frightening and potentially dangerous behavior disturbances. Anticholinergic drugs such as belladona, trihexyphenidyl, and Jimson weed produce similar effects.

LSD. LSD is the most potent hallucinogen (Tables 10–7 and 10–8). It produces a dramatic change in visual perceptions and visual hallucinations. It is a typically ingested orally as a liquid, and effects last approximately 12 hours. Untoward symptoms include depersonalization, panic, disorientation, tremors, dizziness, and nausea. Its primary action in the CNS is to block serotonin receptors. The prominent effects of LSD on behavior as well as the effects of amphetamine derivatives such as MDMA suggest that serotonergic innervation of the brain plays an important functional role.[119] Patients who are intoxicated with LSD or other hallucinogens should be placed in a quiet room and someone should be assigned to provide reassurance. Severe agitation can be treated with diazepam or haloperidol.

PCP. PCP was originally developed in the 1950s as a "dissociative" anesthetic agent, but unacceptable adverse effects prevented its clinical use. The agent has sympathomimetic, anticholinergic, and dopaminergic actions and interacts with CNS opiate receptors.[5,147] It is also a specific noncompetitive antagonist of the NMDA-type EAA receptor channel complex (see Chapter 1). Aside from being a CNS depressant and analgesic, the drug also has CNS stimulant and hallucinogenic properties (see Table 10–7). These latter characteristics, plus the ease with which it can be illicitly synthesized, have made it a widely abused street drug. It may be ingested as a tablet, smoked, or "snorted".

PCP overdose may present as coma (Table 10–9). In a review of 1000 cases of PCP intoxication,[111,112] 10.6% of patients were comatose at initial evaluation in the emergency room. Unconsciousness typically followed delirium, or violent or bizarre behavior. There were 55 cases in which coma was due to PCP alone. Most patients had nystagmus, and approximately half were hypertensive and tachycardic. Other neurologic findings are shown in Table 10–9. Respiratory depression occurred in approximately 10% of the cases, but

Table 10–8 SIGNS OF HALLUCINOGEN INTOXICATION

Mental status change: marked anxiety, panic, paranoid ideation
Pupillary dilation
Tachycardia
Sweating
Palpitations
Blurred vision
Tremors
Uncoordination

Table 10–9 SIGNS OF PHENCYCLIDINE INTOXICATION

Mental status change: agitation, coma, belligerence, impaired judgment, coma
Nystagmus (vertical or horizontal)
Increased blood pressure
Tachycardia, cardiac arrhythmias
Flushing, increased sweating
Reduced sensitivity to pain
Ataxia
Dysarthria
Muscle rigidity, dystonia
Seizures
Hyperacusis
Pupillary constriction (variable)
Decerebrate posturing
Tremor, twitching
Athetosis
Variable reactivity of tendon reflexes
Respiratory depression

was more common in patients also intoxicated with sedative-hypnotics or narcotics. During recovery, many patients were delirious, catatonic, agitated, or psychotic for days to weeks.

In these patients, benzodiazepines may be used for severe agitation.[134] Antipsychotics (chlorpromazine and haloperidol)[42,106] have been used for treatment of psychosis or extreme agitation, but some authorities feel they are contraindicated because they may worsen symptoms or do not help.

INHALANTS

Abuse of inhalants such as model airplane glue, spray paints, cleaning fluids such as Scotchgard, and aerosols used as propellants in deodorants is a problem, especially among children and teenagers in deprived socioeconomic groups.[147] Toluene is the most ubiquitous solvent that is inhaled; it may cause encephalopathy, convulsions, liver damage, and peripheral neuropathy (Table 10–10). Sudden death related to cardiac arrhythmias has been reported after inhalation of halogenated hydrocarbons (Freon), spot removers, and typewriter correction fluids. Although inhaling amyl, butyl, and isobutyl nitrites has been reported to cause headaches, tachycardia and syncope, few long-lasting toxic effects on the nervous system have been reported. Gasoline sniffing may produce a profound encephalopathy and inhalation of leaded gas may lead to acute lead poisoning, producing a cerebellar syndrome with myoclonus. For all these acute intoxications severe enough to produce an altered mental status, general supportive care is needed. There are no specific therapies, other than the use of chelators for acute lead exposure.

EXCITOTOXINS

Although EAA neurotransmitters are important in brain function and appear to have a role in certain neurologic diseases, direct evidence of neurotoxicity produced by EAA is limited. Recently, an outbreak of toxic encephalopathy caused by eating mussels contaminated with the neurotoxic amino acid domoic acid drew attention to this mechanism of neurotoxicity.[172] In Canada in late 1987, there was an outbreak of an acute illness characterized by gastrointestinal symptoms, encephalopathy, oculomotor abnormalities, and seizures among persons who ate cultivated mussels from three river estuaries on the eastern coast of Prince Edward Island. Domoic acid, which acts as an excitatory neurotransmitter and has a structure similar to kainic acid (see Chapter 1), was identified in mussels left uneaten by the patients and mussels sampled from these estuaries. The domoic acid was traced to a form of marine vegetation (*Nitzschia pungens*) growing in the waters. Acute neurologic abnormalities included headache, seizures, hemiparesis, ophthalmoplegia, and mental status abnormalities ranging from agitation to coma. After the acute symptoms and signs had cleared, 12 patients had severe anterograde memory deficits with relative preservation of other cognitive disorders. Eleven patients had clinical and electromyographic evidence of pure motor or sensory motor neuropathy or axonopathy. Neuropathologic studies in four patients who died demonstrated neuron necrosis in the hippocampus and amygdala in a pattern similar to that produced in animals by administration of kainic acid. In the acute phase of illness, the seizures were particularly difficult to control in some patients. In

---

**Table 10–10 SIGNS OF INHALANT
INTOXICATION**

Mental status change: lethargy, coma, impaired judgment, assaultiveness, apathy
Dizziness
Nystagmus
Uncoordination
Slurred speech
Depressed reflexes
Tremor
Blurred vision

three patients, seizures were resistant to phenytoin therapy but responded to intravenous administration of diazepam and phenobarbital. Seizures became progressively less frequent during an 8-week period after ingestion and ceased within 4 months of intoxication in all patients. A similar pattern of hyperexcitation followed by neuron necrosis and loss of function has also been reported in human lathyrism, which is probably caused by the glutamate analogue beta-N-oxalylamino-L-alanine.[172] Therefore naturally occurring excitotoxic amino acid analogues should be added to the list of substances that may produce severe encephalopathy and coma.

SEIZURES CAUSED BY DRUG INTOXICATION

A variety of drugs cause seizures (Table 10–11). The incidence of drug-induced seizures depends on the class of drug and the circumstances in which the drug is used. For instance, the Boston Collaborative Drug Surveillance Program[131] identified 26 cases of drug-induced seizures among 32,812 patients (0.08%) and found the most common drugs to be penicillins, hypoglycemic agents, lidocaine, methylxanthines, and antipsychotics. Messing and colleagues[115] reviewed drug-induced seizures (including those from overdoses) observed at the San Francisco General Hospital emergency room during a 9-year period for problems related to drug abuse (Table 10–12). The drugs of abuse most frequently associated with seizures were cocaine, PCP, and amphetamine.

Drugs play a role in the etiology of status epilepticus as well. One report[1] identified "toxic exogenous" factors as the basis of nine cases of status epilepticus in 239 pediatric patients, although details about these patients were not provided. In adults, another study[4] attributed 10 of 98 cases of status epilepticus to probable drug overdose. The specific agents included isoniazid (n = 3), aminophylline, diphenhydramine, lidocaine, amitriptyline, thioridazine, pentazocine, and cocaine.

These studies suggest that drug toxicity should be a consideration in any pa-

Table 10–11 DRUGS REPORTED TO CAUSE SEIZURES AND STATUS EPILEPTICUS

Aqueous iodinated contrast agents	Mefenamic acid
Anticholinesterase agents (organophosphates, physostigmine)	Methylxanthines
Antihistamines	Metronidazol
Antidepressants	Misonidazole
Antipsychotics	Nalidixic acid
Baclofen	Narcotic analgesics (fentanyl, meperidine, pentazocine, propoxyphene)
Beta blockers (propranolol, oxprenolol)	Oxytocin (secondary to water intoxication)
Camphor	Penicillins
Chlorambucil	Phencyclidine
Cocaine	Phenobarbitol withdrawal
Cycloserine	Phenytoin
Cyclosporin A	Prednisone (with hypocalcemia)
Ergonovine	Sympathomimetics (amphetamines, ephedrine, phenylpropranolamine, terbutaline)
Folic acid	Vitamin K oxide
General anesthetics (ketamine, halothane, althesin, enflurane, propanidid)	
Hyperbaric oxygen	
Hypoglycemic agents	
Hyposmolar parenteral solutions	
Isoniazid	
Local anesthetics (bupivacaine, lidocaine, procaine, etidocaine)	

Source: Adapted from Messing et al,[115] p 1583.

Table 10–12 DRUGS ASSOCIATED WITH GENERALIZED SEIZURES IN 51 PATIENTS

Drugs	Status	No. of Patients with:	
		Two or More Seizures	Single Seizures
Isoniazid	3	7	—
Psychotropic agents	1	6	9
Bronchodilators	1	3	1
Insulin	1	2	2
Stimulants	—	2	3
Lidocaine	2	1	—
Opioid analgesics	—	—	2
Anticholinergics	—	—	2
Cefazolin	—	—	1
Loxapine/benztropine	—	—	1
Thioridazine/pentazocine	—	—	1
Total	8	21	22

Source: Adapted from Messing et al,[115] p 1583.

tient presenting with either a single generalized seizure, multiple seizures, or status epilepticus. Such consideration is especially important with regard to therapy. Patients with an isolated generalized seizure due to drug abuse need not be started on anticonvulsants. Conversely, drug-induced status epilepticus is often difficult to control, and such patients may require especially aggressive anticonvulsant therapy.

Several mechanisms probably account for seizures induced by drugs and toxins. As discussed in detail in Chapter 3, the basic mechanisms for initiation and generation of seizures include a reduction in neuron inhibition, overactivity of excitatory pathways, and abnormalities in the ion gradients that regulate the electrical gradients across membranes. The mechanisms by which specific drugs produce seizures in humans are uncertain but can be hypothesized based on experimental studies with animals. For example, penicillin appears to produce seizures by antagonizing the effect of GABA on the chloride channel. Methylxanthines may cause seizures by antagonizing the effect of the inhibitory transmitter substance adenosine on release of excitatory neurotransmitters. Ethanol may also reduce GABAergic inhibition, and antidepressants and stimulants may

cause seizures by enhancing the activity of aminergic neurotransmitters.

The following sections review seizures related to some of the drugs discussed earlier in the chapter, that is, opioids, ethanol, heterocyclic antidepressants, antipsychotics, and hallucinogens and stimulants.

Opioids

Opioids have both convulsant and anticonvulsant properties, depending on the particular class of agent and experimental model.[44] For example, morphine and certain endogenous opioids have been shown to produce epileptiform activity and seizures when injected into the lateral ventricle of the rat.[44,178] They also alter the threshold to seizures induced by the convulsant flurothyl[174] or electroshock.[31] Naloxone antagonizes the convulsant effect of heroin and propoxyphene, and, to a lesser degree, of meperidine and normeperidine.[50] Opioids with the most anticonvulsant properties appear to act on the mu and delta binding sites.[9,30,156] Furthermore, different regions of the brain mediate the analgesic and convulsant properties of endogenous opioids. Metenkephalin produces analgesia when injected in or near the midbrain periaqueductal gray matter, but provokes seizures when injected into the forebrain dorsomedial nucleus of the thalamus (see Chapter 9).[44,178] Studies of the rat hippocampal formation have also demonstrated that certain opioid peptides provoke epileptogenic activity in pyramidal neurons, presumably through inhibition of inhibitory interneurons.[151]

Clinically, seizures are a particularly common problem with meperidine and pentazocine, and are rarely seen with other opioids. This observation parallels that of Cowan and associates,[30] who classified 20 opioids according to their effect on fluorthyl-induced seizures in rats and found meperidine and pentazocine among the most convulsant.

Seizures following meperidine intoxication are due to the accumulation of normeperidine, an active metabolite formed by N-demethylation of meperidine (see Chapter 9).[83] Normeperidine has significantly more excitatory and less analgesic effects than its parent compound, possibly due to actions on different receptors. Thus, toxicity is characterized by generalized CNS excitation, ranging from tremor to hyperreflexia, myoclonus, and seizures. Accumulation of normeperidine may result from a number of different factors. First, the half-life of normeperidine is 24 to 48 hours, while that of meperidine is 3 to 6 hours. Therefore, repeated doses of meperidine taken for its analgesic effect lead to a gradual increase in normeperidine levels. Second, oral administration favors the formation of normeperidine because of first-pass hepatic metabolism, and also increases the dose required for analgesia compared to the parenteral route. Third, the half-life of normeperidine is significantly prolonged in patients with renal failure.[168] Finally, other drugs that stimulate microsomal enzyme activity, such as phenobarbital, phenytoin, and chlorpromazine, will favor the formation of normeperidine and increase the dose requirement for analgesia.[162]

Normeperidine-induced seizures are usually generalized and short lived.[170]

They are often preceded by other signs of CNS excitability such as myoclonus.[53] Treatment is simply to discontinue the drug. Naloxone, which will antagonize the depressant effects of meperidine, appears to have much less effect on normeperidine, and may actually lower the seizure threshold.[30,50]

The association of pentazocine with seizures was first recognized during its use as an adjunct to general anesthesia,[74] but this was an uncommon adverse effect.[161] More recently, however, pentazocine has been abused in combination with tripelennamine hydrochloride (an antihistamine), and seizures have emerged as an important form of toxicity.[150] This combination of drugs is known as "Ts and Blues" by street addicts, and is used as an alternative to heroin. Generalized seizures may be seen immediately following intravenous injection of the drugs. One report[21] described 13 patients with CNS complications of "Ts and Blues" abuse; 11 had seizures and 2 presented with status epilepticus. Both drugs have epileptogenic characteristics; whether one or the other is the primary cause for seizures remains unknown.

Ethanol

Seizures associated with ethanol abuse are commonly observed during withdrawal (Table 10–13). The effect of modest alcohol use on seizure frequency in epileptics is less clear. A brief report by Mattson[110] recorded the expe-

Table 10–13 SIGNS OF ALCOHOL WITHDRAWAL

Tremor of hands, tongue, eyelids
Nausea, vomiting
Malaise
Tachycardia
Sweating
Elevated blood pressure
Anxiety
Irritability
Hallucinations or illusions
Insomnia

rience of 112 epileptics who used alcohol. When an exacerbation of seizure frequency occurred in the setting of alcohol abuse, the seizure exacerbation occurred "the morning after" in 95% of cases. Fourteen such patients were further studied electroencephalographically following oral administration of 0.5 to 1.0 mL/kg of alcohol. Marked suppression of baseline epileptiform activity occurred during the rise or peak of ethanol levels. In two patients, a rebound increase in spike activity occurred 12 hours later. Thus acute intoxication may produce a transient anticonvulsant effect, although in some patients a rebound phenomenon may follow. A "morning-after" seizure exacerbation is also described in a small group of patients by Victor and Brausch.[181] In a study of 308 patients from Harlem Hospital, however, the risk of seizures increased with increasing current alcohol use. The authors concluded that seizures were a direct result of alcohol use.[123] This observation is based heavily on the authors' statistical analysis, and it requires confirmation.

Heterocyclic Antidepressants

Heterocyclic antidepressants have a biphasic effect in animal models of epilepsy; they are anticonvulsant at low doses and convulsant at higher doses.[89,94] The latter effect has been ascribed to alterations in levels of serotonin, catecholamine, or dopamine in the CNS[175,176,185] and effects on excitable membranes.[94]

The antidepressants cause seizures at therapeutic doses as well as with toxic overdoses. Recent surveys suggest that the incidence is approximately 0.1% to 2% in patients on antidepressant therapy.[72,77,105,129,131] Not surprisingly, patients having a history of CNS disease, especially epilepsy, are at higher risk for antidepressant-induced seizures.[77,105]

Seizures are estimated to occur in 4% to 20% of patients with tricyclic over-

dose; in most cases, the patients are comatose and have multiple convulsions.[16,20,66,124,163,183] Some of the newer antidepressants, such as amoxapine and maprotiline, appear to be significantly more epileptogenic in the setting of an overdose.[14,90,100,171,183] Boenhert and Lovejoy[14] have shown that the QRS duration is a better predictor for risk of convulsions than the serum drug level in acute overdoses. When seizures occur, they are often refractory to standard management and denote a significantly poorer prognosis compared to an overdose without seizures.[20] Diazepam, phenytoin, and (in the case of status epilepticus) high-dose barbiturates have been advocated for therapy.[73,90] We recommend prompt administration of these anticonvulsants in the standard protocol we use for status epilepticus (see Chapter 3).[153] Physostigmine, due to its own convulsant actions, should not be used.[124]

Antipsychotics

Although antipsychotic agents rarely cause coma, their ability to lower the seizure threshold, especially at higher doses, suggests that seizures may be a complication of any overdose involving these drugs. The basis of their convulsant actions is not fully understood. The essential biochemical action of effective antipsychotics is blockade of CNS dopamine transmission; they also have varying degrees of antimuscarinic activity. These two properties appear to have opposite effects on the seizure threshold, in that blockade of dopamine transmission induces seizures, whereas blockade of CNS cholinergic (especially muscarinic) transmission reduces seizures.[136] Attempts have been made to predict which antipsychotics are convulsants by considering their relative effects on dopamine and acetylcholine transmission. Important exceptions exist, however, suggesting that the mechanism is much more complex.

The relative effect of antipsychotics

on seizure thresholds has been studied using various animal models, hippocampal slices,[125] observations of EEG changes,[70] and clinical investigations.[136,173] The results from these studies diverge. Nonetheless, it appears that low-potency phenothiazines, such as chlorpromazine and promazine hydrochloride, are the most epileptogenic, while piperazine phenothiazines (e.g., fluphenazine) and thioxanthenes (e.g., thiothixene) are the least so.[71] The overall incidence of seizures in patients taking antipsychotics appears to be on the order of 1% or 2%. A higher incidence is seen in patients taking larger doses, those exposed to a rapid change in drug dosage or multiple drugs, and those with CNS disease, including epilepsy.[173]

Itil and Soldatos[71] have proposed an algorithm for avoiding the epileptogenic side effects of the antipsychotics. In some cases they advocate anticonvulsants as prophylactic therapy for patients with an abnormal EEG before or during antipsychotic treatment, or for patients with a history or examination suggestive of CNS disease. Seizures in the setting of antipsychotic overdose should be acutely treated using standard measures.

Hallucinogens and Stimulants

In this section, we limit our discussion to seizures related to PCP and cocaine. However, methylxanthines, especially aminophylline, appear to be clinically important stimulants also associated with seizures.[115,146,193] In addition, seizures have been described with both therapeutic use and abuse of amphetamine, methylphenidate, phenylpropanolamine, ephedrine, and terbutaline,[3,115] but they are relatively uncommon.

PCP

Seizures are one of the manifestations of the hyperexcitable state induced by PCP.[5,190] PCP affects multiple neurotransmitter systems, especially the NMDA receptor channel complex, yet the mechanism by which it induces seizures is not known (see Chapter 3). McCarron and associates[112] described generalized convulsions in 31 of 1000 cases of acute PCP intoxication. Of these, 26 patients had single or isolated seizures and 5 had status epilepticus. Of a subgroup of comatose patients in which PCP was thought to be the only drug ingested (55 cases), seizures were observed in 19%.

COCAINE

Seizures related to cocaine abuse have been recognized for more than a century,[45] but this complication has received little attention in the medical literature until recently.[121] This increased attention appears partly due to the fact that the incidence of toxic reactions to cocaine is on the rise. Concurrent with the re-emergence of cocaine as a popular recreational drug during the past decade, there has been a striking increase in the number of patients presenting to hospitals complaining of seizures following cocaine use.[3] A recent report of 474 patients presenting to an inner-city emergency room because of cocaine intoxication found an incidence of 7.9% in patients who had not experienced previous seizures.[128] The incidence was higher (16.9%) in patients who previously had had seizures. This trend may be attributed to a number of factors, including an increase in the number of seizure-susceptible new users, changes in the potency of cocaine, and a shift toward the administration of cocaine by intravenous injection and "freebasing," that is, smoking the pure alkaloid form of cocaine ("crack").[80] An increasing number of young children presenting to emergency rooms with seizures have accidentally ingested cocaine.[140]

The pathophysiologic basis of cocaine-induced seizures has not been fully elucidated. Cocaine has three important neuropharmacologic actions: It is a local anesthetic, it increases mono-amine release, and it blocks mono-amine uptake by neurons (see Table 10–5 and Chapter 1).[48,80] Acutely, the last effects increase norepinephrine and dopamine concentrations at central synapses. Chronically, there is a decrease in these transmitters compared to baseline. Depletion of CNS nor-epinephrine has been shown to decrease the seizure threshold, but cocaine appears to provoke seizures even when norepinephrine levels are very low. Various animal studies have shown that at relatively low doses, cocaine has an anticonvulsant effect,[169] whereas at high doses, it is a convulsant. More recently, kindling studies have demonstrated that low doses of cocaine lower the seizure threshold and increase the speed of propagation of epileptiform activity away from kindled regions, but also decrease the duration of after-discharge potentials and spread. Drugs that have been shown experimentally to antagonize effects of cocaine include alpha-1 receptor blockers, antidopaminergics, chlorpromazine, reserpine, and calcium channel blockers.[128,142,143] In patients with chronic abuse, seizures may also reflect hemorrhagic, ischemic, and chronic neurotoxic effects of cocaine.[96] Cocaine can produce vasospasm and hemorrhage both in adults and in the fetus of a pregnant abuser.[48]

Clinical reports of cocaine-induced seizures emphasize their idiosyncratic and potentially dangerous nature. In a study of the neurologic complications of cocaine abuse at the San Francisco General Hospital,[104] 29 patients were identified who had seizures temporally related to the administration of cocaine. Seizures occurred in both first-time users and the chronic addict and were associated with all modes of administration (i.e., nasal, free-base, intravenous). Dosages ranged from 25 mg (i.e., 1 "line") to 10 g. The seizures were of the generalized tonic-clonic type, usually single, and occurred from minutes up to 12 hours following administration. A few of the patients had repeated episodes of seizures following cocaine use, but most appeared to have single, uncomplicated seizures. Two patients had status epilepticus eventually requiring barbiturate coma for control, and both were left with significant fixed encephalopathies presumed secondary to prolonged seizures. A number of reports have described prolonged convulsions as the preterminal event in patients who are intoxicated with large quantities of cocaine, as well as in "body packers" (i.e., smugglers who have ingested bags, balloons, or condoms filled with cocaine) who experience intraintestinal rupture of the cocaine-filled container.[34,81,117]

In many cases, seizures induced by cocaine are self-limited and do not require specific therapy. Our experience and that of others suggests that seizures due to large cocaine overdoses may be extremely difficult to treat.[143] We advocate aggressive treatment of status epilepticus using standard anti-convulsants,[153] resorting to pentobarbital coma if necessary.[103] The role of such agents as prazosin, chlorpromazine, or calcium channel antagonists in the treatment of cocaine-induced seizures requires further study.[143]

Many patients with seizures experience a wide range of associated psychiatric side effects including anxiety, panic, paranoia, delusions, and psychosis. Benzodiazepines are used to treat milder anxiety, and neuroleptic drugs such as haloperidol or chlorpromazine are useful for treating delusions.

CONCLUSIONS

Intoxication with drugs used therapeutically and drugs of abuse produce a wide range of acute and chronic neurologic effects. The most serious acute effects are coma, respiratory depression, and seizures. Less serious disorders of consciousness are common, including confusion, delirium, and psychiatric disturbances. Although careful evaluation and meticulous supportive therapy lead to recovery in most cases, catastrophic complications such as hypoxic-ischemic encephalopathy following cardiorespiratory arrest from depressant drugs or persistent status epilepticus from cocaine can cause permanent disability. Caring for patients with disorders produced by drug intoxication has become an increasing part of neurologic practice.

ACKNOWLEDGMENT

We wish to express our sincere appreciation to Drs. Michael Aminoff, Michael Charness, and Michael Callaham for their thoughtful review of this manuscript.

REFERENCES

1. Aicardie, J and Chevrie, JJ: Convulsive status epilepticus in infants and children: A study of 239 cases. Epilepsia 11:187–197, 1970.
2. Albiin, N and Eriksson, A: Fatal accidental hypothermia and alcohol. Alcohol 10:13–22, 1984.
3. Alldredge, BK, Lowenstein, DH, and Simon, RP: Seizures associated with recreational drug use. Neurology 39:1037–1039, 1989.
4. Aminoff, MJ and Simon, RP: Status epilepticus: Causes, clinical features, and consequences in 98 patients. Am J Med 69:657–666, 1980.
5. Aniline, O and Pitts, FN: Phencyclidine (PCP): A review. CRC Crit Rev Toxicol 10:145–177, 1982.
6. Arieff, AI and Friedman, EA: Coma following non-narcotic drug overdose. Management of 208 adult patients. Am J Med Sci 266:405, 1973.
7. Bailey, DN: Methaqualone ingestion: Evaluation of present status. J Anal Toxicol 5:270–282, 1981.
8. Barret, LG, Vincent, FM, Arsac, PL, Debru, JL, and Faure, JR: Internuclear ophthalmoplegia in patients with toxic coma: Frequency, prognostic value, diagnostic significance. J Toxicol Clin Toxicol 20:373–379, 1983.
9. Berman, EF and Adler, MW: The anticonvulsant effect of opioid peptide against maximal electroshock seizures in rats. Neuropharmacology 23:367–371, 1984.
10. Bertino, JS and Reed, MD: Barbiturate and nonbarbiturate sedative hypnotic intoxication in children. Pediatr Clin North Am 33:703–722, 1986.
11. Bettinger, J: Cocaine intoxication: Massive oral overdose. Ann Emerg Med 9:429–430, 1980.
12. Bird, TD and Plum, F: Recovery from barbiturate overdose coma with a prolonged isoelectric electroencephalogram. Neurology 18:456–460, 1968.
13. Blackwell, B: Adverse effects of antidepressant drugs. Drugs 21:201–219, 1981.
14. Boehnert, MT and Lovejoy, FH: Value of QRS duration versus the serum drug level in predicting seizures and ventricular arrhythmias after an acute overdose of tricyclic antidepressants. N Engl J Med 313:474–479, 1985.
15. Bradberry, JC and Raebel, MA: Continuous infusion of naloxone in the treatment of narcotic overdosage. Drug Intell Clin Pharm 15:945–950, 1981.
16. Braden, MH, Jackson, JE, and Walson, PD: Tricyclic antidepressant overdose. Pediatr Clin North Am 33:287–297, 1986.
17. Brehmer-Anderson, E and Pederson, NB: Sweat gland necrosis and bullous skin changes in acute drug intoxication. Acta Derm Venereol 49:157–162, 1969.
18. Brown, DG and Hammill, JF: Glutethimide poisoning: Unilateral pupillary abnormalities. N Engl J Med 285:806, 1971.
19. Brown, SS and Goenechea, S: Methaqualone: Metabolic, kinetic and clinical pharmacologic observations. Clin Pharmacol Ther 14:314–324, 1973.
20. Callaham, M and Kassel, D: Epidemiology of fatal tricyclic ingestion: Implications for management. Ann Emerg Med 14:1–9, 1985.
21. Caplan, LR, Thomas, C, and Banks, G: Central nervous system complications of addiction to "T's and Blues." Neurology 32:623–628, 1982.

22. Chan, AWK: Alcoholism and epilepsy. Epilepsia 26:323–333, 1985.
23. Chatrian, GE, White, LW, and Daly, D: Electroencephalographic patterns resembling those of sleep in certain comatose states after injuries to the head. Electroencephalogr Clin Neurophysiol 15:292–280, 1963.
24. Chen, H: Naloxone in shock and toxic coma. Am J Emerg Med 2:444–452, 1984.
25. Chi, ML and Lin, MT: Involvement of adrenergic receptor mechanisms within hypothalamus in the fever induced by amphetamine and thyrotropin-releasing hormone in the rat. J Neural Transm 58:213–222, 1983.
26. Cho, AK: Ice: A new dosage form of an old drug. Science 249:631–634, 1990.
27. Clowes, GHA and O'Donnell, TF: Heat stroke. N Engl J Med 291:564–567, 1974.
28. Cook, FF, Davis, RG, and Russo, LS: Internuclear ophthalmoplegia caused by phenothiazine intoxication. Arch Neurol 38:465–466, 1981.
29. Cotliar, RW, Stringham, LR, and Leavell, UW: Dermographism, erythema and flare: Clinical signs of drug overdose in the comatose patient. South Med J 66:1277–1278, 1973.
30. Cowan, A, Geller, EB, and Adler, MW: Classification of opioids on the basis of change in seizure threshold in rats. Science 206:465–467, 1979.
31. Czuczwar, SJ and Frey, HH: Effect of morphine and morphine-like analgesics on susceptibility to seizures in mice. Neuropharmacology 25:465–469, 1986.
32. Delay, J and Deniker, P: Drug induced extrapyramidal syndromes. In Vinken, PJ and Bruyn, GW (eds): Handbook of Clinical Neurology, Vol 6. Diseases of the Basal Ganglia. North-Holland Publishing, Amsterdam, 1968, pp 248–266.
33. deVillota, EO, Mosquera, JM, Shubin, H, and Weil, MH: Abnormal temperature control after intoxication with short-acting barbiturates. Crit Care Med 9:662–665, 1981.
34. DiMaio, VJM and Garriott, JC: Four deaths due to intravenous injection of cocaine. Forensic Sci Int 12:119–125, 1978.
35. Dole, VP, Fishman, J, Goldfrank, L, Khanna, J, and McGivern, RF: Arousal of ethanol-intoxicated comatose patients with naloxone. Alcohol Clin Exp Res 6:275–279, 1982.
36. Dorwart, WV and Chalmers, L: Comparison of methods for calculating serum osmolality from chemical concentrations and the prognostic value of such calculations. Clin Chem 21:190–194, 1975.
37. Epstein, FB and Eilers, MA: Poisoning. In Rosen, P, Baker, FJ, Braen, GR, Dailey, RH, and Levy, RC (eds): Emergency Medicine—Concepts and Clinical Practice. CV Mosby, St. Louis, 1983, p 225.
38. Estilo, AE and Cottrell JE: Hemodynamic and catecholamine changes after administration of naloxone. Anesth Analg (Paris) 61:349–353, 1982.
39. Fernandez, JP, O'Rourke, RA, and Ewy, GA: Rapid active external rewarming in accidental hypothermia. JAMA 212:153, 1970.
40. Fischbeck, KH and Simon, RP: Neurological manifestations of accidental hypothermia. Ann Neurol 10:384–387, 1981.
41. Fisher, CM: The neurological examination of the comatose patient. Acta Neurol Scand 45(Suppl 36):1–56, 1969.
42. Fox, SM: Haloperidol in the treatment of phencyclidine intoxication. Am J Hosp Pharm 36:448, 1979.
43. Frand, UI, Chang, SS, and Williams, MH: Methadone-induced pulmonary edema. Ann Intern Med 76:975–979, 1972.
44. Frenk, H: Pro and anticonvulsant actions of morphine and the endogenous opioids: Involvement and interactions of multiple opiate and non-opiate systems. Brain Research Review 6:197–210, 1983.
45. Freud, S: The Cocaine Papers. Dunquin Press, Vienna, 1963.
46. Freinkel, N, Singer, DL, Arky, RA, Bleicher, SJ, Anderson, JB, and Silbert, CK: Alcohol hypoglycemia—I. Carbohydrate metabolism of patients with clinical alcohol hypoglycemia and the experimental reproduction of the syn-

drome with pure ethanol. J Clin Invest 42:1112–1133, 1963.

47. Gary, NE and Tresznewsky, O: Barbiturates and a potpourri of other sedatives, hypnotics and tranquilizers. Heart Lung 12:122–127, 1983.

48. Gawin, FH and Ellinwood, EN: Cocaine and other stimulants: Actions, abuse and treatment. N Engl J Med 318:1173–1182, 1988.

49. Gennari, FJ: Serum osmolality: Uses and limitations. N Engl J Med 310:102–105, 1984.

50. Gilbert, PE and Martin, WR: Antagonism of the convulsant effects of heroin, d-propoxyphene, meperidine, normeperidine and thebaine by naloxone in mice. J Pharmacol Exp Ther 192:538–541, 1975.

51. Glasser, L, Sternglanz, PD, Combie, J, and Robinson, A: Serum osmolality and its applicability to drug overdose. Am J Clin Pathol 60:695–699, 1973.

52. Glauser, FL, Smith, WR, Caldwell, A, Hoshiko, M, Dolan, GS, Baer, H, and Olsher, N: Etchlorvynol (Placidyl)-induced pulmonary edema. Ann Intern Med 84:46–48, 1976.

53. Goetting, MG: Neurotoxicity of meperidine. Ann Emerg Med 14:1007–1009, 1985.

54. Goldfrank, LR and Bresnitz, EA: Opioids. In Goldfrank, LR, Flomenbacm, NE, Lewin, NA, Weisman, RS, Howland, MA, and Kulberg, AG (eds): Goldfrank's Toxicologic Emergencies. Appleton-Century-Crofts, Norwalk, Connecticut, 1986, pp 404–423.

55. Greenberg, DG and Simon, RP: Flexor and extensor postures in sedative drug-induced coma. Neurology 32:448–451, 1982.

56. Greenblatt, DJ, Allen, MD, Harmatz, JS, Noel, BJ, and Shader, RI: Correlates of outcome following acute glutethimide overdosage. J Forensic Sci 24:76–86, 1978.

57. Greenblatt, DJ, Allen, MD, Noel, BJ, and Shader, RI: Acute overdosage with benzodiazepine derivatives. Clin Pharmacol Ther 21:497–514, 1977.

58. Greenblatt, DJ, Allen, MD, Harmatz, JS, Noel, BJ, and Shader, RI: Overdosage with pentobarbital and secobarbital: Assessment of risk factors related to outcome. J Clin Pharmacol 19:658–768, 1979.

59. Guerin, JM and Friedberg, G: Naloxone and ethanol intoxication. Ann Intern Med 97:932, 1982.

60. Haddad, J, Johnson, K, Smith, S, Price, L, and Giardina, E: Acute barbiturate intoxication: Concepts of management. JAMA 209:893–900, 1969.

61. Hadden, LM and Winchester, JF: Clinical Management of Poisoning and Drug Overdose. WB Saunders, Philadelphia, 1983.

62. Helliwell, M, Hampel, G, Sinclair, E, Huggett, A, and Flanagan, RJ: Value of emergency toxicological investigations in differential diagnosis of coma. Br Med J 2:819–821, 1979.

63. Henderson, LW and Merrill, JP: Treatment of barbiturate intoxication. Ann Intern Med 64:876, 1966.

64. Hepler, BR, Sutheimer, CA, and Sunshine, I: The role of the toxicology laboratory in emergency medicine. J Toxicol Clin Toxicol 19:353–365, 1982.

65. Holt, S, Stewart, IC, Dixon, JW, Elton, RA, Taylor, TV, and Little, K: Alcohol and the emergency service patient. Br Med J 281:638–640, 1980.

66. Hulten, B and Heath, A: Clinical aspects of tricyclic antidepressant poisoning. Acta Med Scand 213:275–278, 1983.

67. Hunt, WA: The effect of ethanol on GABAergic transmission. Neurosci Biobehav Rev 7:87–95, 1983.

68. Huttunen, P and Myers, RD: Release of norepinephrine from the rat's hypothalamus perfused with alcohol: Relation to body temperature. Alcohol 2:683–691, 1985.

69. Isbell, H, Altshul, S, Kornetsky, CH, Eisenman, AJ, Flanary, HG, and Fraser, HF: Chronic barbiturate intoxication: Experimental study. Archives of Neurology and Psychiatry 64:1–28, 1950.

70. Itil, TM and Meyers, JP: Epileptic and antiepileptic properties of psychotropic drugs. In Mercier, J (ed): International Encyclopedia of Pharmacology and Therapeutics, Vol 2. Pergamon Press, Oxford, 1973, pp 599–622.

71. Itil, TM and Soldatos, C: Epileptogenic side effects of psychotropic drugs: Practical recommendations. JAMA 244: 1460–1463, 1980.

72. Jabbari, B, Bryan, GE, Marsh, EE, and Gunderson, CH: Incidence of seizures with tricyclic and tetracyclic antidepressants. Arch Neurol 42:480–481, 1985.

73. Jackson, JE and Bressler, R: Prescribing tricylic antidepressants. Part III: Management of overdose. Drug Ther Bull 12:49–63, 1982.

74. Jackson, SH, Dueker, C, and Grace, L: Seizures induced by pentazocine. Anesthesiology 35:92–95, 1971.

75. Jacobsen, D, Bredsen, JE, Eide, I, and Ostborg, J: Anion and osmolal gaps in the diagnosis of methanol and ethylene glycol poisoning. Acta Med Scand 212:17–20, 1982.

76. Jefferys, DB and Volans, GN: An investigation of the role of the specific opioid antagonist naloxone in clinical toxicology. Human Toxicology 2:227–231, 1983.

77. Jick, H, Dinan, BJ, Hunter, JR, Stergachis, A, Ronning, A, Perera, DR, Modsen, S, and Nudelman, PM: Tricyclic antidepressants and convulsions. Journal of Clinical Psychopharmacology 3:182–185, 1983.

78. Johnson, DA, Friedman, HJ, Cooke, R, and Lee, MN: Adaptation of brain lipid bilayers to ethanol-induced fluidization. Biochem Pharmacol 24:1673–1676, 1980.

79. Johnson, RA, Noll, EC, and MacMillan, R: Survival after a serum ethanol concentration of 1½%. Lancet 2:1394, 1982.

80. Johanson, CE and Fischman, MW: The pharmacology of cocaine related to its abuse. Pharmacol Rev 41:3–52, 1989.

81. Jonsson, S, O'Meara, M, and Young, AB: Acute cocaine poisoning: Importance of treating seizures and acidosis. Am J Med 75:1061–1064, 1983.

82. Jordon, SC and Hampson, F: Amphetamine poisoning associated with hyperpyrexia. Br Med J 2:844, 1960.

83. Kaiko, RF, Foley, KM, Gabrinski, PY, Heidrich G, Rogers, AG, Inturrisi, CE, and Reidenberg, MM: Central nervous system excitatory effects of meperidine in cancer patients. Ann Neurol 13:180–185, 1983.

84. Kalant, H and Le, AD: Effects of ethanol on thermoregulation. Pharmacol Ther 23:313–364, 1983.

85. Kendrick, WC, Hull, AR, and Knochel, JP: Rhabdomyolysis and shock after intravenous amphetamine administration. Ann Intern Med 86:381–387, 1977.

86. Khantzian, EJ and McKenna, GJ: Acute toxic withdrawal reactions associated with drug use and abuse. Ann Intern Med 90:361–372, 1979.

87. Knight, ME and Roberts, RJ: Phenothiazine and butyrophenone intoxication in children. Pediatr Clin North Am 33:299–309, 1986.

88. Knudsen, K and Heath, A: Effects of self poisoning with maprotiline. Br Med J 288:601–602, 1984.

89. Koella, WP, Glatt, A, Klebs, K, and Durst, T: Epileptic phenomena induced in the cat by the antidepressant maptrotiline, imipramine, clomipramine and amitriptyline. Biol Psychiatry 14:485–497, 1979.

90. Kulig, K, Rumack, BH, Sullivan, JB, Brandt, H, Spyker, DA, Duffy, JP, and Shipe, JR: Amoxapine overdose: Coma and seizures without cardiotoxic effects. JAMA 248:1092–1094, 1982.

91. Kulonen, E: Ethanol and GABA. Med Biol 61:147–167, 1983.

92. Kuroiwa, Y, Furukawa, T, and Inaki, K: Recovery from drug-induced alpha coma. Neurology 31:1359–1361, 1981.

93. Kurtz, D: The EEG in acute and chronic drug intoxications. In Glase, GH (ed): Handbook of Electroencephalography and Clinical Neurophysiology, Vol 15, Part C. Elsevier, Amsterdam, 1976, pp 88–104.

94. Lange, SC, Julien, RM, and Fowler, GW: Biphasic effects of imipramine in experimental models of epilepsy. Epilepsia 17:183–196, 1976.

95. Leavell, UW: Sweat gland necrosis in barbiturate poisoning. Arch Dermatol 100:218–221, 1969.

96. Levine, SR, Brust, JCM, Fatrell, N, Ho, K-L, Blake, D, Millikan, CH, Brass, LM,

Fayad, P, Schultz, LR, Selwa, JF, and Welch, KMA: Cerebrovascular complications of the use of "crack" cocaine form of alkaloidal cocaine. N Engl J Med 323:699–704, 1990.

97. Lin, MT, Chandra, A, Chern, YF, and Tsay, BL: Effects of intracerebroventricular injection of d-amphetamine on metabolic, respiratory and vasomotor activities and body temperatures in the rat. Can J Physiol Pharmacol 58:903–908, 1980.

98. Linton, AL and Ledingham, I: Severe hypothermia with barbiturate intoxication. Lancet 1:24–26, 1966.

99. Lipton, JM, Payne, H, Garza, HR, and Rosenberg, RN: Thermolability in Wernicke's encephalopathy. Arch Neurol 35:750–753, 1978.

100. Litovitz, TL and Troutman, WG: Amoxapine overdose: Seizures and fatalities. JAMA 250:1069–1071, 1983.

101. Loeb, JN: The hyperosmolar state. N Engl J Med 284:1253–1255, 1974.

102. Lovinger, DM, White, G, and Weight, FF: Ethanol inhibits NMDA-activated ion current in hippocampal neurons. Science 243:1721–1724, 1989.

103. Lowenstein, DH, Aminoff, MJ, and Simon, RP: Barbiturate anesthesia in the treatment of status epilepticus: Clinical experience with 14 patients. Neurology 38:395–400, 1988.

104. Lowenstein, DH, Massa, SM, Rowbotham, MC, Collins, SD, McKinney, HW, and Simon, RP: Acute neurologic and psychiatric complications associated with cocaine abuse. Am J Med 83:841–846, 1987.

105. Lowry, MR and Dunner, FJ: Seizures during tricyclic therapy. Am J Psychiatry 137:1461–1462, 1980.

106. Luisada, PV: The phencyclidine psychosis: Phenomenology and treatment. In Petersen, RC, Stillman, RC (eds): PCP Phencyclidine Abuse: An Appraisal. National Institute on Drug Abuse. Department New Publication No (ADM) 78-728, U.S. Govt. Printing Office, Washington, DC, 1978, pp 244–253.

107. Mackenzie, AI: Naloxone in alcohol intoxication. Lancet 1:733–734, 1979.

108. Mandy, S and Ackerman, AB: Characteristic trauma skin lesions in drug-induced coma. JAMA 213:253–256, 1970.

109. Marshall, JB and Forker, AD: Cardiovascular effects of tricyclic antidepressant drugs: Therapeutic usage, overdose and management of complications. Am Heart J 103:401–414, 1982.

110. Mattson, RH, Sturman, JK, Gronowski, ML, and Goico, N: Effect of alcohol intake in nonalcoholic epileptics. Neurology 25(4):361–362, 1975.

111. McCarron, MM, Schulze, BW, Thompson, GA, Conder, MC, and Goetz, WA: Acute phencyclidine intoxication: Incidence of clinical findings in 1,000 cases. Ann Emerg Med 10:237–242, 1981.

112. McCarron, MM, Schulze, BW, Thompson, GA, Conder, MC, and Goetz, WA: Acute phencyclidine intoxication: Clinical patterns, complications and treatment. Ann Emerg Med 10:290–297, 1981.

113. McCarron, MM, Schulze, BW, Walberg, CB, Thompson, GA, and Ansari, A: Short-acting barbiturate overdosage—Correlation of intoxication score with serum barbiturate concentration. JAMA 248:55–61, 1982.

114. McCarron, MM: The use of toxicology tests in emergency room diagnosis. J Anal Toxicol 7:131–136, 1983.

115. Messing, RO, Closson, RG, and Simon, RP: Drug-induced seizures: A 10-year experience. Neurology 34:1582–1586, 1984.

116. Mitchell, AA, Lovejoy, FH, and Foldman, P: Drug ingestions associated with miosis in comatose children. J Pediatr 89:303–305, 1976.

117. Mittleman, RE and Wetli, CV: Deaths caused by recreational cocaine use: An update. JAMA 252:1889–1893, 1984.

118. Mladinich, EK and Carlow, TJ: Total gaze paresis in amitriptyline overdose. Neurology 17:695, 1977.

119. Molliver, ME, Berger, UV, Mamounas, LA, Molliver, DC, O'Hearn, E, Wilson, MA: Neurotoxicity of MDMA and related compounds: Anatomic studies. Ann NY Acad Sci 600:640–664, 1990.

120. Moore, RA, Rumack, BH, Conner, CS, and Peterson, RG: Naloxone: Underdo-

sage after narcotic poisoning. Am J Dis Child 134:156–157, 1980.

121. Myers, JA and Earnest, MP: Generalized seizures and cocaine abuse. Neurology 34:675–676, 1984.

122. Myers, RR and Stockard, JJ: Neurologic and electroencephalographic correlates in glutethimide intoxication. Clin Pharmacol Ther 17:212–220, 1975.

123. Ng, SKC, Hauser, WA, Brust, JCM, and Susser, M: Alcohol consumption and withdrawal in new-onset seizures. N Engl J Med 319:666–673, 1988.

124. Noble, J and Matthew, H: Acute poisoning by tricyclic antidepressants: Clinical features and management of 100 patients. Clin Toxicol 2:403–421, 1969.

125. Oliver, AP, Luchins, DJ, and Wyatt, RJ: Neuroleptic-induced seizures: An *in vitro* technique for assessing relative risk. Arch Gen Psychiatry 39:206–209, 1982.

126. Olson, KR and Benowitz, NL: Environmental and drug-induced hyperthermia: Recognition and management. Emerg Med Clin North Am 2:459–474, 1984.

127. Pan, HYM and Huang, CY: Alternating skew deviation associated with Mandrax overdosage. Aust NZ J Med 14:265–266, 1984.

128. Pascual-Leone, A, Dhuna, A, Altafullah, I, and Anderson, DC: Cocaine-induced seizures. Neurology 40:404–407, 1990.

129. Peck, AW, Stern, WC, and Watkinson, C: Incidence of seizures during treatment with tricyclic antidepressant drugs and bupropion. J Clin Psychiatry 44:197–201, 1983.

130. Plum, F and Posner, JB: The Diagnosis of Stupor and Coma, ed. 3. FA Davis, Philadelphia, 1980, pp. 348–365.

131. Porter, J and Jick, H: Drug-induced convulsions, deafness and extrapyramidal symptoms. Lancet 1:587–588, 1977.

132. Pulst, SM and Lombroso, CT: External ophthalmoplegia, alpha and spindle coma in imipramine overdose: Case report and review of the literature. Ann Neurol 14:587–590, 1983.

133. Quastel, DMJ, Hackett, JT, and Okamoto, K: Presynaptic action of central depressant drugs: Inhibition of depolarization-secretion coupling. Can J Physiol Pharmacol 50:279–284, 1972.

134. Rappolt, RT, Gay, GR, and Farris, RD: Emergency management of phencyclidine intoxication. Journal of the American College of Emergency Physicians 8:68–76, 1979.

135. Reed, CE, Driggs, MF, and Foote, CC: Acute barbiturate intoxication: Study of 300 cases based on physiologic system of classification of severity of intoxication. Ann Intern Med 27:290–303, 1952.

136. Remick, RA and Fine, SH: Antipsychotic drugs and seizures. J Clin Psychiatry 40:78–80, 1979.

137. Reuler, JB: Hypothermia: Pathophysiology, clinical settings and management. Ann Intern Med 89:519–527, 1978.

138. Ricaurte, G, Bryan, G, Strauss, L, Seiden, L, and Schuster, C: Hallucinogenic amphetamine selectively destroys brain serotonin nerve terminals. Science 229:986–988, 1985.

139. Richards, CD: On the mechanism of barbiturate anesthesia. J Physiol (Lond) 227:749–767, 1972.

140. Rivkin, M and Gilmore, HE: Generalized seizures in an infant due to environmentally acquired cocaine. Pediatrics 84:1100–1102, 1987.

141. Rosenbaum, JL, Kramer, MS, and Raja, R: Resin hemoperfusion for acute drug intoxication. Arch Intern Med 136:263–265, 1976.

142. Rosenberg, J, Pentel, P, Pond, S, Benowitz, N, and Olson, K: Hyperthermia associated with drug intoxication. Crit Care Med 14:964–969, 1986.

143. Rowbotham, MC, Jones, RT, Benowitz, NL, and Jacob, P: Trazadone-oral cocaine interactions. Arch Gen Psychiatry 41:895–899, 1984.

144. Sarnquist, F and Larson, CP: Drug-induced heat stroke. Anesthesiology 39:348–350.

145. Schottstaedt, MW, Nicotra, B, and Rivera, M: Placidyl abuse: A dimorphic picture. Crit Care Med 9:677–679, 1981.

146. Schwartz, MS and Scott, DF: Aminophylline-induced seizures. Epilepsia 15:501–505, 1974.

147. Schonberg, SK (ed): Substance abuse: A guide for health professionals. American Academy of Pediatrics, Elk Grove Village, Ill, 1988.

148. Scollo-Lavizzari, G: First clinical investigation of the benzodiazepine antagonist RO 15-1788 in comatose patients. Eur Neurol 22:7–11, 1983.

149. Sellers, EM and Kalant, H: Alcohol intoxication and withdrawal. N Engl J Med 294:757–761, 1976.

150. Showalter, CV: T's and blues: Abuse of pentazocine and tripelennamine. JAMA 244:1224–1225, 1980.

151. Siggins, GR, Henriksen, SJ, Chavkin, C, and Gruol, D: Opioid peptides and epileptogenesis in the limbic system: Cellular mechanisms. In Delgado-Escueta, AV, Wasterlain, CG, Treiman, DM, and Porter, RJ (eds): Advances in Neurology, Vol 44. Raven Press, New York, 1986, pp 501–512.

152. Simon, RP: Forced downward ocular deviation: Occurrence during oculovestibular testing in sedative drug-induced coma. Arch Neurol 35:456–458, 1978.

153. Simon, RP: Management of status epilepticus: In Pedly, TA and Meldrum, BS (eds): Recent Advances in Epilepsy. Churchill Livingstone, London, 1985.

154. Simon, RP, Benowitz, N, Hedlund, R, and Copeland, J: The influence of the blood-brain pH gradient on brain phenobarbital uptake during status epilepticus. J Pharmacol Exp Ther 234:830–835, 1985.

155. Simpson, DL and Rumack, BH: Methylenedioxyamphetamine: Clinical description of overdose death and review of pharmacology. Arch Intern Med 141:1507–1509, 1981.

156. Snead, OC: Opiate-induced seizures: A study of mu and delta specific mechanisms. Exp Neurol 93:348–358, 1986.

157. Sorensen, BF: Skin symptoms in acute narcotic intoxication. Dan Med Bull 10:130–131, 1963.

158. Sorenson, SC and Mattison, I: Naloxone as an antagonist in severe alcohol intoxication. Lancet 2:688–689, 1978.

159. Spector, RH and Schnapper, R: Amitriptyline-induced ophthalmoplegia. Neurology 31:1188–1190, 1981.

160. Stahl, SM and Kasser, IS: Pentazocine overdose. Ann Emerg Med 12:28–31, 1983.

161. Staiman, A and Seeman, P: The impulse blocking concentrations of anesthetics, alcohols, anticonvulsants, barbiturates and narcotics on phrenic and sciatic nerves. Can J Physiol Pharmacol 52:535–550, 1974.

162. Stambaugh, JE and Wainer, IW: Drug interaction: Meperidine and chlorpromazine, a toxic combination. J Clin Pharmacol 21:140–146, 1981.

163. Starkey, IR and Lawson, AA: Poisoning with tricyclic and related antidepressants—A ten-year review. Q J Med 193:33–49, 1980.

164. Steinberg, A and Karliner, JS: The clinical spectrum of heroin pulmonary edema. Arch Intern Med 122:122–127, 1968.

165. Stern, TA, O'Gara, PT, Mulley, AG, Singer, DE, and Thibault, GE: Complications after overdose with tricyclic antidepressants. Crit Care Med 13:672–674, 1985.

166. Stockard, JJ, Werner, SS, Aalbers, JA, and Chiappa, KH: Electroencephalographic findings in phencyclidine intoxication. Arch Neurol 33:200–203, 1976.

167. Suzdak, PD, Glowa, JR, Crawley, JN, Schwartz, RD, Skolnick, P, and Paul, SM: A selective imidazobenzodiazepine antagonist of ethanol in the rat. Science 234:1243–1247, 1986.

168. Szeto, HH, Inturrisi, CE, Houde, R, Saul, S, Cheigh, J, and Reidenberg, MM: Accumulation of normeperidine, an active metabolite of meperidine, in patients with renal failure or cancer. Ann Intern Med 86:738–741, 1977.

169. Tanaka, K: Anticonvulsant properties of procaine, cocaine, adephinine and related structures. Proc Soc Exp Biol Med 90:192–195, 1955.

170. Tang, R, Shimomura, SK, and Rotblatt, M: Meperidine-induced seizures in sickle cell patients. Hospital Formulary 15:764–772, 1980.

171. Tasset, JJ and Pesce, AJ: Amoxapine in human overdose. J Anal Toxicol 8:124–128, 1984.

172. Teitelbaum, JS, Zatorre, RJ, Carpenter, S, Gendron, D, Evans, AC, Gjeddle, A, and Cashman, NR: Neurologic sequelae of domoic acid intoxication due to the ingestion of contaminated mussels. N Engl J Med 322:1781–1787, 1990.

173. Toone, BK and Fenton, GW: Epileptic seizures induced by psychotropic drugs. Psychol Med 7:265–270, 1977.

174. Tortella, FC, Cowan, A, and Adler, MW: Studies on excitatory and inhibitory influence of intracerebroventricularly injected opioids on seizure thresholds in rats. Neuropharmacology 23:749–754, 1984.

175. Trimble, M, Anlezark, G, and Meldrum, BS: Seizure activity in photosensitive baboons following antidepressant drugs and the role of serotonergic mechanisms. Psychopharmacology 51:159–164, 1977.

176. Trimble, M: Non-monoamine oxidase inhibitory antidepressants and epilepsy: A review. Epilepsia 19:241–250, 1978.

177. Tucker, HSG and Porter, WB: Hypoglycemia following alcoholic intoxication. Am J Med Sci 204:559–566, 1942.

178. Urca, G, Frenk, N, Liebeskind, JC, and Taylor, AN: Morphine and enkephaline: Analgesic and epileptic properties. Science 197:83–86, 1977.

179. Vale, JA: The immediate care of cases of poisoning. Anesthesiology 32:483–493, 1977.

180. Victor, M and Laureno, R: Neurologic complications of alcohol abuse: Epidemiologic aspects. In Schoenberg, BS (ed): Advances in Neurology, Vol 19. Raven Press, New York, 1978, pp 603–617.

181. Victor, M and Brausch, C: The role of abstinence in the genesis of alcoholic epilepsy. Epilepsia 8:1–20, 1967.

182. Ward, A, Chaffman, MO, and Sorkin, EM: Dantrolene: A review of its pharmacodynamic and pharmacokinetic properties and therapeutic use in malignant hyperthermia, the neuroleptic malignant syndrome and an update of its use in muscle spasticity. Drugs 21:130–168, 1986.

183. Wedin, GP, Oderda, GM, Klein-Schwartz, W, and Gorman, RL: Relative toxicity of cyclic antidepressants. Ann Emerg Med 15:797–804, 1986.

184. Westerfield, BT and Blouin, R: Ethchlorvynol intoxication. South Med J 70:1019–1020, 1977.

185. Westheimer, R and Klawans, HL: The role of serotonin in the pathophysiology of myoclonic seizures associated with acute imipramine toxicity. Neurology 24:1175–1177, 1984.

186. Weymann, AE and Goodman, RM: Severe accidental hypothermia in an alcoholic population. Am J Med 56:13–21, 1974.

187. Wiltbank, TB, Sine, ME, and Brady, BB: Are emergency toxicology measurements really used? Clin Chem 20:116–120, 1974.

188. Winchester, JF and Gelfand, MC: Hemoperfusion in drug intoxication: Clinical and laboratory aspects. Drug Metab Rev 8:69–104, 1978.

189. Winters, W and Grace, W: Prolonged coma caused by glutethimide. Clin Pharmacol Ther 2:40–44, 1961.

190. Yago, KB, Pitts, FN, Burgoyne, RW, Aniline, O, Yago, LS, and Pitts, AF: The urban epidemic of phencyclidine (PCP) use: Clinical and laboratory evidence from a public psychiatric hospital emergency service. J Clin Psychiatry 42:193–196, 1981.

191. Zalis, EG, Lundberg, GD, and Knutson, RA: The pathophysiology of acute amphetamine poisoning with pathologic correlation. J Pharmacol Exp Ther 158:115–127, 1967.

192. Zalis, EG and Parmley, LF: Fatal amphetamine poisoning. Arch Intern Med 112:822–826, 1963.

193. Zwillich, CW, Sutton, FD, and Neff, TA: Theophylline-induced seizures in adults: Correlation with serum concentrations. Ann Intern Med 82:784–787, 1987.

APPENDIX: SOURCES OF DRUG INFORMATION

Current information about new drugs and use of old drugs is available from a variety of sources. Some of the best are listed here with a brief description.

DRUG INFORMATION CENTERS

A network of pharmacist-operated drug information centers is located throughout the United States and Europe. Most are associated with large university hospitals. They were surveyed in Rosenberg, JM, Martino, FP, Kirshenbaum, HL, and Robbins, J: Pharmacist-operated drug information centers in the United States — 1986. Am J Hosp Pharm 44:337, 1987. Another list is updated yearly in Drug Topics Redbook, Medical Economics Publishers; Oradell, NJ, 1990. (This book lists the prices of all drugs and is available through pharmacies).

COMPUTER DATABASES

A number of commercial database services are available to search the medical literature about drugs. GRATEFUL MED, prepared by the National Library of Medicine (NLM), offers direct access to the Library's collection from a personal computer. After the software (for the IBM-PC or Apple Macintosh) has been obtained, a suitably equipped computer will call the NLM computer, log on with the user code and password, enter the search request, store references, disconnect from the NLM computer, and present references. The software allows someone to perform searches with minimal training. An average search costs $3.00. It also allows access to a number of useful databases including TOXNET, TOXLINE, and TOXLIT on toxicology, and CHEMLINE, about chemical substances. For information about ordering the software ($29.95 + $3.00 handling) call 1-800-638-8480 or 301-496-6193 or write to:

US Department of Commerce, National Technical Information Service, 5285 Port Royal Road, Springfield, VA 22161. Telephone: 703-487-4650. For ordering by FAX: 703-321-8547 (only for orders using credit card or purchase order).

COMPENDIA AND HANDBOOKS

Facts and Comparisons: J. B. Lippincott, Philadelphia, PA. A useful reference for general prescribing information for all US-marketed drugs, updated monthly.

AHFS Drug Information: American Society of Hospital Pharmacists, Bethesda, MD, 1990. A very comprehensive source of evaluation of drug information.

Physicians' Desk Reference: Medical Economics, Oradell, NJ. Annual. A reference containing information on selected drug products. The information provided about these drugs is essentially that which is found in the package insert. This is a good reference for Food and Drug Administration-approved indications, available dosage forms, normal dosage ranges, and pictures of selected drug products for use in identification.

Drug Interactions: Hansten, PD, ed 6, Lea & Febiger, Philadelphia, 1989.

Manual of Neurologic Therapeutics: Samuels, MA (Ed), Little Brown, Boston, 1986. Good "quick reference" for therapeutics.

The Harriet Lane Handbook: Greene, MG (Ed), ed 12, Year Book Medical Publishers, Chicago, 1990. A handbook reference for drug doses and other information about therapeutics in children.

The Pediatric Drug Handbook: Benitz, WE and Tatro, DS, Year Book Medical Publishers, Chicago, 1988. A comprehensive guide to drug doses in children.

DRUG EVALUATIONS Subscription: American Medical Association, Chicago. Current evaluations of prescription drugs, in looseleaf format, updated quarterly. Also available in book form, without updates. Telephone: 1-800-621-8335.

Index

An "f" following a page number indicates a figure; a "t" following a page number indicates a table.